Endovascular Aortic Interventions and Aneurysm Repair: Recent Advances and Future Prospects

Endovascular Aortic Interventions and Aneurysm Repair: Recent Advances and Future Prospects

Editors

Martin Teraa
Constantijn E.V.B. Hazenberg

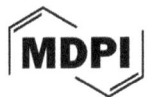

Basel • Beijing • Wuhan • Barcelona • Belgrade • Novi Sad • Cluj • Manchester

Editors
Martin Teraa
University Medical Center Utrecht
Utrecht
The Netherlands

Constantijn E.V.B. Hazenberg
University Medical Center Utrecht
Utrecht
The Netherlands

Editorial Office
MDPI
St. Alban-Anlage 66
4052 Basel, Switzerland

This is a reprint of articles from the Special Issue published online in the open access journal *Journal of Clinical Medicine* (ISSN 2077-0383) (available at: https://www.mdpi.com/journal/jcm/special_issues/endovascular_aneurysm).

For citation purposes, cite each article independently as indicated on the article page online and as indicated below:

Lastname, A.A.; Lastname, B.B. Article Title. *Journal Name* **Year**, *Volume Number*, Page Range.

ISBN 978-3-7258-0531-0 (Hbk)
ISBN 978-3-7258-0532-7 (PDF)
doi.org/10.3390/books978-3-7258-0532-7

© 2024 by the authors. Articles in this book are Open Access and distributed under the Creative Commons Attribution (CC BY) license. The book as a whole is distributed by MDPI under the terms and conditions of the Creative Commons Attribution-NonCommercial-NoDerivs (CC BY-NC-ND) license.

Contents

Preface vii

Martin Teraa and Constantijn E. V. B. Hazenberg
The Current Era of Endovascular Aortic Interventions and What the Future Holds
Reprinted from: *J. Clin. Med.* **2022**, *11*, 5900, doi:10.3390/jcm11195900 1

Denis Skrypnik, Marius Ante, Katrin Meisenbacher, Dorothea Kronsteiner, Matthias Hagedorn, Fabian Rengier, et al.
Dynamic Morphology of the Ascending Aorta and Its Implications for Proximal Landing in Thoracic Endovascular Aortic Repair
Reprinted from: *J. Clin. Med.* **2023**, *12*, 70, doi:10.3390/jcm12010070 5

Tomoaki Kudo, Toru Kuratani, Yoshiki Sawa and Shigeru Miyagawa
Effectiveness and Minimal-Invasiveness of Zone 0 Landing Thoracic Endovascular Aortic Repair Using Branched Endograft
Reprinted from: *J. Clin. Med.* **2022**, *11*, 6981, doi:10.3390/jcm11236981 15

Petar Zlatanovic, Aleksa Jovanovic, Paolo Tripodi and Lazar Davidovic
Chimney vs. Fenestrated Endovascular vs. Open Repair for Juxta/Pararenal Abdominal Aortic Aneurysms: Systematic Review and Network Meta-Analysis of the Medium-Term Results
Reprinted from: *J. Clin. Med.* **2022**, *11*, 6779, doi:10.3390/jcm11226779 25

Tim Wittig, Arsen Sabanov, Andrej Schmidt, Dierk Scheinert, Sabine Steiner and Daniela Branzan
Feasibility and Safety of Percutaneous Axillary Artery Access in a Prospective Series of 100 Complex Aortic and Aortoiliac Interventions
Reprinted from: *J. Clin. Med.* **2023**, *12*, 1959, doi:10.3390/jcm12051959 40

Sinead Gormley, Oliver Bernau, William Xu, Peter Sandiford and Manar Khashram
Incidence and Outcomes of Abdominal Aortic Aneurysm Repair in New Zealand from 2001 to 2021
Reprinted from: *J. Clin. Med.* **2023**, *12*, 2331, doi:10.3390/jcm12062331 51

Petra Z. Bachrati, Guglielmo La Torre, Mohammed M. Chowdhury, Samuel J. Healy, Aminder A. Singh and Jonathan R. Boyle
A State-of-the-Art Review of Intra-Operative Imaging Modalities Used to Quality Assure Endovascular Aneurysm Repair
Reprinted from: *J. Clin. Med.* **2023**, *12*, 3167, doi:10.3390/jcm12093167 66

Taeouk Kim, Nic S. Tjahjadi, Xuehuan He, JA van Herwaarden, Himanshu J. Patel, Nicholas S. Burris and C. Alberto Figueroa
Three-Dimensional Characterization of Aortic Root Motion by Vascular Deformation Mapping
Reprinted from: *J. Clin. Med.* **2023**, *12*, 4471, doi:10.3390/jcm12134471 80

Merel Verhagen, Daniel Eefting, Carla van Rijswijk, Rutger van der Meer, Jaap Hamming, Joost van der Vorst and Jan van Schaik
Increased Aortic Exclusion in Endovascular Treatment of Complex Aortic Aneurysms
Reprinted from: *J. Clin. Med.* **2023**, *12*, 4921, doi:10.3390/jcm12154921 97

Xun Yuan, Xiaoxin Kan, Zhihui Dong, Xiao Yun Xu and Christoph A. Nienaber
Nonsurgical Repair of the Ascending Aorta: Why Less Is More
Reprinted from: *J. Clin. Med.* **2023**, *12*, 4771, doi:10.3390/jcm12144771 108

Khamin Chinsakchai, Thana Sirivech, Frans L. Moll, Sasima Tongsai and Kiattisak Hongku
The Correlation of Aortic Neck Angle and Length in Abdominal Aortic Aneurysm with Severe Neck Angulation for Prediction of Intraoperative Neck Complications and Postoperative Outcomes after Endovascular Aneurysm Repair
Reprinted from: *J. Clin. Med.* **2023**, *12*, 5797, doi:10.3390/jcm12185797 119

Nicola Leone, Magdalena Anna Broda, Jonas Peter Eiberg and Timothy Andrew Resch
Systematic Review and Meta-Analysis of the Incidence of Rupture, Repair, and Death of Small and Large Abdominal Aortic Aneurysms under Surveillance
Reprinted from: *J. Clin. Med.* **2023**, *12*, 6837, doi:10.3390/jcm12216837 130

Wojciech Kazimierczak, Natalia Kazimierczak and Zbigniew Serafin
Review of Clinical Applications of Dual-Energy CT in Patients after Endovascular Aortic Repair
Reprinted from: *J. Clin. Med.* **2023**, *12*, 7766, doi:10.3390/jcm12247766 148

Preface

This Special Issue, entitled "Endovascular Aortic Interventions and Aneurysm Repair: Recent Advances and Future Prospects", focuses on the advancements that have been made in endovascular aortic repair and the expected future developments. We, as the Guest Editors, aim to provide an insight into some of the contemporary issues that are encountered in endovascular aortic repairs and lay the foundation for some future research questions. We truly appreciate and are very grateful to all the authors that contributed to this Special Issue and made it a great success.

Martin Teraa and Constantijn E.V.B. Hazenberg
Editors

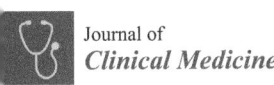

Editorial

The Current Era of Endovascular Aortic Interventions and What the Future Holds

Martin Teraa * and Constantijn E. V. B. Hazenberg

Department of Vascular Surgery, University Medical Center Utrecht, 3584 CX Utrecht, The Netherlands
* Correspondence: m.teraa@umcutrecht.nl; Tel.: +31-887556965; Fax: +31-887555017

Today, more than 30 years after the first endovascular aneurysm repair (EVAR) by Juan Parodi and Julio Palmaz [1], endovascular aortic interventions have become the preferred treatment modality for a wide range of aortic pathologies. We have long passed the era in which endovascular aortic interventions were confined to simple infrarenal abdominal aortic aneurysms (AAA); nowadays, complex aortic pathologies, such as juxtarenal AAA, extensive thoraco-abdominal aneurysms, AAAs with challenging neck or access anatomies, aortic dissections, and even pathology of the aortic arch, can be treated via a complete or hybrid endovascular approach. Despite important advantages, endovascular (aortic) interventions, compared with traditional vascular surgery, also bring new challenges and demands for further innovation to achieve the best outcome for the patient and the treating physician. This applies for the complete course of the treatment of patients with aortic disease, i.e., the pre-operative, peri-operative, and post-operative phases.

1. Pre-Operative Phase and Planning

Patient selection has changed, and the indications for endovascular aortic interventions have broadened over the past decade, which goes hand in hand with more complex pathologies being treated with minimally invasive procedures. For example, patients unfit for open repair of an arch aneurysm can be treated with a complete endovascular or hybrid approach. Accurate knowledge of all (endovascular) options and their corresponding advantages and drawbacks is essential. Consequently, the question has been raised as to whether these complex interventions should be performed in all centers equipped with modern hybrid operation rooms (ORs) or only in high-volume centers. In line with what has been repeatedly shown for major surgical procedures, mortality and major complications after complex endovascular interventions, such as fenestrated (FEVAR) and branched EVAR (BEVAR), are substantially higher (up to 4 times higher) in low-volume than high-volume centers [2–4]. These results underline the importance of the centralization of these complex interventions, which is likely to become even more important in the near future.

Intervention-related decision making based on pre-operative planning and stent graft sizing and selection has evolved enormously in recent decades, these factors directly influence initial technical success, the durability of aortic interventions, as well as the risk of complications [5,6]. Dynamic properties of the aorta during the cardiac cycle and dimensional changes due to hemodynamic shifts make sizing in aortic interventions challenging, especially in acute aortic syndromes such as blunt traumatic aortic injury (BTAI). To optimize outcomes, methods to guide treatment planning are mandatory. For instance, it has been shown that the real-time assessment of aortic diameters using intravascular ultrasound (IVUS) to support stent graft selection in acute aortic syndromes improves post-operative outcomes. Other promising technologies that are increasingly used in different medical fields, such as machine learning and artificial intelligence (AI), have still to be proven in the routine management of patients with aortic pathology. Although, its role in fully automated volume segmentation [7] and treatment planning [8] has been shown in infrarenal AAA, its value in pre-operative planning and stent graft selection and sizing is yet to be established. Furthermore, patient selection and screening, per-operative guidance,

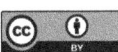

and individual patient's post-operative follow-up planning could benefit from AI methods. Therefore, AI or deep learning algorithms will become indispensable tools in the future management of patients with aortic disease.

2. Per-Procedural Phase

Per-operative image guidance is an essential element in the chain of endovascular interventions and especially complex aortic procedures. Image guidance has evolved enormously in recent years and, consequently, endovascular navigation during complex endovascular aorta interventions has improved. However, this requires fluoroscopy. Fluoroscopically guided endovascular interventions have some important limitations: (1) the acquired images are a two-dimensional (2D) conversion of three-dimensional (3D) structures and movements, (2) images are projected only in gray scale, and importantly (3) it requires radiation exposure. Increasing attention has been paid to these important drawbacks of fluoroscopy and, importantly, the awareness of occupational radiation exposure during these interventions has increased. This increased awareness is reflected by the 2023 clinical practice guidelines on radiation safety by the European Society for Vascular Surgery (ESVS) [9], which give firm recommendations and expose knowledge gaps regarding radiation safety during endovascular (aortic) interventions.

A state-of-the-art hybrid OR has options to perform image fusion, which enables merging pre- or per-operative imaging, such as CTA or MRA, with the real-life images on the hybrid OR. Image fusion enables navigation within a 3D roadmap and easier and more accurate navigation. It has been shown that the use of image fusion reduces contrast volume, fluoroscopy and procedure time in complex EVAR, but influence on radiation dose has not been substantial [10]. In order to reduce or even banish radiation from the OR, radiation-free techniques must be investigated and developed to pursue radiation-free endovascular surgery. Promising techniques are IVUS, electromagnetic tracking (EM) robotic navigation, and Fiber Optic RealShape (FORS).

Fully IVUS-assisted EVAR has been shown to be feasible in twenty-seven cases and to significantly reduce the amount of radiation exposure and contrast volume during EVAR procedures [11,12]. Although IVUS in itself is not novel, its application in aortic interventions is still very limited, but it could be one of the methods to reduce radiation exposure during aortic interventions significantly.

EM-tracking systems consist of a low-magnetic-field generator and EM position coils integrated within the tip of the used catheter or guidewire. Information about the EM field within the EM coils at the tip of the devices is analyzed in a control box that converts this information into a 3D position of the coil. In combination with navigation software, the system can visualize the 3D position and orientation of the devices relative to the anatomy, segmented from a preoperative CTA. Most articles describing EM tracking have reported results of in vitro and animal studies [13]; however, its feasibility and potential in endovascular aortic surgery have been shown in small clinical studies [14–16]. Larger studies have yet to confirm the additional value and radiation-reducing capacity of EM tracking during complex aortic procedures.

Finally, an important and promising innovation that should ease 3D navigation and reduce radiation exposure in endovascular interventions is FORS technology [17]. FORS technology makes use of special designed guidewires and catheters with an integrated optical fiber. Positional changes in the devices alter the optical signal and the FORS software visualizes the actual position of the devices in real time. FORS technology can be combined with image fusion. Important advantages of FORS include a better appreciation of 3D movements, visualization in bright colors, the option of simultaneous biplane view, and real-time navigation without the use of fluoroscopy. FORS technology has been successfully adopted in complex endovascular aortic repair programs in selected high-volume aortic centers, and initial results show encouraging success rates and high potential for radiation reduction [18].

Although most of the abovementioned methods are still not routinely available in daily practice, they will help us to shape the radiation-free hybrid ORs and angiosuites of the future. In addition to imaging and radiation-reducing innovations, the development of a new generation of endografts enables the treatment of wider and more complex aortic pathologies (e.g., hostile necks or atherosclerotic iliac access). These innovations require tight collaboration between vascular surgeons and broad groups of specialists, such as technicians, IT specialists, basic and clinical scientists, and industry representatives. This will fuel these innovations and speed up the translation of these novel techniques towards our ORs.

3. Post-Operative Phase and Follow-Up

Compared with traditional aortic reconstructions, endovascular aortic interventions also differ in post-operative follow-up. For instance, endoleaks are the Achilles heel of EVAR, and have varying consequences depending on the type and presence of aneurysm sac expansion. Especially, the role and importance of type 2 endoleaks remain a matter of debate, and it would be significant if we could identify clinically relevant endoleaks, as less than 1% of patients with a type 2 endoleak will eventually develop a ruptured aneurysm. It has been shown that machine learning algorithms are able to reliably predict those endoleaks related to significant aneurysm sac expansion [19], as these aneurysms are more prone to rupture than the stable ones. Thus, this could help with the selection of patients in whom the type 2 endoleak should be treated. Furthermore, similar techniques have been able to predict reinterventions after thoracic endovascular aortic repair (TEVAR) for type B aortic dissection [20]. Methods to inform tailor-made follow-up and guide reinterventions will further improve the long-term results of endovascular aortic interventions, prevent unnecessary imaging and reinterventions, and ultimately reduce costs.

4. Conclusions

In conclusion, this Special Issue addresses important aspects of modern endovascular aortic interventions, some of which have been discussed in this Editorial, and casts a view on future developments in this fast-moving field. We sincerely hope that this Special Issue will help to increase insight in endovascular aortic interventions and fuel the next steps in innovation and personalized care. This will ultimately help to improve outcomes for both the patients, suffering from serious and often life-threatening aortic pathologies, and for us, as vascular surgeons and interventional radiologists, by attempting to reduce and finally banish radiation exposure and achieve durable results.

We would like to thank all reviewers for their insightful comments and help to further improve the manuscripts included in this Special Issue and the *JCM* team for their support. Additionally, foremost, we heartily thank the authors for their valuable and high-quality contributions which have shaped this Special Issue and will help to shape the future of endovascular aortic surgery.

Funding: This research received no external funding.

Conflicts of Interest: The Division of Surgical specialties of the University Medical Center Utrecht has a research and consultancy agreement with Philips Medical Systems Netherlands B.V. The department of Vascular surgery is part of the Division of Surgical Specialties. M.T. is or has been a consultant for Cook Medical Inc. and Pluristem Therapeutics Inc. C.E.V.B.H. is or has been a consultant for Cook Medical Inc., W.L. Gore & Associates, Inc., Medtronic and Terumo Aortic.

References

1. Parodi, J.; Palmaz, J.; Barone, H. Transfemoral Intraluminal Graft Implantation for Abdominal Aortic Aneurysms. *Ann. Vasc. Surg.* **1991**, *5*, 491–499. [CrossRef] [PubMed]
2. Alberga, A.J.; von Meijenfeldt, G.C.I.; Rastogi, V.; de Bruin, J.L.; Wever, J.J.; van Herwaarden, J.A.; Hamming, J.F.; Hazenberg, C.E.V.B.; van Schaik, J.; Mees, B.M.E.; et al. Association of Hospital Volume with Perioperative Mortality of Endovascular Repair of Complex Aortic Aneurysms. *Ann. Surg.* **2021**, *75*, 1492. [CrossRef] [PubMed]

3. Locham, S.; Hussain, F.; Dakour-Aridi, H.; Barleben, A.; Lane, J.S.; Malas, M. Hospital Volume Impacts the Outcomes of Endovascular Repair of Thoracoabdominal Aortic Aneurysms. *Ann. Vasc. Surg.* **2019**, *67*, 232–241.e2. [CrossRef] [PubMed]
4. Sawang, M.; Paravastu, S.; Liu, Z.; Thomas, S.D.; Beiles, B.; Mwipatayi, B.P.; Verhagen, H.J.; Verhoeven, E.L.; Varcoe, R.L. The Relationship Between Aortic Aneurysm Surgery Volume and Peri-Operative Mortality in Australia. *Eur. J. Vasc. Endovasc. Surg.* **2018**, *57*, 510–519. [CrossRef] [PubMed]
5. Teraa, M.; Hazenberg, C.E.; Houben, I.B.; Trimarchi, S.; van Herwaarden, J.A. Important issues regarding planning and sizing for emergent TEVAR. *J. Cardiovasc. Surg.* **2021**, *61*, 708–712. [CrossRef] [PubMed]
6. Rychla, M.; Dueppers, P.; Meuli, L.; Rancic, Z.; Menges, A.-L.; Kopp, R.; Zimmermann, A.; Reutersberg, B. Influence of measurement and sizing techniques in thoracic endovascular aortic repair on outcome in acute complicated type B aortic dissections. *Interact. Cardiovasc. Thorac. Surg.* **2021**, *34*, 628–636. [CrossRef] [PubMed]
7. Caradu, C.; Spampinato, B.; Vrancianu, A.M.; Bérard, X.; Ducasse, E. Fully automatic volume segmentation of infrarenal abdominal aortic aneurysm computed tomography images with deep learning approaches versus physician controlled manual segmentation. *J. Vasc. Surg.* **2020**, *74*, 246–256.e6. [CrossRef] [PubMed]
8. Raffort, J.; Adam, C.; Carrier, M.; Ballaith, A.; Coscas, R.; Jean-Baptiste, E.; Hassen-Khodja, R.; Chakfé, N.; Lareyre, F. Artificial intelligence in abdominal aortic aneurysm. *J. Vasc. Surg.* **2020**, *72*, 321–333.e1. [CrossRef] [PubMed]
9. Modarai, B.; Haulon, S.; Hertault, A.; Wanhainen, A.; Patel, A.; Böckler, D.; Vano, E.; Ainsbury, E.; Van Herzeele, I.; van, J.; et al. European Society for Vascular Surgery (ESVS) 2023 Clinical Practice Guidelines on Radiation Safety. *Eur. J. Vasc. Endovasc. Surg.* **2022**, in press. [CrossRef] [PubMed]
10. Doelare, S.A.N.; Smorenburg, S.P.M.; van Schaik, T.G.; Blankensteijn, J.D.; Wisselink, W.; Nederhoed, J.H.; Lely, R.J.; Hoksbergen, A.W.J.; Yeung, K.K. Image Fusion During Standard and Complex Endovascular Aortic Repair, to Fuse or Not to Fuse? A Meta-analysis and Additional Data From a Single-Center Retrospective Cohort. *J. Endovasc. Ther.* **2020**, *28*, 78–92. [CrossRef] [PubMed]
11. Illuminati, G.; Nardi, P.; Fresilli, D.; Sorrenti, S.; Lauro, A.; Pizzardi, G.; Ruggeri, M.; Ulisse, S.; Cantisani, V.; D'Andrea, V. Fully Ultrasound-Assisted Endovascular Aneurysm Repair (EVAR): Preliminary report. *Ann. Vasc. Surg.* **2022**, *84*, 55–60. [CrossRef] [PubMed]
12. Pecoraro, F.; Bracale, U.M.; Farina, A.; Badalamenti, G.; Ferlito, F.; Lachat, M.; Dinoto, E.; Asti, V.; Bajardi, G. Single-Center Experience and Preliminary Results of Intravascular Ultrasound in Endovascular Aneurysm Repair. *Ann. Vasc. Surg.* **2019**, *56*, 209–215. [CrossRef] [PubMed]
13. de Ruiter, Q.M.; Moll, F.L.; van Herwaarden, J.A. Current state in tracking and robotic navigation systems for application in endovascular aortic aneurysm repair. *J. Vasc. Surg.* **2015**, *61*, 256–264. [CrossRef] [PubMed]
14. Manstad-Hulaas, F.; Tangen, G.A.; Dahl, T.; Hernes, T.A.N.; Aadahl, P. Three-Dimensional Electromagnetic Navigation vs. Fluoroscopy for Endovascular Aneurysm Repair: A Prospective Feasibility Study in Patients. *J. Endovasc. Ther.* **2012**, *19*, 70–78. [CrossRef] [PubMed]
15. Cochennec, F.; Kobeiter, H.; Gohel, M.; Marzelle, J.; Desgranges, P.; Allaire, E.; Becquemin, J.P. Feasibility and Safety of Renal and Visceral Target Vessel Cannulation Using Robotically Steerable Catheters During Complex Endovascular Aortic Procedures. *J. Endovasc. Ther.* **2015**, *22*, 187–193. [CrossRef] [PubMed]
16. Perera, A.; Riga, C.; Monzon, L.; Gibbs, R.; Bicknell, C.; Hamady, M. Robotic Arch Catheter Placement Reduces Cerebral Embolization During Thoracic Endovascular Aortic Repair (TEVAR). *Eur. J. Vasc. Endovasc. Surg.* **2017**, *53*, 362–369. [CrossRef] [PubMed]
17. van Herwaarden, J.A.; Jansen, M.M.; Vonken, E.-J.P.; Bloemert-Tuin, T.; Bullens, R.W.; de Borst, G.J.; Hazenberg, C.E. First in Human Clinical Feasibility Study of Endovascular Navigation with Fiber Optic RealShape (FORS) Technology. *Eur. J. Vasc. Endovasc. Surg.* **2020**, *61*, 317–325. [CrossRef] [PubMed]
18. Panuccio, G.; Schanzer, A.; Rohlffs, F.; Heidemann, F.; Wessels, B.; Schurink, G.W.; van Herwaarden, J.A.; Kölbel, T. Endovascular Navigation with Fiber Optic RealShape (FORS) Technology. *J. Vasc. Surg.* **2022**, in press. [CrossRef]
19. Charalambous, S.; Klontzas, M.E.; Kontopodis, N.; Ioannou, C.V.; Perisinakis, K.; Maris, T.G.; Damilakis, J.; Karantanas, A.; Tsetis, D. Radiomics and machine learning to predict aggressive type 2 endoleaks after endovascular aneurysm repair: A proof of concept. *Acta Radiol.* **2021**, *63*, 1293–1299. [CrossRef] [PubMed]
20. Dong, Y.; Que, L.; Jia, Q.; Xi, Y.; Zhuang, J.; Li, J.; Liu, H.; Chen, W.; Huang, M. Predicting reintervention after thoracic endovascular aortic repair of Stanford type B aortic dissection using machine learning. *Eur. Radiol.* **2021**, *32*, 355–367. [CrossRef] [PubMed]

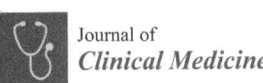

Article

Dynamic Morphology of the Ascending Aorta and Its Implications for Proximal Landing in Thoracic Endovascular Aortic Repair †

Denis Skrypnik [1,*], Marius Ante [1], Katrin Meisenbacher [1], Dorothea Kronsteiner [2], Matthias Hagedorn [1], Fabian Rengier [3], Florian Andre [4], Norbert Frey [4], Dittmar Böckler [1] and Moritz S. Bischoff [1]

1. Department of Vascular and Endovascular Surgery, University Hospital Heidelberg, 69120 Heidelberg, Germany
2. Institute of Medical Biometry and Informatics, University of Heidelberg, 69117 Heidelberg, Germany
3. Clinic for Diagnostic and Interventional Radiology, University Hospital Heidelberg, 69120 Heidelberg, Germany
4. Clinic for Cardiology, Angiology and Pneumology, University Hospital Heidelberg, 69120 Heidelberg, Germany
* Correspondence: denis.skrypnik@med.uni-heidelberg.de; Tel.: +49-6221-563-79-84; Fax: +49-6221-565-423
† Meeting presentation: This study was accepted for presentation at the Annual Meeting of the Austrian, German, and Swiss Society for Vascular Surgery (DREILÄNDERTAGUNG 2022 der Österreichischen, Deutschen und Schweizerischen Gesellschaft für Gefäßchirurgie), Vienna, Austria, 19–22 October 2022.

Abstract: In this study, we assessed the dynamic segmental anatomy of the entire ascending aorta (AA), enabling the determination of a favorable proximal landing zone and appropriate aortic sizing for the most proximal thoracic endovascular aortic repair (TEVAR). **Methods:** Patients with a non-operated AA (diameter < 40 mm) underwent electrocardiogram-gated computed tomography angiography (ECG-CTA) of the entire AA in the systolic and diastolic phases. For each plane of each segment, the maximum and minimum diameters in the systole and diastole phases were recorded. The Wilcoxon signed-rank test was used to compare aortic size values. **Results:** A total of 100 patients were enrolled (53% male; median age 82.1 years; age range 76.8–85.1). Analysis of the dynamic plane dimensions of the AA during the cardiac cycle showed significantly higher systolic values than diastolic values ($p < 0.001$). Analysis of the proximal AA segment showed greater distal plane values than proximal plane values ($p < 0.001$), showing a reversed funnel form. At the mid-ascending segment, the dynamic values did not notably differ between the distal plane and the proximal segmental plane, demonstrating a cylindrical form. At the distal segment of the AA, the proximal plane values were larger than the distal segmental plane values ($p < 0.001$), thus generating a funnel form. **Conclusions:** The entire AA showed greater systolic than diastolic aortic dimensions throughout the cardiac cycle. The mid-ascending and distal-ascending segments showed favorable forms for TEVAR using a regular cylindrical endograft design. The most proximal segment of the AA showed a pronounced conical form; therefore, a specific endograft design should be considered.

Keywords: TEVAR of ascending aorta; endograft of ascending aorta; dynamic morphology of ascending aorta; landing zone morphology; thoracic endovascular aortic repair

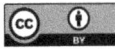

1. Introduction

Thoracic endovascular aortic repair (TEVAR) with landing in the ascending aorta (AA) is a treatment option for a variety of proximal aortic pathologies in selected patients for whom open surgery carries high risk [1–5]. The outcome of any TEVAR procedure critically depends on the morphology of the proximal landing zone (PLZ), with non-optimal aortic sizing and endograft sizing reportedly associated with increasing rates of endoleaks (ELs), endograft migration, and reintervention [6–10]. The pulsatile morphology of the AA, and its variable segmental geometry during the cardiac cycle, may be disadvantageous for proximal endograft alignment and may thereby lead to poor TEVAR outcomes [11–13]. Few studies have reported the dynamic slice anatomy and motility of selected parts of the AA and aortic arch, and the segmental anatomy of the entire AA remains under-reported [14–17]. TEVAR in the AA shows promising outcomes but is associated with high rates of ELs and substantial rates of retrograde aortic dissection (RAD) and conversion [2,4,18,19]. Thus, the dynamic segmental anatomy of the AA must be further investigated to advance TEVAR in the AA and to improve the current clinical and technical outcomes of this procedure.

The objective of the present study was to assess the dynamic segmental anatomy of the entire AA, enabling the determination of a favorable PLZ and appropriate aortic sizing for the most proximal TEVAR.

2. Materials and Methods

2.1. Study Design and Patient Population

We conducted a single-center, retrospective analysis of prospectively collected clinical and computer tomography (CT)-based imaging data. CT examinations were clinically indicated due to the critical stenosis of the aortic valve, for the planning of transcatheter aortic valve implantation (TAVI). The retrospective scientific data analyses were approved by the local ethics committee (S-620/2018).

This study included patients with an indication for TAVI, admitted between 1 July and 8 October 2020, who underwent preoperative electrocardiogram-gated computed tomography angiography (ECG-CTA) (Philips IQon; Philips, Best, The Netherlands) of the entire AA. All the included patients had a non-operated AA. Patients were excluded if they exhibited AA pathology (e.g., aneurysm or dissection), dilatation of the AA of >40 mm, a left ventricular ejection fraction of <30%, or incomplete CTA presentation of the AA. The study did not include patients with connective tissue disease, previous surgery of the left ventricle, or with AA calcinosis of >30% of the circumference (Figure 1).

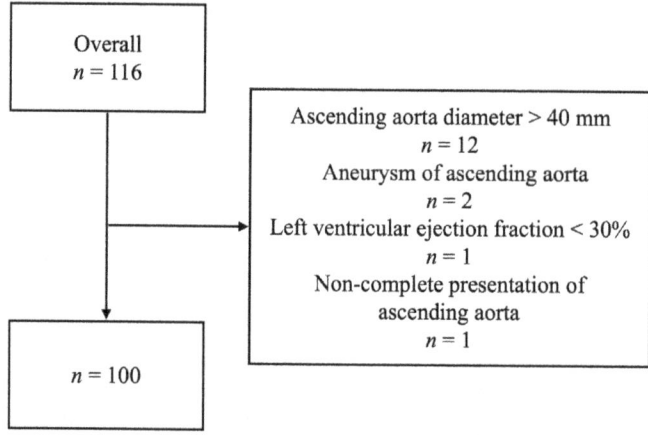

Figure 1. Flowchart of patient inclusion. The chart demonstrates selection of patients in terms of inclusion/exclusion criteria.

2.2. Image Acquisition

Image acquisition was performed using a 64-slice CT scanner (Philips IQon; Philips, Best, The Netherlands) in the supine position with an inspiratory breath-hold. We retrospectively obtained the results for ECG-gated CTA examinations of the heart, the ascending aorta, and the aortic arch with the following protocol parameters: tube potential of 120 kVp, automated tube current modulation, and 80 mL of iodinated contrast medium followed by a 50 mL saline bolus. The images were reconstructed at 5% steps of the RR interval, with a slice thickness of 0.67 mm, a slice increment of 0.33 mm, and the IMR 1, cardiac routine kernel. The reconstruction at 40% of the RR interval was defined as the diastolic phase and the reconstruction at 75% of the RR interval was considered the systolic phase.

2.3. Segmentation and Image Analysis

We analyzed the ECG-CTA of the entire AA in the systolic and diastolic phases. The CTA image series was uploaded from the institutional database to a separate workstation equipped with the "3mensio Vascular" postprocessing software (Pie Medical Imaging BV, Maastricht, The Netherlands). After a three-dimensional centerline reconstruction of the systolic and diastolic image series of the entire AA (from the sinotubular junction to the brachiocephalic trunk), manual aortic segmentation was performed (Figure 2). For this segmentation, a 25 mm centerline length of each AA segment was obtained, based on the recommended length of the proximal landing zone for TEVAR in the proximal thoracic aorta [2]. Each plane of each segment was automatically set perpendicular to the centerline. The proximal plane of segment A was at the sinotubular junction, the middle of the length of segment B was at the middle of the AA, and the distal border of segment C was at the proximal circumference of the brachiocephalic trunk (Figure 2). For each plane of each segment, the area and maximum and minimum diameters in the systole and diastole phases were automatically recorded (Figure 3). All image series were analyzed by two independent study collaborators.

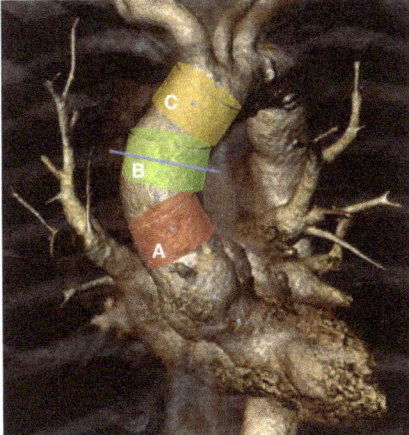

Figure 2. Segmentation of the ascending aorta: Segment A: 2.5 cm distally to the sinotubular junction. Segment B: middle of the segment is on the middle line of the ascending aorta. Segment C: 2.5 cm proximally to the brachiocephalic trunk. All segments had a 25 mm centerline length. Dashed blue line is the centerline. Solid transverse blue line is the middle of the ascending aorta.

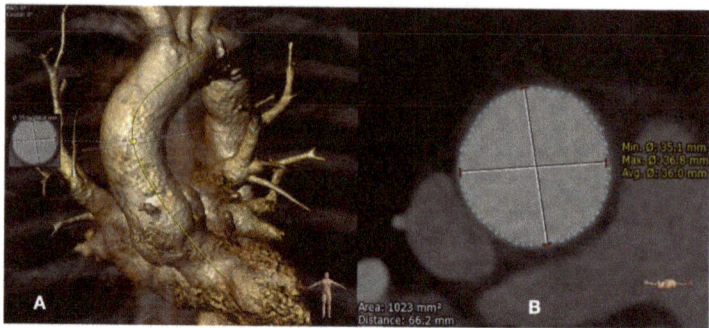

Figure 3. Screenshot of the "3mensio Vascular" program: (**A**) a 3D reconstruction of the ascending aorta. Solid yellow line is the centerline; (**B**) axial presentation of the mid-ascending plane of the ascending aorta with automatically measured size values.

3. Definitions

The centerline length of the AA was between the sinotubular junction and the proximal border of the brachiocephalic trunk. Segmental pulsatility was defined as the radial change in the aortic lumen during the cardiac cycle and was calculated as the largest difference between the systole and diastole values in both area and diameter [11]. The segmental shapes of aortic segments were determined based on the difference between the distal and proximal sizes of the aortic planes in the systole and diastole phases. Segmental strain was determined as follows: (maximum systolic diameter−maximum diastolic diameter)/maximum diastolic diameter (%) [20]. The aortic plane was defined as a 2D aortic slice positioned perpendicular to the centerline. The aortic segment was defined as a cylindrical/conical/reversed conical 3D part of the AA between the proximal and distal segmental plane.

4. Statistical Analysis

All the collected data were descriptively analyzed using median and Q1–Q3 for continuous variables and absolute and relative numbers for categorical variables. Intraclass correlation coefficients (ICC3), including 95% confidence intervals (CIs), were used to assess the inter-rater reliability, with the rater considered a fixed effect, since ICC2 caused unstable models. These models only represented the reliability between these raters and do not apply to other raters. The Wilcoxon signed-rank test was used to compare the aortic size values between the systole and diastole phases and between the proximal and distal aortic plane dimensions. We also calculated the non-parametric 95% CIs for the median values. An explorative significance level of $p < 0.05$ was used, but p values are descriptive only.

5. Results

This study enrolled 100 patients, including 53 males (53%), with a median age of 82.1 years (range 76.8–85.1 years), and median BMI of 25.8 kg/m^2 (range 23.1–29.79 kg/m^2). All the patients showed critical aortic stenosis. The leading cardiovascular risk factors were arterial hypertension (89%, 89/100), coronary heart disease (92%, 92/100), and hyperlipoproteinemia (64%, 64/100). Table 1 presents patient demographics.

5.1. Aortic Dimensions

The median AA length was 69.3 mm (Q1–Q3, 63.75–75.4 mm). The aortic diameter (D) and area showed considerable variation during the heart cycle (Table 2). The smallest systolic and diastolic D and area were at the proximal plane of segment A: systolic D_{min} 26.2 mm (Q1–Q3, 24.4–28.1 mm); systolic D_{max} 29.6 mm (Q1–Q3, 27.9–31.5 mm); systolic area 618 mm^2 (Q1–Q3, 539–701 mm^2); diastolic D_{min} 25.9 mm (Q1–Q3, 24.1–28.2 mm);

diastolic D_{max} 29.2 mm (Q1–Q3, 27.4–31.1 mm); and diastolic area 614.5 mm^2 (Q1–Q3, 516–696.5 mm^2).

5.2. The 2D Form of Aortic Planes

All the cross-sections of the AA were oval, with a relative difference of approximately 10% between the maximum and minimum diameter, which was constant throughout the cardiac cycle (Table 3). Analysis of the dynamic plane dimensions of the AA during the cardiac cycle revealed that systolic values were significantly higher than diastolic values ($p < 0.001$) (Table 4). The systolic D of segment A was 0.3 mm larger than the diastolic D on the proximal plane (95% CI 0.15–0.55) and the distal plane (95% CI 0.25–0.55). Similarly, on the proximal and distal planes of segment B, the systolic D was 0.5 mm (95% CI 0.35–0.6) larger than the diastolic D. At segment C, the dimension variability during the cardiac cycle was more pronounced on the distal segmental plane (0.5 mm, 95% CI 0.4–0.75) than on the proximal segmental plane (0.3 mm, 95% CI 0.2–0.5). Similar to the plane diameter, the segmental area was larger in the systole phase than in the diastole phase ($p < 0.001$) (Table 4).

Table 1. Patient demographic data [a].

Variable	Median [Q1–Q3]; % (n/N)
Age, years	82.1 [76.8–85.1]
Male	53 (53/100)
Female	47 (47/100)
BMI, kg/m^2	25.8 [23.1–29.7]
Hypertension	89 (89/100)
Coronary heart disease	92 (92/100)
PTCA	34 (34/100)
AF	39 (39/100)
Previous stroke/TIA	14 (14/100)
COPD	13 (13/100)
Diabetes	28 (28/100)
Adipositas (BMI > 30)	22 (22/100)
Chronic renal insufficiency (Creatinine > 1.2 mg/dL)	18 (18/100)
History of smoking	29 (29/100)
Hyperlipoproteinemia	64 (64/100)
Stenosis of aortic valve	100 (100/100)

Abbreviations: BMI, body mass index; PTCA, percutaneous transluminal coronary angioplasty; AF, atrial fibrillation; TIA, transient ischemic attack; COPD, chronic obstructive pulmonary disease. [a] Categorical data are presented as absolute numbers and percentages; continuous data are presented as medians and interquartile ranges (N = 100).

Table 2. Segmental area and systolic/diastolic diameter values [a].

Segment	A		B		C	
Plane	Proximal Plane	Distal Plane	Proximal Plane	Distal Plane	Proximal Plane	Distal Plane
Systolic D_{min}, mm	26.2 (24.4–28.1)	32.3 (30–34.7)	31.4 (29.6–34.5)	32.2 (29.9–34.1)	32.3 (30.2–34)	30.4 (28.3–32.2)
Systolic D_{max}, mm	29.6 (27.9–31.5)	35.1 (32.75–37)	34.3 (32–36.75)	34.7 (32.5–36.5)	34.8 (32.7–36.5)	33.5 (31.4–35.5)
Area systolic, mm^2	618 (539–701)	890 (777–1016)	847.5 (755.4–997)	876.5 (765–992)	883 (783–980.3)	803 (697.5–900)
Diastolic D_{min}, mm	25.9 (24.1–28.2)	32.1 (30–34.1)	31.3 (29.1–34)	31.8 (29.25–34)	32.2 (30–34)	30.3 (27.9–31.6)
Diastolic D_{max}, mm	29.2 (27.4–31.1)	34.9 (32.2–36.4)	33.8 (31.75–36.3)	34.3 (31.5–36)	34.5 (32–36.2)	33.2 (30.75–35.2)
Area diastolic, mm^2	614.5 (516–696.5)	875.5 (753–986)	833.5 (732.5–974)	862.5 (740.5–978)	875 (757.5–965)	783 (679–874.5)

[a] Data are presented as medians and quantiles (Q1, Q3) (N = 100).

Table 3. The predominance of larger over smaller diameters of the aortic planes [a].

Segment	Proximal Segmental Plane	Distal Segmental Plane	Proximal Segmental Plane	Distal Segmental Plane
	Systole		Diastole	
A	0.1 (0.1, 0.1)	0.1 (0.1, 0.1)	0.1 (0.1, 0.1)	0.1 (0, 0.1)
B	0.1 (0.1, 0.1)	0.1 (0.1, 0.1)	0.1 (0, 0.1)	0.1 (0.1, 0.1)
C	0.1 (0.1, 0.1)	0.1 (0.1, 0.1)	0.1 (0, 0.1)	0.1 (0.1, 0.1)

The table shows that maximum diameter of each aortic plane was larger than a smaller diameter for 10% during the cardiac cycle, thus demonstrating an oval-shaped rather than round 2D morphology. [a] The predominance of larger over smaller diameter was calculated for each plane as $(D_{max} - D_{min})/D_{max}$ in the systole and diastole phases; data are presented as medians and quantiles (Q1, Q3) (N = 100).

Table 4. Difference between maximum systolic and maximum diastolic diameters and areas [a].

Segment	Proximal Segmental Plane, mm	p-Value	Proximal Segmental Plane, mm^2	p-Value	Distal Segmental Plane, mm	p-Value	Distal Segmental Plane, mm^2	p-Value
A	0.3 (0.15, 0.55)	0.001	10 (5.5, 19)	<0.001	0.3 (0.25, 0.55)	<0.001	15 (13, 23)	<0.001
B	0.5 (0.35, 0.6)	<0.001	18 (14, 25.5)	<0.001	0.5 (0.35, 0.6)	<0.001	18 (16.5, 25.5)	<0.001
C	0.3 (0.2, 0.5)	<0.001	15 (11, 20)	<0.001	0.5 (0.4, 0.75)	<0.001	19 (15.5, 24)	<0.001

[a] Differences between maximum systolic and diastolic diameters and areas are presented as medians and 95% CIs (N = 100).

5.3. The 3D Form of Aortic Segments

The 3D segmental form was described using a comparison between the distal and proximal plane sizes of each AA segment, considering that all the segments lied on the centerline and had a fixed length (25 mm). Analysis of segment A revealed larger distal plane values than proximal plane values ($p < 0.001$) (Table 5). Therefore, segment A of the AA had a reversed funnel form. In segment B, the dynamic values did not notably differ between the distal plane and the proximal segmental plane, thus resulting in a cylindrical form for segment B of the AA during the cardiac cycle (Table 5). In segment C, during the cardiac cycle, the proximal plane values were larger than the distal segmental plane values ($p < 0.001$); therefore, segment C had a funnel form (Table 5).

Table 5. Segmental shapes of ascending aorta during the heart cycle [a].

Segment	D Systolic Max, mm	p-Value	Area Systolic, mm²	p-Value	D Diastolic Max, mm	p-Value	Area Diastolic, mm²	p-Value
A	5.5 (4.9, 5.8)	<0.001	293 (259, 306)	<0.001	5.3 (4.8, 5.7)	<0.001	265 (252, 293)	<0.001
B	0 (−0.3, 0.35)	0.947	1.7 (−13, 21) [b]	0.653	0 (−0.35, 0.35)	0.99	5 (−16, 16)	0.99
C	−1 (−1.35, −0.85)	<0.001	−78 (−87.4, −59.5)	<0.001	−1.4 (−1.6, 1)	<0.001	−82 (−97, −70)	<0.001

[a] Differences between distal and proximal maximum plane diameters and areas are presented as medians and 95% CIs ($N = 100$). [b] Negative values show that distal diameters and areas are smaller than proximal diameters and areas.

The aortic strain was above 5% in all the planes of the AA (Table 6). The greatest variation was observed in the strain at the distal plane of segment C ($1.8 \pm 2.9\%$) on the border of the aortic arch.

Table 6. Segmental strain of ascending aorta during the cardiac cycle [a].

Segment	Proximal Segmental Plane, %	Distal Segmental Plane, %
A	1.2 ± 3.7	1.2 ± 2.6
B	1.4 ± 2.5	1.4 ± 2.0
C	1.0 ± 2.3	1.8 ± 2.9

[a] Strain was calculated as (D_{max} systolic − D_{max} diastolic)/D_{max} diastolic (%) and is presented as mean $\pm$ SD ($N = 100$).

Image quality was sufficient for reliable measurements in all the cases ($N = 100$). The intraclass correlation coefficient was >0.91, indicating high similarity between the measured values and good reproducibility for all the measurements.

6. Discussion

The current study shows a predominance of the systolic over diastolic diameter during the whole cardiac cycle at all levels of the ascending aorta. Each aortic plane demonstrated an oval-shaped 2D morphology with a 10% predominance of maximum plane diameters over small diameters. Furthermore, our analysis revealed a cylindrical form for the mid-ascending aortic segment, a slightly funneled form for the distal-ascending segments, and a pronounced conical form for most proximal segments of the AA.

The currently available reports in the literature highlight the pulsatility of some segments of the AA. De Heer et al. found that the aortic diameter at the sinotubular junction is larger in the systole phase than in the diastole phase (D_{max} systolic 32.4 ± 3.8 mm, D_{max} diastolic 31.5 ± 3.9 mm, $p < 0.001$) [17]. Jian-ping et al. reported significant changes in the aortic diameter of the distal AA during the cardiac cycle, with greater aortic size in the systole phase than in the diastole phase (3.26 ± 0.24 mm and 3.18 ± 0.27 mm, respectively, $p < 0.01$) [13]. Rengier et al. showed the prominent mid-ascending pulsatility of the AA in healthy volunteers, where the systolic aortic dimension was over 10% greater than the diastolic aortic dimension [14]. In line with these prior reports, our current findings showed a wide range of variability in the cross-sectional dimensions of the aorta during the cardiac cycle, with clearly larger systolic dimensions than diastolic dimensions at all levels of the AA ($p \leq 0.001$).

Satriano et al. performed a 3D reconstruction of the ECG-CTA series and reported asymmetrical distension in the AA during the cardiac cycle, which was more prominent along the greater curvature of the AA, consistent with the jet flow direction during heart output [21]. Other reports have described non-circular shapes for some aortic planes during the cardiac cycle [11,13,22].

Liu et al. analyzed the precise sizing for TEVAR in the AA and reported that if the diameters differed by >5%, the real aortic diameter should be calculated as an average between the maximum and minimum diameters, to avoid retrograde aortic dissection [22]. Our present findings confirmed the oval shape of the segmental planes at all levels of the

AA, with a relative difference of approximately 10% between the maximum and minimum diameter throughout the cardiac cycle. Thus, it seems appropriate to use the average diameter for the precise measurement of the AA diameter.

In our current study, we observed increased aortic diameter in the systole phase compared with that in the diastole phase and showed an AA strain of up to 5%. Satriano et al. reported a 10.2 ± 6.0% peak principal strain amplitude for the entire AA [21]. Redheuil et al. reported a similar AA strain (8 ± 4%) in patients over 70 years old and found an AA strain of up to 15 ± 8% in patients 40–49 years old [23]. Thus, the published literature and the data from our current study support the use of a systolic CTA series for the most precise sizing of TEVAR in the AA, wherein 5–15 of the aortic diameter size may be balanced out compared with CTA in the diastolic phase, independent of the patient's age.

In a recent systematic review, Muetterties et al. reported an 18.6% rate of early-term EL Ia after TEVAR in the AA [4]. Similarly, a meta-analysis by Baikoussis et al. revealed a high pooled rate of late EL Ia (16.4%) after TEVAR in the AA [2]. These results are most likely related to the inappropriate alignment of the endograft to the aortic wall [4]. Accordingly, it is crucial to understand the 3D shape of the PLZ to improve outcomes.

A study by van Prehn et al. reported the dynamic plane morphology at the three AA levels and described the 3D motions of 2D aortic planes. However, the authors did not consider the 3D segmental morphology of AA, which is essential for understanding the volume geometry of a potential proximal landing zone [24].

In the current study, we observed that the mid-ascending segment of the AA retained its cylindrical shape throughout the cardiac cycle; therefore, the common cylindrical design of the endograft seems appropriate in this setting. The distal AA segment showed a funnel form; however, the diameter size difference of 1.5 mm between the proximal and distal segmental planes does not seem to be relevant for practical sizing; therefore, a cylindrical endograft design could also be considered here. In contrast, most proximal AA segments showed a reversed funnel (conical) form, which is reportedly unfavorable for aortic endograft alignment [25–27]. Moreover, the difference of >5 mm between the proximal (smaller) and distal (larger) diameters of segmental planes corresponds to an 18% (5.5/29.6 mm) systolic diameter difference between the proximal and distal segmental planes. Therefore, the conventional cylindrical endograft design may not be suitable for use in such cases.

7. Limitations

The present study has several limitations. First, we included patients with significant aortic stenosis, which may influence aortic asymmetry throughout the power and direction of jets during the cardiac cycle. However, previously published studies reported increased arterial stiffness for the whole arterial tree, including the AA, due to severe aortic stenosis; however, a reduced distensibility (a function of change in AA diameter and arterial pressure) of non-calcified AA was not observed compared with patients without several aortic stenoses if cardiac output and stroke volume were saved [28,29]. Furthermore, evenly distributed AA stiffness may introduce bias in terms of absolute diameter and area numbers. However, this is unlikely to result in any change in the aortic plane size ratios. Thus, the volumetric form of the AA segments would probably stay the same.

Second, our patient cohort included those with advanced age and atherosclerosis, which may influence aortic distensibility. One may speculate that AA compliance may be higher in younger subjects. Third, this study did not investigate the longitudinal motions, side deviations, or angulation of the AA during the cardiac cycle, which may be relevant for a complete description of 3D aortic geometry during the cardiac cycle.

8. Conclusions

The entire AA showed variable dynamic anatomy during the cardiac cycle. Precise AA sizing, using the average aortic diameter and systolic CTA series, may be considered. The mid-ascending and distal-ascending segments showed favorable forms for TEVAR using a regular cylindrical endograft design. The most proximal segment of the AA showed a pronounced conical form; therefore, a specific endograft design should be considered.

Author Contributions: Conceptualization and study design, D.S., M.A. and M.S.B.; data analysis and interpretation, D.S., M.A., K.M., M.H., F.R., F.A. and D.K.; data collection, D.S., M.A., M.H., F.R. and F.A.; writing—original draft preparation, D.S., M.S.B., F.R. and F.A.; writing—review and editing, D.S., M.S.B., N.F. and D.B.; statistical analysis, D.K. All authors equally contributed to revising the final manuscript. All authors have read and agreed to the published version of the manuscript.

Funding: The authors received no financial support for the research, authorship, and/or publication of this article.

Institutional Review Board Statement: This study was conducted according to the guidelines of the Declaration of Helsinki and approved by the Institutional Review Board (or Ethics Committee) of the University of Heidelberg (protocol code S-620/2018, date of approval 12 January 2021).

Informed Consent Statement: Informed consent was obtained from all subjects involved in the study.

Data Availability Statement: Not applicable.

Conflicts of Interest: Dittmar Böckler is a consultant for W.L. Gore and Associates and Siemens AG, and has received speaker honoraria and educational and research grants from Gore. Moritz S. Bischoff has received speaker honoraria from W.L. Gore and Associates. All the other authors have no conflict of interest to declare.

Abbreviations

TEVAR	Thoracic endovascular aortic repair
AA	Ascending aorta
PLZ	Proximal landing zone
EIs	Endoleaks
RAD	Retrograde aortic dissection
CT	Computer tomography
TAVI	Transcatheter aortic valve implantation
ECG-CTA	Electrocardiogram-gated computed tomography angiography
ICC3	Intraclass correlation coefficients
CI	Confidence interval
D	Aortic diameter

References

1. Czerny, M.; Schmidli, J.; Adler, S.; Van Den Berg, J.C.; Bertoglio, L.; Carrel, T.; Chiesa, R.; E Clough, R.; Eberle, B.; Etz, C.; et al. Current options and recommendations for the treatment of thoracic aortic pathologies involving the aortic arch: An expert consensus document of the European Association for Cardio-Thoracic surgery (EACTS) and the European Society for Vascular Surgery (ESVS). *Eur. J. Cardiothorac. Surg.* **2019**, *55*, 133–162. [PubMed]
2. Baikoussis, N.G.; Antonopoulos, C.N.; Papakonstantinou, N.A.; Argiriou, M.; Geroulakos, G. Endovascular stent grafting for ascending aorta diseases. *J. Vasc. Surg.* **2017**, *66*, 1587–1601. [CrossRef] [PubMed]
3. Tsilimparis, N.; Drewitz, S.; Detter, C.; Spanos, K.; von Kodolitsch, Y.; Rohlffs, F.; Reichenspurner, H.; Debus, E.S.; Kölbel, T. Endovascular Repair of Ascending Aortic Pathologies with Tubular Endografts: A Single-Center Experience. *J. Endovasc. Ther.* **2019**, *26*, 439–445. [CrossRef]
4. Muetterties, C.E.; Menon, R.; Wheatley, G.H., III. A systematic review of primary endovascular repair of the ascending aorta. *J. Vasc. Surg.* **2018**, *67*, 332–342. [CrossRef] [PubMed]
5. Lescan, D.M. Endovascular treatment of complex thoracic aortic pathologies with arch involvement. Patient selection, planning and technical features in Ishimaru zone 0. *Gefäßchirurgie* **2021**, *4*, 270–277. [CrossRef]
6. Yoon, W.J.; Mell, M.W. Outcome comparison of thoracic endovascular aortic repair performed outside versus inside proximal landing zone length recommendation. *J. Vasc. Surg.* **2020**, *72*, 1883–1890. [CrossRef]
7. Kudo, T.; Kuratani, T.; Shimamura, K.; Sawa, Y. Determining the Optimal Proximal Landing Zone for TEVAR in the Aortic Arch: Comparing the Occurrence of the Bird-Beak Phenomenon in Zone 0 vs Zones 1 and 2. *J. Endovasc. Ther.* **2020**, *27*, 368–376. [CrossRef]
8. Sternbergh, W.C., III; Money, S.R.; Greenberg, R.K.; Chuter, T.A. Influence of endograft oversizing on device migration, endoleak, aneurysm shrinkage, and aortic neck dilation: Results from the Zenith Multicenter Trial. *J. Vasc. Surg.* **2004**, *39*, 20–26. [CrossRef]

9. Hakimi, M.; Bischoff, M.S.; Meisenbacher, K.; Ante, M.; Böckler, D. Der Aortenbogen—Was ist bei der endovaskulären Versorgung zu beachten? *Gefässchirurgie* **2016**, *21*, 224–231. [CrossRef]
10. Skrypnik, D.; Kalmykov, E.; Bischoff, M.S.; Meisenbacher, K.; Klotz, R.; Hagedorn, M.; Kalkum, E.; Probst, P.; Dammrau, R.; Böckler, D. Late Endograft Migration After Thoracic Endovascular Aortic Repair: A Systematic Review and Meta-analysis. *J. Endovasc. Ther.* **2022**, Online ahead of print. [CrossRef]
11. Muhs, B.E.; Vincken, K.L.; van Prehn, J.; Stone, M.K.; Bartels, L.W.; Prokop, M.; Moll, F.L.; Verhagen, H.J. Dynamic cine-CT angiography for the evaluation of the thoracic aorta; insight in dynamic changes with implications for thoracic endograft treatment. *Eur. J. Vasc. Endovasc. Surg.* **2006**, *32*, 532–536. [CrossRef] [PubMed]
12. Plonek, T.; Berezowski, M.; Kurcz, J.; Podgorski, P.; Sąsiadek, M.; Rylski, B.; Mysiak, A.; Jasinski, M. The evaluation of the aortic annulus displacement during cardiac cycle using magnetic resonance imaging. *BMC Cardiovasc. Disord* **2018**, *18*, 154. [CrossRef] [PubMed]
13. Guo, J.P.; Jia, X.; Sai, Z.; Ge, Y.Y.; Wang, S.; Guo, W. Thoracic Aorta Dimension Changes During Systole and Diastole: Evaluation with ECG-Gated Computed Tomography. *Ann. Vasc. Surg.* **2016**, *35*, 168–173. [CrossRef]
14. Rengier, F.; Weber, T.F.; Henninger, V.; Bockler, D.; Schumacher, H.; Kauczor, H.U.; von Tengg-Kobligk, H. Heartbeat-related distension and displacement of the thoracic aorta in healthy volunteers. *Eur. J. Radiol.* **2012**, *81*, 158–164. [CrossRef] [PubMed]
15. Weber, T.F.; Ganten, M.K.; Böckler, D.; Geisbüsch, P.; Kopp-Schneider, A.; Kauczor, H.U.; von Tengg-Kobligk, H. Assessment of thoracic aortic conformational changes by four-dimensional computed tomography angiography in patients with chronic aortic dissection type b. *Eur. Radiol.* **2009**, *19*, 245–253. [CrossRef]
16. Weber, T.F.; Ganten, M.K.; Böckler, D.; Geisbüsch, P.; Kauczor, H.U.; von Tengg-Kobligk, H. Heartbeat-related displacement of the thoracic aorta in patients with chronic aortic dissection type B: Quantification by dynamic CTA. *Eur. J. Radiol.* **2009**, *72*, 483–488. [CrossRef] [PubMed]
17. de Heer, L.M.; Budde, R.P.; Mali, W.P.; de Vos, A.M.; van Herwerden, L.A.; Kluin, J. Aortic root dimension changes during systole and diastole: Evaluation with ECG-gated multidetector row computed tomography. *Int. J. Cardiovasc. Imaging* **2011**, *27*, 1195–1204. [CrossRef]
18. Chen, D.; Luo, M.; Fang, K.; Shu, C. Endovascular repair for acute zone 0 intramural hematoma with most proximal tear or ulcer-like projection in the descending aorta. *J. Vasc. Surg.* **2021**, *75*, 1561–1569. [CrossRef]
19. Roselli, E.E.; Atkins, M.D.; Brinkman, W.; Coselli, J.; Desai, N.; Estrera, A.; Johnston, D.R.; Patel, H.; Preventza, O.; Vargo, P.R.; et al. ARISE: First-In-Human Evaluation of a Novel Stent Graft to Treat Ascending Aortic Dissection. *J. Endovasc. Ther.* **2022**, Online ahead of print. [CrossRef] [PubMed]
20. Csobay-Novák, C.; Fontanini, D.M.; Szilágyi, B.; Szeberin, Z.; Kolossváry, M.; Maurovich-Horvat, P.; Hüttl, K.; Sótonyi, P. Thoracic Aortic Strain is Irrelevant Regarding Endograft Sizing in Most Young Patients. *Ann. Vasc. Surg.* **2017**, *38*, 227–232. [CrossRef]
21. Satriano, A.; Guenther, Z.; White, J.A.; Merchant, N.; Di Martino, E.S.; Al-Qoofi, F.; Lydell, C.P.; Fine, N.M. Three-dimensional thoracic aorta principal strain analysis from routine ECG-gated computerized tomography: Feasibility in patients undergoing transcatheter aortic valve replacement. *BMC Cardiovasc. Disord* **2018**, *18*, 76. [CrossRef] [PubMed]
22. Liu, L.; Zhang, S.; Lu, Q.; Jing, Z.; Zhang, S.; Xu, B. Impact of Oversizing on the Risk of Retrograde Dissection After TEVAR for Acute and Chronic Type B Dissection. *J. Endovasc. Ther.* **2016**, *23*, 620–625. [CrossRef] [PubMed]
23. Redheuil, A.; Yu, W.C.; Wu, C.O.; Mousseaux, E.; de Cesare, A.; Yan, R.; Kachenoura, N.; Bluemke, D.; Lima, J.A. Reduced ascending aortic strain and distensibility: Earliest manifestations of vascular aging in humans. *Hypertension* **2010**, *55*, 319–326. [CrossRef] [PubMed]
24. van Prehn, J.; Vincken, K.L.; Muhs, B.E.; Barwegen, G.K.; Bartels, L.W.; Prokop, M.; Moll, F.L.; Verhagen, H.J. Toward endografting of the ascending aorta: Insight into dynamics using dynamic cine-CTA. *J. Endovasc. Ther.* **2007**, *14*, 551–560. [CrossRef] [PubMed]
25. Marone, E.M.; Freyrie, A.; Ruotolo, C.; Michelagnoli, S.; Antonello, M.; Speziale, F.; Veroux, P.; Gargiulo, M.; Gaggiano, A. Expert Opinion on Hostile Neck Definition in Endovascular Treatment of Abdominal Aortic Aneurysms (a Delphi Consensus). *Ann. Vasc. Surg.* **2020**, *62*, 173–182. [CrossRef] [PubMed]
26. Jordan, W.D., Jr.; Ouriel, K.; Mehta, M.; Varnagy, D.; Moore, W.M., Jr.; Arko, F.R.; Joye, J.; de Vries, J.P. Outcome-based anatomic criteria for defining the hostile aortic neck. *J. Vasc. Surg.* **2015**, *61*, 1383–1390.e1381. [CrossRef] [PubMed]
27. Pitoulias, G.A.; Valdivia, A.R.; Hahtapornsawan, S.; Torsello, G.; Pitoulias, A.G.; Austermann, M.; Gandarias, C.; Donas, K.P. Conical neck is strongly associated with proximal failure in standard endovascular aneurysm repair. *J. Vasc. Surg.* **2017**, *66*, 1686–1695. [CrossRef]
28. Plunde, O.; Bäck, M. Arterial Stiffness in Aortic Stenosis and the Impact of Aortic Valve Replacement. *Vasc. Health Risk Manag.* **2022**, *18*, 117–122. [CrossRef]
29. Voges, I.; Jerosch-Herold, M.; Hedderich, J.; Pardun, E.; Hart, C.; Gabbert, D.D.; Hansen, J.H.; Petko, C.; Kramer, H.H.; Rickers, C. Normal values of aortic dimensions, distensibility, and pulse wave velocity in children and young adults: A cross-sectional study. *J. Cardiovasc. Magn. Reson.* **2012**, *14*, 77. [CrossRef]

Disclaimer/Publisher's Note: The statements, opinions and data contained in all publications are solely those of the individual author(s) and contributor(s) and not of MDPI and/or the editor(s). MDPI and/or the editor(s) disclaim responsibility for any injury to people or property resulting from any ideas, methods, instructions or products referred to in the content.

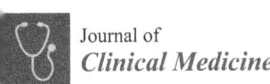

Article

Effectiveness and Minimal-Invasiveness of Zone 0 Landing Thoracic Endovascular Aortic Repair Using Branched Endograft

Tomoaki Kudo [1,*], Toru Kuratani [2], Yoshiki Sawa [1] and Shigeru Miyagawa [1]

[1] Department of Cardiovascular Surgery, Osaka University Graduate School of Medicine, Suita 5650871, Osaka, Japan
[2] Department of Minimally Invasive Cardiovascular Medicine, Osaka University Graduate School of Medicine, Suita 5650871, Osaka, Japan
* Correspondence: tkudoh0217@gmail.com; Tel.:+81-6-6879-3154

Abstract: Background: Zone 0 landing thoracic endovascular aortic repair (TEVAR) for the treatment of aortic arch diseases has become a topic of interest. This study aimed to verify whether branced TEVAR (bTEVAR) is an effective and a more minimally invasive treatment by comparing the outcomes of bTEVAR and hybrid TEVAR (hTEVAR) in landing zone 0. Methods: This retrospective, single-center, observational cohort study included 54 patients (bTEVAR, $n = 25$; hTEVAR, $n = 29$; median age, 78 years; median follow-up period, 5.4 years) from October 2012 to June 2018. The logistic Euro-SCORE was significantly higher in the bTEVAR group than in the hTEVAR group (38% vs. 21%, $p < 0.001$). Results: There was no significant difference the in-hospital mortality between the bTEVAR and hTEVAR groups (0% vs. 3.4%, $p = 1.00$). The operative time (220 vs. 279 min, $p < 0.001$) and length of hospital stay (12 vs. 17 days, $p = 0.013$) were significantly shorter in the bTEVAR group than in the hTEVAR group. The 7-year free rates of aorta-related deaths (bTEVAR [95.5%] vs. hTEVAR [86.9%], Log-rank $p = 0.390$) and aortic reintervention (bTEVAR [86.3%] vs. hTEVAR [86.9%], Log-rank $p = 0.638$) were not significantly different. Conclusions: The early and mid-term outcomes in both groups were satisfactory. bTEVAR might be superior to hTEVAR in that it is less invasive. Therefore, bTEVAR may be considered an effective and a more minimally invasive treatment for high-risk patients.

Keywords: thoracic endovascular aortic repair; stroke; endoleak

1. Introduction

Conventional open surgery is the most commonly performed procedure for aortic arch diseases. However, the treatment of aortic arch pathologies is complicated to treat because conventional open surgeries are highly invasive and complex [1,2]. In some reports, the short-term results of hybrid thoracic endovascular aortic repair (TEVAR) were superior to those of conventional open surgery, whereas the long-term outcomes were equivalent [3–5]. Recently, hybrid TEVAR (hTEVAR) has gained increasing attention for the treatment of aortic arch pathologies, especially for high-risk patients [6–8]. Conventional zone 0 landing hTEVAR is moderately invasive surgical procedure because it requires median sternotomy and aorto-cervical bypasses but does not necessitate cardiopulmonary bypass [9–11]. To reduce the invasiveness, we have performed TEVAR using a branched stent-graft, in which complex aorto-cervical bypass or graft replacement is not required [12]. The purpose of this study was to verify whether branched (bTEVAR) is an effective and a more minimally invasive treatment by comparing the outcomes of bTEVAR and hTEVAR in the landing zone (LZ) 0.

2. Materials and Methods

2.1. Ethics Statement and Study Design

All protocols of TEVAR using branched endografts in this study were approved by the Medical Ethics Committee of Osaka University School of Medicine (No. 15087). Informed

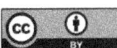

consent was obtained from all patients before the procedures. This study was conducted as a single-center, retrospective, and observational cohort study.

2.2. Preoperative Measurements and Treatment Strategy

All patients underwent contrast-enhanced multidetector computed tomography (MDCT) using a slice thickness of ≤ 1 mm. Three-dimensional reconstructions were performed on an image processing workstation (Aquarius Intuition; TeraRecon, Foster City, CA, USA) to evaluate the adequacy of the proximal and distal LZs, the inflow artery, the aortic arch, and the access vessels before the procedure. The indications for surgical intervention were aortic diameter expansion by ≥ 5 mm in six months, a maximum aortic diameter of >55 mm, aortic rupture, any size of saccular aneurysm, a malperfusion syndrome, or an initial diameter of >40 mm in type B aortic dissection. We did not perform a hTEVAR with a zone 0 landing in patients with suitable LZs at zones 1 and 2. In the treatment strategy, we ensured the following preprocedural conditions: proximal LZ diameter was ≤ 42 mm, and atheroma grade of the proximal LZ and the cervical arteries was 1 or 2, as described previously [6,7].

2.3. Surgical Procedure

2.3.1. Branched TEVAR

First, the patients received an extra-anatomical bypass from the right axillary artery (AxA) to the left AxA or from the right AxA to the left common carotid artery (CCA) and the left AxA using a ringed 8 mm expanded polytetrafluoroethylene graft. To protect against embolization, the left subclavian artery (LSA) was occluded using the balloon catheter.

A curved super-stiff wire was advanced to the left ventricle. The custom-made Bolton Relay NBS stent-graft (Bolton Medical, Inc., Sunrise, FL, USA) device was inserted through the femoral artery. We confirmed the precise match between the orifices of the cervical arteries and the device gate by performing standard angiography and 3D mapping using the Dyna-CT. Rapid pacing (heart rate > 160 bpm) was started, and the main device was deployed at a constant speed. Next, the wire was advanced to the posterior tunnel from the right CCA, and the stent-graft for the brachiocephalic artery (BCA) was inserted into the tunnel and deployed. The stent-graft deployment in the left CCA was performed by the same procedure. Lastly, we performed coiling of the left subclavian artery. Aortography was conducted to check for endoleaks and bypass patency, as described previously [12].

2.3.2. Hybrid TEVAR

After median sternotomy, end-to-side anastomosis was performed using a woven Dacron trifurcated graft on the greater curvature of the ascending aorta with a partial occlusion clamp without cardiopulmonary bypass. Subsequently, the BCA and left CCA were anastomosed to the branch of the graft in an end-to-end manner. The LSA was anastomosed side-to-end. The BCA was occluded by suturing, the left CCA was clipped, and the LSA was clipped or embolized with a coil. In the case of banding the ascending aorta, a woven Dacron graft was cut to the target length, and the ascending aorta was shrunk. After the supra-aortic vessels were rerouted, stent-graft devices were deployed, as described previously [7].

2.3.3. Follow-Up

Follow-up was performed at our department during regular patient visits at least once every 3 months for the first year and every 6 months or annually thereafter. MDCT was performed before discharge, at 6 months after the procedure, and yearly thereafter. Patients were followed up until death, the details of which were confirmed through telephonic interviews with their families.

Aortic events included known or suspected events such as aortic diameter enlargement >5 mm, any endoleaks, stent-graft migration, aneurysm rupture, aortic dissection, bypass graft occlusion, and prosthetic infection. Aorta-related deaths were defined as death due to aortic reinterventions.

2.4. Statistical Analyses

Results are expressed as mean ± standard deviation and median (interquartile range [IQR]) according to the normality of distribution as assessed using the Shapiro–Wilk test and were compared using the Mann–Whitney U test. Categorical variables, presented as counts and percentages, were analyzed using the chi-square test or the Fisher's exact test. The curves for overall survival and freedom from aorta-related death, aortic events, and aortic reintervention were estimated using the Kaplan–Meier product-limiting method and compared using the *Log-rank* test. Estimates were provided with 95% confidence intervals (CIs). All *p*-values were two-sided, and $p < 0.05$ was considered to indicate statistical significance. All statistical analyses were performed using JMP statistical software, version 16.0.0 for MacOS X (SAS Institute Inc., Cary, NC, USA).

3. Results

3.1. Study Population

The patient flow diagram is shown in Figure 1. Of 123 patients who underwent zone 0 landing TEVAR from October 2012 to June 2018, 54 underwent zone 0 landing TEAVR were included in this study: bTEVAR ($n = 25$, 46.3%) in patients with incapable of median sternotomy and hTEVAR ($n = 29$, 53.7%) in patients with capable of median sternotomy. We excluded cases with zone 0 landing TEVAR with graft replacement of the ascending aorta, chimney technique, graft replacement of the ascending aorta for aneurysm and type A dissection, and concomitant procedures. No patients were lost to follow-up, and all patient data were available.

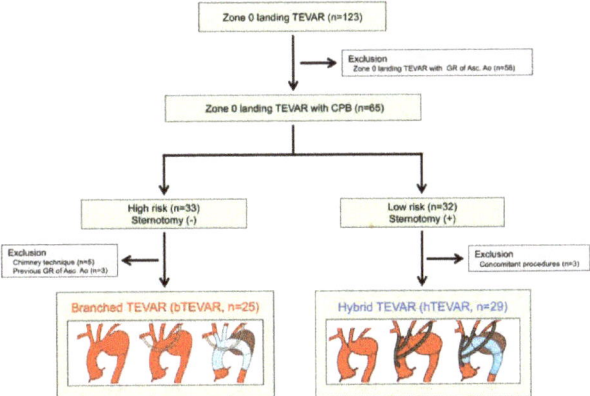

Figure 1. Treatment algorithm of this study. TEVAR: thoracic endovascular aortic repair; GR: graft replacement; Asc. Ao: ascending aorta; bTEVAR: branched TEVAR; hTEVAR: hybrid TEVAR.

3.2. Patients' Characteristics

The patient characteristics are listed in Table 1. The median follow-up period was 5.4 years (IQR, 3.2–7.8 years). The median patient age at surgery was 78 years (IQR, 73–82 years), 22 (40.7%) patients were older than 80 years, and 12 (22.2%) patients were female. None of the patients underwent emergent procedures. The pathologies were attributed to dissecting aortic aneurysms in five (9.3%) patients; however, no patients had a patent false lumen. Thirteen (24.1%) patients had a history of cardiovascular surgery, however, no patients had previous median sternotomy. The median logistic Euro-SCORE was 32% (IQR, 20–40%). The logistic Euro-SCORE was significantly higher in the bTEVAR group (38%; IQR, 34–56%) than in the hTEVAR group (21%; IQR, 13–30%) ($p < 0.001$).

Table 1. Patients' characteristics and preoperative measurements.

	All n = 54	bTEVAR n = 25 (46.3%)	hTEVAR n = 29 (53.7%)	*p*-Value
Patients' characteristics				
Age (years)	78 (73–82)	81 (76–84)	77 (69–80)	0.023
Age $\geq$ 80 years, n (%)	22 (40.7)	15 (60.0)	7 (24.1)	0.007
Female, n (%)	12 (22.2)	9 (36.0)	3 (10.3)	0.046
Emergency, n (%)	0	0	0	1.00
Aortic pathologies				
Degenerative aortic aneurysm, n (%)	49 (90.7)	22 (88.0)	27 (93.1)	0.653
Dissecting aortic aneurysm, n (%)	5 (9.3)	3 (12.0)	2 (6.9)	0.653
Dissection with patent false lumen, n (%)	0	0	0	1.00
Medical history				
Cerebrovascular disease, n (%)	12 (22.2)	7 (28.0)	5 (7.2)	0.513
Coronary artery disease, n (%)	11 (20.4)	7 (28.0)	4 (13.8)	0.310
CKD stage $\geq$ 4, n (%)	12 (22.2)	6 (24.0)	6 (20.7)	0.771
COPD, n (%)	14 (25.9)	12 (48.0)	2 (6.9)	0.001
EF (%)	66 (60–73)	65 (59–72)	68 (60–74)	0.419
Previous cardiovascular surgery, n (%)	13 (24.1)	10 (40.0)	3 (10.3)	0.023
Prior median sternotomy, n (%)	0	0	0	1.00
Logistic Euro SCORE (%)	32 (20–40)	38 (34–56)	21 (13–30)	<0.001

Data are represented as median (IQR: interquartile range). bTEVAR; branched TEVAR; hTEVAR; hybrid TEVAR; TEVAR: thoracic endovascular aortic repair; CKD: chronic kidney disease; COPD: chronic obstructive pulmonary disease; EF: ejection fraction.

3.3. Preoperative Measurements and Stent-Grafts

The preoperative measurements obtained by contrast-enhanced MDCT are shown in Table 2. The median maximum aneurysmal diameter was 58 mm (IQR, 53–65 mm). The median length and diameter of the proximal LZ were 33.6 ± 6.8 mm and 33.6 ± 3.0 mm, respectively. The mean length of the proximal LZ was significantly longer in the bTEVAR group (35.6 ± 1.3 mm) than in the hTEVAR group (31.9 ± 5.4 mm) (p = 0.049). The mean diameter of the proximal LZ was significantly greater in the bTEVAR group (39.4 ± 3.5 mm) than in the hTEVAR group (32.5 ± 2.0 mm) (p = 0.003).

Table 2. Preoperative measurements and stent-grafts.

	All n = 54	bTEVAR n = 25 (46.3%)	hTEVAR n = 29 (53.7%)	*p* Value
Preoperative measurements				
Maximum aneurysm diameter (mm)	58 (53–65)	57 (54–62)	60 (52–74)	0.335
Length of proximal LZ (mm)	33.6 ± 6.8	35.6 ± 1.3	31.9 ± 5.4	0.049
Diameter of proximal LZ (mm)	33.6 ± 3.0	34.9 ± 3.5	32.5 ± 2.0	0.003
Diameter of distal LZ (mm)	28.5 ±3.2	29.3 ± 3.4	27.8 ± 3.0	0.109
Atheroma grade				
Ascending aorta $\geq$ 2, n (%)	13 (24.1)	9 (36.0)	4 (13.8)	0.109
Aortic arch $\geq$ 3, n (%)	47 (87.0)	21 (84.0)	26 (89.7)	0.692
Descending aorta $\geq$ 3, n (%)	9 (16.7)	7 (28.0)	2 (6.9)	0.065
BCA $\geq$ 2, n (%)	14 (25.9)	6 (24.0)	8 (27.6)	0.764
Left CCA $\geq$ 2, n (%)	5 (9.3)	4 (16.0)	1 (3.5)	0.170
Stent-grafts				
Number of stent-graft, n (%)	1.5 ± 0.5	1.1 ± 0.3	1.8 ± 0.4	<0.001
Type of proximal stent-grafts				
Bolton Relay NBS, n (%)	25 (46.3)	25 (100)	0	
Bolton Relay Plus, n (%)	2 (3.7)	0	2 (6.9)	
Gore TAG, n (%)	10 (18.5)	0	10 (34.5)	
Gore CTAG, n (%)	16 (29.6)	0	16 (55.2)	
Cook Zenith TX2, n (%)	1 (1.9)	0	1 (3.4)	
Proximal stent-grafts				
Diameter (mm)	39.2 ± 3.8	41.9 ± 3.3	36.9 ± 2.4	<0.001
Oversizing rate (%)	16.9 ± 8.1	20.7 ± 8.1	13.7 ± 6.6	0.001
Distal stent-grafts				
Diameter (mm)	34.0 ± 3.9	34.4 ± 4.7	33.7 ± 3.1	0.531
Oversizing rate (%)	19.7 ± 8.6	17.6 ± 9.4	21.5 ± 7.4	0.097

Data are represented as mean ± standard deviation and median (IQR: interquartile range). bTEVAR; branched TEVAR; hTEVAR; hybrid TEVAR; TEVAR: thoracic endovascular aortic repair; LZ: landing zone; BCA: brachiocephalic artery; CCA: common carotid artery.

The numbers of patients with an atheroma grade of ≥2 in the ascending aorta and BCA were 13 (24.1%) and 14 (25.9%), respectively. These numbers were not significantly different between the two groups.

For proximal stent grafting, the custom-made branched Relay NBS was used in 25 (46.3%) patients in the bTEVAR group. The Bolton Relay Plus (Bolton Medical, Inc.) was used in two (3.7%) patients, Gore TAG (W.L. Gore & Associates, Inc., Flagstaff, AZ, USA) in 10 (18.5%) patients, Gore CTAG (W.L. Gore & Associates, Inc.) in 16 (29.6%) patients, and Cook Zenith TX2 (Cook Medical, Inc., Bloomington, IN, USA) in one (1.9%) patient in the hTEVAR group. The mean size of the proximal stent-graft was 39.2 ± 3.8 mm, and the mean oversizing rate was 16.9 ± 8.1%. The mean size of the proximal stent-graft was significantly larger in the bTEVAR group (41.9 ± 3.3 mm) than of the hTEVAR group (36.9 ± 2.4 mm) ($p < 0.001$), and the mean oversizing rate of the proximal stent-graft was significantly larger in the bTEVAR group (20.7 ± 8.1 %) than of the hTEVAR group (13.7 ± 6.6%) ($p < 0.001$).

3.4. Operative and in-Hospital Outcomes

The operative and in-hospital data are shown in Table 3. All procedures were successful, and the median operative time was 255 min (IQR, 217–290 min). The operative time was significantly longer in the hTEAVR group (220 min; IQR, 193–257 min) than in the bTEVAR group (279 min; IQR, 246–328 min) ($p < 0.001$). The median postoperative hospital stay was 16 days (IQR, 12–25 days). The postoperative hospital stay was significantly longer in the hTEVAR group (17 days; IQR, 14–26 days) than in the bTEVAR group (12 days; IQR, 9–22 days) ($p = 0.013$).

Table 3. Operative and in-hospital outcomes.

	All n = 54	bTEVAR n = 25 (46.3%)	hTEVAR n = 29 (53.7%)	p-Value
Procedure success (%)	100	100	100	1.00
Operative time (minutes)	255 (217–290)	220 (193–257)	279 (246–328)	<0.001
Postoperative hospital stay (days)	16 (12–25)	12 (9–22)	17 (14–26)	0.013
In-hospital mortality				
RTAD, n (%)	1 (1.9)	0	1 (3.4) *	1.00
Aortic complication, n (%)				
PND, n (%)	2 (3.7)	2 (8.0)	0	0.210
Spinal cord injury, n (%)	0	0	0	1.00
Abdominal embolic event, n (%)	0	0	0	1.00
New dialysis, n (%)	1 (1.9)	0	1 (3.4)	1.00
RTAD, n (%)	1 (1.9)	0	1 (3.4) *	1.00
Aneurysm enlargement, n (%)	0	0	0	1.00
Aneurysm rupture, n (%)	0	0	0	1.00
Endoleaks, n (%)				
Type 1a, n (%)	0	0	0	1.00
Type 1b, n (%)	0	0	0	1.00
Type 1c, n (%)	0	0	0	1.00
Type 2, n (%)	0	0	0	1.00
Type 3, n (%)	0	0	0	1.00

Data are represented as median (IQR: interquartile range). bTEVAR; branched TEVAR; hTEVAR; hybrid TEVAR; TEVAR: thoracic endovascular aortic repair; PND: permanent neurological dysfunction; RTAD: retrograde type A dissection, *: same patient.

One (1.9%) patient in the hTEVAR group had 30-day mortality due to retrograde type A dissection (RTAD). Two (3.7%) patients experienced permanent neurological dysfunction (PND). There were no patients with endoleaks. One (1.9%) patient in the hTEVAR group had in-hospital aortic event due to retrograde type A dissection (RTAD). However, the patient died at 11 days after hTEVAR.

3.5. Late Outcomes

The late outcomes are presented in Table 4. Aneurysm rupture was detected in two (3.7%) patients in the bTEVAR group. Those two patients had stent-graft migration, which was the cause of type 1b and 3 endoleaks. Of these two patients, the one patient with type 3 endoleak survived, whereas the other did not. Type 1a endoleak and RTAD were not observed in the late stage. Four (7.4%) cases had aortic events due to two (3.7%) aneurysm ruptures and two (3.7%) prosthetic infections.

Table 4. Late aortic events.

	All n = 54	bTEVAR n = 25 (46.3%)	hTEVAR n = 29 (53.7%)	p-Value
Aortic complication, n (%)				
PND, n (%)	0	0	0	1.00
RTAD, n (%)	0	0	0	1.00
Aneurysm enlargement, n (%)	0	0	0	1.00
Aneurysm rupture, n (%)	2 (3.7)	2 (8.0) *,+	0	0.210
Distal SINE, n (%)	0	0	0	1.00
Prosthetic infection, n (%)	2 (3.7)	0	2 (6.9)	0.493
Branched endograft occlusion, n (%)	0	0	0	1.00
Bypass graft occlusion, n (%)	0	0	0	1.00
Endoleaks, n (%)				
Type 1a, n (%)	0	0	0	1.00
Type 1b, n (%)	1 (1.9)	1 (4.0) *	0	0.463
Type 1c, n (%)	0	0	0	1.00
Type 2, n (%)	0	0	0	1.00
Type 3, n (%)	1 (1.9)	1 (4.0) +	0	0.463

bTEVAR; branched TEVAR; hTEVAR; hybrid TEVAR; TEVAR: thoracic endovascular aortic repair; PND: permanent neurological dysfunction; RTAD: retrograde type A dissection; SINE: stent graft-induced new entry, *: same patient, +: same patient.

3.6. Survival

The Kaplan–Meier curve indicating the cumulative survival is presented in Figure 2A. The survival rates at 1, 3, 5, and 7 years were 94.4% (95% CI: 84.1–98.2%), 90.6% (95% CI: 79.3–96.0%), 86.0% (95% CI: 73.3–93.2%), and 70.4% (95% CI: 53.7–83.0%), respectively. Figure 2B shows that the survival rates at 7 years were 71.5% (95% CI: 47.6–87.4%) and 71.0% (95% CI: 47.3–87.0%) for bTEVAR and hTEVAR groups, respectively, which were not significantly different (Log-rank p = 0.958).

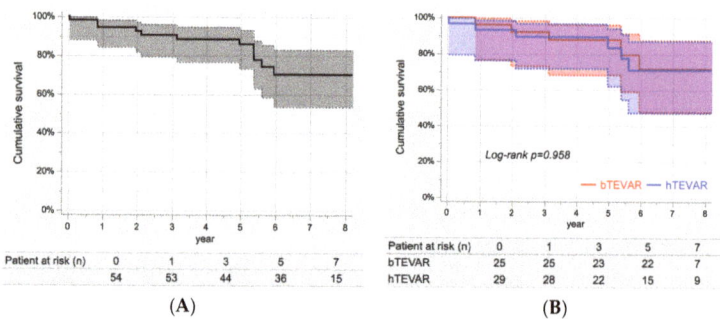

Figure 2. Cumulative survival. (**A**) Cumulative survival of the entire study group. The cumulative survival rates at 1, 3, 5, and 7 years were 94.4% (95% CI:84.1–98.2%), 90.6% (79.3–96.0%), 86.0% (73.3–93.2%), and 70.4% (53.7–83.0%), respectively. (**B**) Cumulative survival of each group. The 7-year survival rates in the bTEVAR group and the hTEVAR group were 71.5% (47.6–87.4%) and 71.0% (47.3–87.0%), respectively. There were no significant differences between the two groups (Log-rank p = 0.958).

3.7. Aorta-Related Death

Figure 3A shows the Kaplan–Meier curve indicating aorta-related death for the entire study group. The event-free rates at 1, 3, 5, and 7 years were 96.3% (95% CI: 86.2–99.1%), 94.2% (95% CI: 83.5–98.1%), 90.8% (95% CI: 77.2–96.7%), and 90.8% (95% CI: 77.2–96.7%), respectively. During the follow-up period, there were four aorta-related deaths, including one patient in the bTEVAR group who developed aneurysm rupture due to a type 1b endoleak, and in the hTEVAR group, one patient who had RTAD and two patients had the prosthetic infection. Figure 3B shows that the aorta-related death-free rates at 7 years for the bTEVAR and hTEVAR groups were 95.5% (95% CI: 73.9–99.4%) and 86.9% (95% CI: 64.8–96.0%), respectively, which were not significantly different (Log-rank p = 0.390).

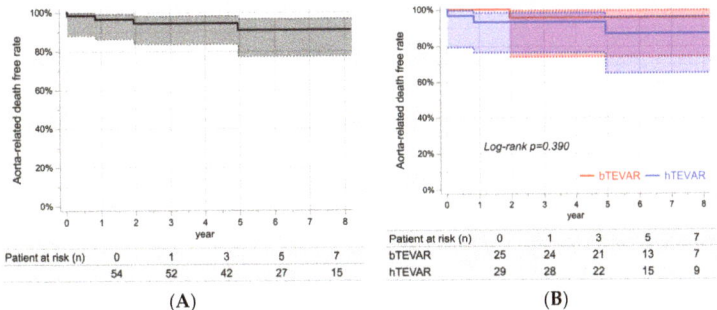

Figure 3. Freedom from aorta-related death. (**A**) Freedom from aorta-related deaths in the entire study group. The event-free rates at 1, 3, 5, and 7 years were 96.3% (95% CI: 86.2–99.1%), 94.2% (95% CI: 83.5–98.1%), 90.8% (95% CI: 77.2–96.7%), and 90.8% (95% CI: 77.2–96.7%), respectively. (**B**) Freedom from aorta-related deaths in each group. The aorta-related death free rates at 7 years for the bTEVAR and hTEVAR groups were 95.5% (95% CI: 73.9–99.4%) and 86.9% (95% CI: 64.8–96.0%), respectively, which were not significantly different (Log-rank p = 0.390).

3.8. Aortic Events

Figure 4A shows the Kaplan–Meier curve indicating aortic events for the entire study group. The event-free rates at 1, 3, 5, and 7 years were 92.6% (95% CI: 81.9–97.2%), 90.6% (95% CI: 79.4–96.0%), 87.9% (95% CI: 75.2–94.5%), and 83.3% (95% CI: 67.1–92.4%), respectively. Seven patients had aortic events: two had PND and one had RTAD in the early phase, and two had aneurysm rupture due to type 1b and 3 endoleaks and two had prosthetic infection in the late phase. Figure 4B shows the Kaplan–Meier event-free curves stratified by group. The aortic event-free rates at 7 years for the bTEVAR and hTEVAR groups were 78.9% (95% CI: 52.7–92.6%) and 86.9% (95% CI: 64.8–96.0%), respectively, with no significant differences (Log-rank p = 0.614).

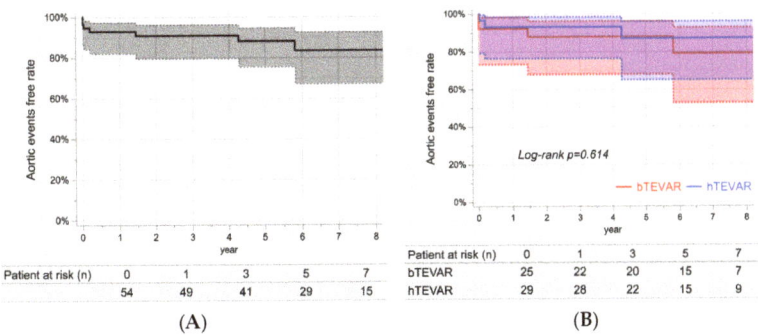

Figure 4. Freedom from aortic events. (**A**) The event-free rates at 1, 3, 5, and 7 years were 92.6% (95% CI: 81.9–97.2%), 90.6% (95% CI: 79.4–96.0%), 87.9% (95% CI: 75.2–94.5%), and 83.3% (95% CI: 67.1–92.4%), respectively. (**B**) The aortic events-free rates at 7 years for the bTEVAR and hTEVAR groups were 78.9% (95% CI: 52.7–92.6%) and 86.9% (95% CI: 64.8–96.0%), respectively, with no significant differences (Log-rank p = 0.614).

4. Discussion

For over a half of a century, the conventional total arch replacement has been considered the gold standard for the surgical treatment of aortic arch diseases [13–15]. However, this treatment is difficult for high-risk patients due to its complexity and substantial invasiveness, thus yielding unsatisfactory outcomes such as an in-hospital mortality rate of 5.0–11.3%, as reported by some studies [9,16–18]. TEVAR was introduced as a minimally invasive technique, while hTEVAR was reported as a potential alternative to conventional total arch replacement in high-risk patients [3,6–8,19–21]. Milewski et al. [22] stated that the high-risk patients aged >75 years had significantly lower in-hospital mortality after hybrid TEVAR. Consequently, the indications for hybrid TEVAR have been gradually expanded. The previously reported the in-hospital mortality after zone 0 landing TEVAR was 5.0–12% [9,23–25]. In fact, some reports from institutions performing both conventional arch repair and hTEVAR stated that the in-hospital mortalities were not significantly different [9,19,24,26]. In this study, early results were satisfactory because the in-hospital mortality was 1.6% ($n = 1$).

Because bTEVAR had a shorter operation time and postoperative hospital stay (bTEVAR: 12 days vs. hTEVAR: 17 days; $p = 0.013$), bTEVAR is considered to be less invasive than hTEVAR. In addition, bTEVAR could be cosidered an effective and a more minimally invasive treatment despite its use in high-risk patients, because the early and mid-term results of bTEVAR and hTEVAR are not significantly different. The PND rates in the bTEVAR and hTEVAR groups were 8.0% ($n = 2$) and 0%, respectively. The PND rate in the bTEVAR group reported by previous articles was equal to that of zone 0 landing hTEVAR (5–17%); however, it was higher than that reported in previous studies with conventional arch repair (2–9%) [10,18–24]. In addition, the 7-year aorta-related death-free and aortic event-free rates were 90.8% (bTEVAR: 95.5% and hTEVAR: 86.9%, Log-rank $p = 0.390$) and 83.3% (bTEVAR: 78.9% and hTEVAR: 86.9%, Log-rank $p = 0.614$), which were equal to those of conventional arch repair [13,14]. In the future, it will be possible to reduce the invasiveness of the surgery by performing bTEVAR; however, PND and aortic reintervention due to endoleak should be prevented.

As for PND, preoperative evaluation of aorta properties, such as shagginess, is important, as reported in other studies [27]. We reported that the risk factor for PND in bTEVAR is an atheroma grade ≥ 2 in the BCA, and we recommend hTEVAR instead of bTEVAR for such patients [12].

Type 1a endoleaks are a fatal complication to be avoided, with few practical alternatives to endovascular treatment. In previous reports, the rates of type 1a endoleak ranged from 2.3–22.6% [21,25,28,29]. In addition, one (1.6%) patient in the hTEVAR group experienced RTAD and died. RTAD originated from a partially clamped site of the ascending aorta and was not induced by the stent-graft. In some reports, an ascending aorta diameter of >40 mm and a stent-graft diameter of ≥ 42 mm are considered risk factors for RTAD [30–32]. Thus, we believe that using stent-grafts with a diameter of ≥ 42 mm is a risk factor for RTAD. However, patients in the bTEVAR group at high risk for median sternotomy reluctantly used 42–46 mm stent-grafts, none of whom had RTAD. The other endoleaks were observed in the bTEVAR group; however, we believe that these endoleaks could be prevented. Regarding bTEVAR, a shorter and stricter follow-up time seem necessary.

bTEVAR can be considered more minimally invasive because of its short operating time and postoperative hospital stay. Although bTEVAR may be effective for high-risk patients who are not candidates for median sternotomy due to its low risk of aorta-related death and aortic events, preventing cerebral infarction in these patients will be an important issue in the future.

Limitations

This study has some biases as follows: (1) it was a retrospective single-center study with a relatively small sample size, (2) some patients had relatively short follow-up periods, and (3) the patients were carefully selected. Therefore, a prospective multicenter study with long-term follow-up is required to confirm our findings. Moreover, the findings of this study need to be validated through further clinical investigations.

5. Conclusions

We achieved satisfactory early and mid-term results of zone 0 landing bTEVAR and hTEVAR. bTEVAR might be superior to hTEVAR in that it is less invasive. bTEVAR may be considered an effective and more minimally invasive treatment for high-risk patients.

Author Contributions: Conceptualization, T.K. (Tomoaki Kudo) and T.K. (Toru Kuratani); Data curation, T.K. (Tomoaki Kudo); Formal analysis, T.K. (Tomoaki Kudo) and T.K. (Toru Kuratani); Supervision, T.K. (Toru Kuratani), Y.S. and S.M.; Validation, T.K. (Tomoaki Kudo), T.K. (Toru Kuratani), Y.S. and S.M.; Writing—original draft, T.K. (Tomoaki Kudo); Writing—review and editing, T.K. (Tomoaki Kudo), T.K. (Toru Kuratani), Y.S. and S.M. All authors have read and agreed to the published version of the manuscript.

Funding: This research received no external funding.

Institutional Review Board Statement: All protocols of TEVAR using branched endografts in this study were approved by the Medical Ethics Committee of Osaka University School of Medicine (No. 15087).

Informed Consent Statement: Informed consent was obtained from all patients before the procedures.

Data Availability Statement: Data cannot be shared for ethical/privacy reasons. The data underlying this article cannot be shared publicly due to the privacy of individuals that participated in the study. On reasonable request, the data will be available from the corresponding author after approval from the Ethical Committee of the University of Osaka.

Conflicts of Interest: The authors declare no conflict of interest.

References

1. Iafrancesco, M.; Ranasinghe, A.M.; Dronavalli, V.; Adam, D.J.; Claridge, M.W.; Riley, P.; McCafferty, I.; Mascaro, J.G. Open aortic arch replacement in high-risk patients: The gold standard. *Eur. J. Cardiothorac. Surg.* **2016**, *49*, 646–651; discussion 651. [CrossRef] [PubMed]
2. Tanaka, Y.; Mikamo, A.; Suzuki, R.; Kurazumi, H.; Kudo, T.; Takahashi, M.; Ikenaga, S.; Shirasawa, B.; Hamano, K. Mortality and morbidity after total aortic arch replacement. *Ann. Thorac. Surg.* **2014**, *97*, 1569–1575. [CrossRef] [PubMed]
3. Shirakawa, Y.; Kuratani, T.; Shimamura, K.; Torikai, K.; Sakamoto, T.; Shijo, T.; Sawa, Y. The efficacy and short-term results of hybrid thoracic endovascular repair into the ascending aorta for aortic arch pathologies. *Eur. J. Cardiothorac. Surg.* **2014**, *45*, 298–304; discussion 304. [CrossRef]
4. Lotfi, S.; Clough, R.E.; Ali, T.; Salter, R.; Young, C.P.; Bell, R.; Modarai, B.; Taylor, P. Hybrid repair of complex thoracic aortic arch pathology: Long-term outcomes of extra-anatomic bypass grafting of the supra-aortic trunk. *Cardiovasc. Intervent. Radiol.* **2013**, *36*, 46–55. [CrossRef]
5. Murashita, T.; Matsuda, H.; Domae, K.; Iba, Y.; Tanaka, H.; Sasaki, H.; Ogino, H. Less invasive surgical treatment for aortic arch aneurysms in high-risk patients: A comparative study of hybrid thoracic endovascular aortic repair and conventional total arch replacement. *J. Thorac. Cardiovasc. Surg.* **2012**, *143*, 1007–1013. [CrossRef] [PubMed]
6. Kudo, T.; Kuratani, T.; Shimamura, K.; Sakamoto, T.; Kin, K.; Masada, K.; Shijo, T.; Torikai, K.; Maeda, K.; Sawa, Y. Type 1a endoleak following Zone 1 and Zone 2 thoracic endovascular aortic repair: Effect of bird-beak configuration. *Eur. J. Cardiothorac. Surg.* **2017**, *52*, 718–724. [CrossRef]
7. Kudo, T.; Kuratani, T.; Shimamura, K.; Sakaniwa, R.; Sawa, Y. Long-term results of hybrid aortic arch repair using landing zone 0: A single-centre study. *Eur. J. Cardiothorac. Surg.* **2021**, *59*, 1227–1235. [CrossRef]
8. Kudo, T.; Kuratani, T.; Shimamura, K.; Sawa, Y. Determining the Optimal Proximal Landing Zone for TEVAR in the Aortic Arch: Comparing the Occurrence of the Bird-Beak Phenomenon in Zone 0 vs. Zones 1 and 2. *J. Endovasc. Ther.* **2020**, *27*, 368–376. [CrossRef]
9. Preventza, O.; Garcia, A.; Cooley, D.A.; Haywood-Watson, R.J.; Simpson, K.; Bakaeen, F.G.; Cornwell, L.D.; Omer, S.; de la Cruz, K.I.; Price, M.D.; et al. Total aortic arch replacement: A comparative study of zone 0 hybrid arch exclusion versus traditional open repair. *J. Thorac. Cardiovasc. Surg.* **2015**, *150*, 1591–1598; discussion 1598–1600. [CrossRef]
10. Preventza, O.; Tan, C.W.; Orozco-Sevilla, V.; Euhus, C.J.; Coselli, J.S. Zone zero hybrid arch exclusion versus open total arch replacement. *Ann. Cardiothorac. Surg.* **2018**, *7*, 372–379. [CrossRef]
11. Shimizu, H.; Hirahara, N.; Motomura, N.; Miyata, H.; Takamoto, S. Current status of cardiovascular surgery in Japan, 2015 and 2016: Analysis of data from Japan Cardiovascular Surgery Database. 4-Thoracic aortic surgery. *Gen. Thorac. Cardiovasc. Surg.* **2019**, *67*, 751–757. [CrossRef] [PubMed]

12. Kudo, T.; Kuratani, T.; Shimamura, K.; Sawa, Y. Early and midterm results of thoracic endovascular aortic repair using a branched endograft for aortic arch pathologies: A retrospective single-center study. *JTCVS Tech.* **2020**, *4*, 17–25. [CrossRef]
13. Okita, Y.; Miyata, H.; Motomura, N.; Takamoto, S.; Japan Cardiovascular Surgery Database Organization. A study of brain protection during total arch replacement comparing antegrade cerebral perfusion versus hypothermic circulatory arrest, with or without retrograde cerebral perfusion: Analysis based on the Japan Adult Cardiovascular Surgery Database. *J. Thorac. Cardiovasc. Surg.* **2015**, *149*, S65–S73. [CrossRef] [PubMed]
14. Minatoya, K.; Inoue, Y.; Sasaki, H.; Tanaka, H.; Seike, Y.; Oda, T.; Omura, A.; Iba, Y.; Ogino, H.; Kobayashi, J. Total arch replacement using a 4-branched graft with antegrade cerebral perfusion. *J. Thorac. Cardiovasc. Surg.* **2019**, *157*, 1370–1378. [CrossRef] [PubMed]
15. Kurazumi, H.; Mikamo, A.; Kudo, T.; Suzuki, R.; Takahashi, M.; Shirasawa, B.; Zempo, N.; Hamano, K. Aortic arch surgery in octogenarians: Is it justified? *Eur. J. Cardiothorac. Surg.* **2014**, *46*, 672–677. [CrossRef]
16. Leshnower, B.G.; Kilgo, P.D.; Chen, E.P. Total arch replacement using moderate hypothermic circulatory arrest and unilateral selective antegrade cerebral perfusion. *J. Thorac. Cardiovasc. Surg.* **2014**, *147*, 1488–1492. [CrossRef]
17. Misfeld, M.; Leontyev, S.; Borger, M.A.; Gindensperger, O.; Lehmann, S.; Legare, J.F.; Mohr, F.W. What is the best strategy for brain protection in patients undergoing aortic arch surgery? A single center experience of 636 patients. *Ann. Thorac. Surg.* **2012**, *93*, 1502–1508. [CrossRef]
18. De Rango, P.; Ferrer, C.; Coscarella, C.; Musumeci, F.; Verzini, F.; Pogany, G.; Montalto, A.; Cao, P. Contemporary comparison of aortic arch repair by endovascular and open surgical reconstructions. *J. Vasc. Surg.* **2015**, *61*, 339–346. [CrossRef]
19. Iba, Y.; Minatoya, K.; Matsuda, H.; Sasaki, H.; Tanaka, H.; Oda, T.; Kobayashi, J. How should aortic arch aneurysms be treated in the endovascular aortic repair era? A risk-adjusted comparison between open and hybrid arch repair using propensity score-matching analysis. *Eur. J. Cardiothorac. Surg.* **2014**, *46*, 32–39. [CrossRef]
20. Bavaria, J.; Vallabhajosyula, P.; Moeller, P.; Szeto, W.; Desai, N.; Pochettino, A. Hybrid approaches in the treatment of aortic arch aneurysms: Postoperative and midterm outcomes. *J. Thorac. Cardiovasc. Surg.* **2013**, *145*, S85–S90. [CrossRef]
21. Vallejo, N.; Rodriguez-Lopez, J.A.; Heidari, P.; Wheatley, G.; Caparrelli, D.; Ramaiah, V.; Diethrich, E.B. Hybrid repair of thoracic aortic lesions for zone 0 and 1 in high-risk patients. *J. Vasc. Surg.* **2012**, *55*, 318–325. [CrossRef] [PubMed]
22. Milewski, R.K.; Szeto, W.Y.; Pochettino, A.; Moser, G.W.; Moeller, P.; Bavaria, J.E. Have hybrid procedures replaced open aortic arch reconstruction in high-risk patients? A comparative study of elective open arch debranching with endovascular stent graft placement and conventional elective open total and distal aortic arch reconstruction. *J. Thorac. Cardiovasc. Surg.* **2010**, *140*, 590–597. [CrossRef] [PubMed]
23. Kent, W.D.; Appoo, J.J.; Bavaria, J.E.; Herget, E.J.; Moeller, P.; Pochettino, A.; Wong, J.K. Results of type II hybrid arch repair with zone 0 stent graft deployment for complex aortic arch pathology. *J. Thorac. Cardiovasc. Surg.* **2014**, *148*, 2951–2955. [CrossRef] [PubMed]
24. Narita, H.; Komori, K.; Usui, A.; Yamamoto, H.; Banno, H.; Kodama, A.; Sugimoto, M. Postoperative Outcomes of Hybrid Repair in the Treatment of Aortic Arch Aneurysms. *Ann. Vasc. Surg.* **2016**, *34*, 55–61. [CrossRef]
25. Czerny, M.; Weigang, E.; Sodeck, G.; Schmidli, J.; Antona, C.; Gelpi, G.; Friess, T.; Klocker, J.; Szeto, W.Y.; Moeller, P.; et al. Targeting landing zone 0 by total arch rerouting and TEVAR: Midterm results of a transcontinental registry. *Ann. Thorac. Surg.* **2012**, *94*, 84–89. [CrossRef]
26. Tokuda, Y.; Oshima, H.; Narita, Y.; Abe, T.; Araki, Y.; Mutsuga, M.; Fujimoto, K.; Terazawa, S.; Yagami, K.; Ito, H.; et al. Hybrid versus open repair of aortic arch aneurysms: Comparison of postoperative and mid-term outcomes with a propensity score-matching analysis. *Eur. J. Cardiothorac. Surg.* **2016**, *49*, 149–156. [CrossRef]
27. Maeda, K.; Ohki, T.; Kanaoka, Y.; Shukuzawa, K.; Baba, T.; Momose, M. A Novel Shaggy Aorta Scoring System to Predict Embolic Complications Following Thoracic Endovascular Aneurysm Repair. *Eur. J. Vasc. Endovasc. Surg.* **2020**, *60*, 57–66. [CrossRef]
28. He, X.; Liu, W.; Li, Z.; Liu, X.; Wang, T.; Ding, C.; Zeng, H. Hybrid Approach to Management of Complex Aortic Arch Pathologies: A Single-Center Experience in China. *Ann. Vasc. Surg.* **2016**, *31*, 23–29. [CrossRef]
29. Melissano, G.; Tshomba, Y.; Bertoglio, L.; Rinaldi, E.; Chiesa, R. Analysis of stroke after TEVAR involving the aortic arch. *Eur. J. Vasc. Endovasc. Surg.* **2012**, *43*, 269–275. [CrossRef]
30. Gandet, T.; Canaud, L.; Ozdemir, B.A.; Ziza, V.; Demaria, R.; Albat, B.; Alric, P. Factors favoring retrograde aortic dissection after endovascular aortic arch repair. *J. Thorac. Cardiovasc. Surg.* **2015**, *150*, 136–142. [CrossRef]
31. Williams, J.B.; Andersen, N.D.; Bhattacharya, S.D.; Scheer, E.; Piccini, J.P.; McCann, R.L.; Hughes, G.C. Retrograde ascending aortic dissection as an early complication of thoracic endovascular aortic repair. *J. Vasc. Surg.* **2012**, *55*, 1255–1262. [CrossRef] [PubMed]
32. Yammine, H.; Briggs, C.S.; Stanley, G.A.; Ballast, J.K.; Anderson, W.E.; Nussbaum, T.; Madjarov, J.; Frederick, J.R.; Arko, F.R., 3rd. Retrograde type A dissection after thoracic endovascular aortic repair for type B aortic dissection. *J. Vasc. Surg.* **2019**, *69*, 24–33. [CrossRef] [PubMed]

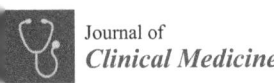

Review

Chimney vs. Fenestrated Endovascular vs. Open Repair for Juxta/Pararenal Abdominal Aortic Aneurysms: Systematic Review and Network Meta-Analysis of the Medium-Term Results

Petar Zlatanovic [1,*], Aleksa Jovanovic [2], Paolo Tripodi [3] and Lazar Davidovic [1,4]

1. Clinic for Vascular and Endovascular Surgery, University Clinical Centre of Serbia, 11000 Belgrade, Serbia
2. Institute of Epidemiology, Faculty of Medicine, University of Belgrade, 11000 Belgrade, Serbia
3. Vascular Surgery Division, Hospital Clinic Universitari Sagrat Cor, University of Barcelona, 08007 Barcelona, Spain
4. Faculty of Medicine, University of Belgrade, 11000 Belgrade, Serbia
* Correspondence: petar91goldy@gmail.com

Abstract: **Abstract Introduction:** This systematic review with network meta-analysis aimed at comparing the medium-term results of open surgery (OS), fenestrated endovascular repair (FEVAR), and chimney endovascular repair (ChEVAR) in patients with juxta/pararenal abdominal aortic aneurysms (JAAAs/PAAAs). **Materials and methods:** MEDLINE, SCOPUS, and Web of Science were searched from inception date to 1st July 2022. Any studies comparing the results of two or three treatment strategies (ChEVAR, FEVAR, or OS) on medium-term outcomes in patients with JAAAs/PAAAs were included. Primary outcomes were all-cause mortality, aortic-related reintervention, and aortic-related mortality, while secondary outcomes were visceral stent/bypass occlusion/occlusion, major adverse cardiovascular events (MACEs), new onset renal replacement therapy (RRT), total endoleaks, and type I/III endoleak. **Results:** FEVAR (OR = 1.53, 95%CrI 1.03–2.11) was associated with higher medium-term all-cause mortality than OS. Sensitivity analysis including only studies that analysed JAAA showed that FEVAR (OR = 1.65, 95%CrI 1.08–2.33) persisted to be associated with higher medium-term mortality than OS. Both FEVAR (OR = 8.32, 95%CrI 3.80–27.16) and ChEVAR (OR = 5.95, 95%CrI 2.23–20.18) were associated with a higher aortic-related reintervention rate than OS. No difference between different treatment options was found in terms of aortic-related mortality. FEVAR (OR = 13.13, 95%CrI 2.70–105.2) and ChEVAR (OR = 16.82, 95%CrI 2.79–176.7) were associated with a higher rate of medium-term visceral branch occlusion/stenosis compared to OS; however, there was no difference found between FEVAR and ChEVAR. **Conclusions:** An advantage of OS compared to FEVAR and ChEVAR after mid-term follow-up aortic-related intervention and vessel branch/bypass stenosis/occlusion was found. This suggests that younger, low-surgical-risk patients might benefit from open surgery of JAAA/PAAA as a first approach.

Keywords: abdominal aortic aneurysm (AAA); juxtarenal; pararenal; endovascular aneurysm repair (EVAR); fenestrated EVAR (FEVAR); chimney EVAR (ChEVAR); open surgery; medium-term

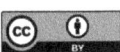

1. Introduction

The complexity of abdominal aortic aneurysm (AAA) repair depends mainly on anatomical detail relating to the segment of non-dilated aorta between renal arteries and the aneurysm, referred to as the aneurysm 'neck'. Some 40–60% of aneurysms fall within the category of infrarenal AAA with adequate neck characteristics [1,2], and there is a wealth of comparative effectiveness evidence relating to such patients [3]. Aneurysms that have a neck that is too short or otherwise unsuitable for standard endovascular aneurysm repair (EVAR) within instructions for use (IFUs) are referred to as "complex aneurysms".

Juxta/pararenal abdominal aortic aneurysms (JAAAs/PAAAs) are a frequent variation of complex abdominal aortic aneurysms (AAAs). JAAA is defined by European Society for Vascular Surgery guidelines and Society for Vascular Surgery reporting standards as "AAA which extends up to renal arteries but does not involve them", while PAAA is defined as "AAA where at least one or both renal arteries derive from AAA itself, but does not involve the superior mesenteric artery" [4–6].

Recent systematic reviews and meta-analyses have demonstrated the short-term benefit of fenestrated and chimney endovascular aneurysm repair (FEVAR/ChEVAR) in comparison with open surgery (OS) [7]; however, medium/long-term results are scarce. Previous reviews performed on the subject were either scoping in nature and lacked an analytical approach, or incorporated studies contributing data from only a single approach [8,9]. Others included also patients with suprarenal and paravisceral AAAs and thoracoabdominal AAAs [10].

This systematic review and network meta-analysis aimed at comparing the medium-term results of OS, FEVAR, and ChEVAR for patients with juxta/pararenal abdominal aortic aneurysms.

2. Methods

We performed a systematic review following the Preferred Reporting Items for Systematic Reviews and Meta-Analyses (PRISMA) and assessing the methodological quality of systematic reviews (AMSTAR) guidelines [11,12]. MEDLINE, SCOPUS, and Web of Science were searched from their inception to 1 July 2022 for studies reporting comparative outcomes for patients with JAAAs/PAAAs undergoing two or more treatment modalities: OS, FEVAR, OR ChEVAR. No restrictions were placed in terms of publication type. Grey literature was not searched. The full search strategy is available in Appendix SA. The study was registered on PROSPERO on 11 August 2021 (record number CRD42021267189).

2.1. Screening and Study Selection

We included studies comparing the results of two or three treatment strategies (OS, FEVAR, and ChEVAR) on medium-term clinical outcomes for patients with JAAAs/PAAAs. Medium-term was defined as a follow-up period of at least 6 months, ranging up to 60 months. Studies with standard infrarenal AAAs, AAAs with long but hostile neck characteristics (excessive thrombus, excessive angulation, conical shape, or calcifications) where standard infrarenal EVAR outside instructions for use has been performed, infected AAAs, ruptured AAA patients, thoracoabdominal aortic aneurysms (ThAAAs), suprarenal AAAs involving visceral segment at the level of the superior mesenteric artery and celiac trunk, connective-tissue-related aneurysms, studies containing less than 10 patients per treatment arm (to ensure enough experience in the treatment of this complex AAA pathology), performed before 2010 (to reduce the number of different stent graft generations in the comparison), and those having less than 6 months of follow-up were excluded from the analysis. Systematic reviews with or without meta-analysis, traditional reviews, comments, editorials and letters, and case reports were excluded, as well as any animal studies. A hand search of systematic reviews was also performed. Non-English articles were excluded unless they had an English abstract with extractable data. Two reviewers (P.Z. and P.T.) independently screened titles and abstracts as well as full texts of potentially eligible studies. Disagreements were resolved by discussion or consulting the third and fourth authors (A.J. and L.D.). The Rayyan systematic review web application (Available from www.rayyan.ai, accessed on 12 August 2022) was used for abstract screening.

2.2. Data Extraction and Definitions

Two authors independently extracted data, and any disagreements were resolved by the third and fourth authors. The following data were extracted from each study: study characteristics, study demographics, and periprocedural data (Appendix SB).

2.3. Outcomes Measures

Outcome measures were decided a priori. The mean follow-up time point was 31.4 months and was considered to be a medium-term interval.

Primary medium-term outcomes:

All-cause mortality, aortic-related reintervention, and aortic-related mortality.

Secondary medium-term outcomes:

Visceral stent/bypass occlusion/occlusion; major adverse cardiovascular events (MACEs) that were defined as a composite endpoint of cardiac death, myocardial infarction, coronary artery revascularisation, stroke, and hospitalisation because of heart failure; new onset renal replacement therapy (RRT); total endoleaks; and type I/III endoleak (including persistent gutter type Ia endoleak in ChEVAR group).

2.4. Quality Assessment

No RCTs that fulfilled the inclusion criteria were found after the screening of the manuscripts. The Risk of Bias in Non-randomized Studies—of Interventions (ROBINS-I) tool was used to assess the quality of included observational studies [13]. The Grading of Recommendation Assessment, Development, and Evaluation (GRADE) system was used to analyse the overall quality of evidence and strength of recommendation for each of the outcomes [14]. The quality of evidence can be rated as "high", "moderate", "low", or "very low". Two reviewers (P.Z. and A.J.) independently performed the methodological quality assessment using the GRADEpro GDT software (available from gradepro.org) and risk of bias summaries generated using the robvis web tool [15].

2.5. Statistical Analysis

A network meta-analysis (NMA) within a Bayesian framework was performed using WinBUGS14 software, with codes adapted from Dias et al. [16]. The parameters were estimated using the Markov Chain Monte Carlo (MCMC) method. Results are based on 50,000 iterations using three chains, with an initial (burn-in) chain of 20,000. Model fit was assessed using posterior mean residual deviances and deviance information criteria (DIC). The transitivity assumption was assessed by observing the distribution of pre-operative characteristics in the studies, as well as the study designs. Odds ratios (ORs) with 95% credible intervals (95%CrI) were computed. Sensitivity analysis was performed for all primary outcomes—including studies reporting exclusively on JAAA.

3. Results

A total of 1723 publications were identified, and after abstract screening, 63 were deemed relevant and read in full text. The network meta-analysis included 16 studies [17–32]. The PRISMA flow diagram for study selection is presented in Figure 1.

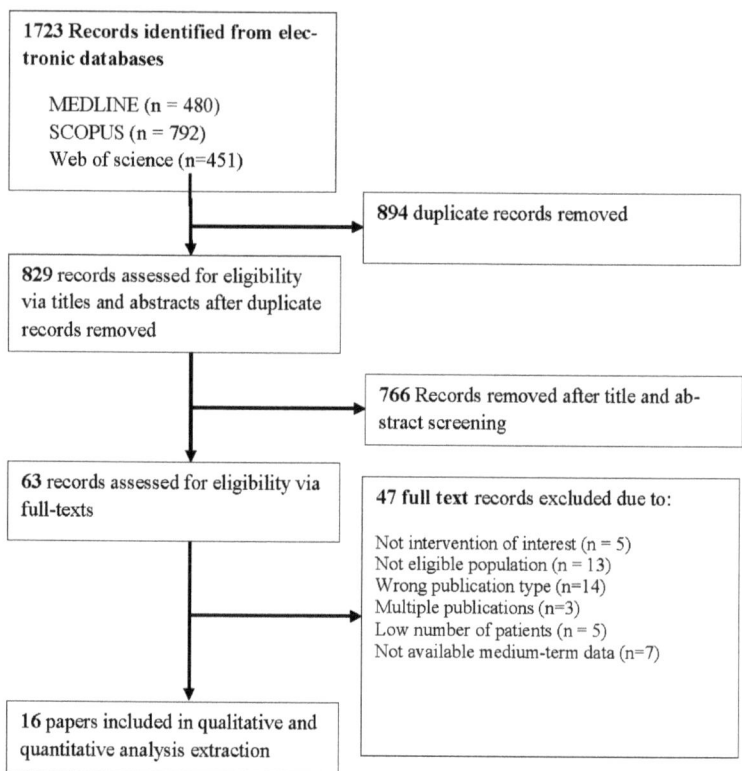

Figure 1. PRISMA flow diagram showing selection of included studies.

3.1. Study Characteristics

The characteristics of the studies included in the network meta-analysis are presented in Table 1. A total of 4369 patients were included, with 2581 undergoing OS, 1498 FEVAR, and 290 undergoing ChEVAR. Most studies included patients with JAAAs [17–20,22–26,28–32]—only one study reported on patients with JAAAs/PAAAs [21], and one reported outcomes for PAAA [27].

Table 2 shows the procedural data of the included studies. Most patients had suprarenal proximal clamp position in the OS group, while the proximal clamping time ranged from 22 to 48 min. Zenith (Cook Medical, Bloomington, IN, USA) was the most frequent stent graft manufacturer in the studies where FEVAR was performed, while it was Endurant (Medtronic, Minneapolis, MN, USA) for ChEVAR. The most commonly used bridging stent graft in FEVAR and chimney graft in the ChEVAR group was Advanta V12 (Atrium Medical, Hudson, NH, USA). The most commonly present design for FEVAR/ChEVAR was with two fenestrations/chimney stent grafts, while the mean number of fenestrations or chimney stent grafts in endovascular interventions ranged from 1.4 to 2.8. The range of the duration of follow-up was 6–60 months.

Table 1. Baseline clinical characteristics of patients in included studies.

First Author (Year of Publication)	Study Design	AAA Type	Follow-Up Duration (Months)	Intervention	Sample Size	Mean AGE (years)	Female Gender (%)	Smoking (%)	HTN (%)	HLP (%)	Diabetes (%)	COPD (%)	CAD (%)	CVD (%)	CKD (%)	AAA Size (mm)	Previous Aortic Intervention
Donas et al. (2012) [17]	Retrospective observational	Juxtarenal	14.2	ChEVAR	30	74	10	-	-	-	-	33.3	33.3	-	23.3	62	11
				FEVAR	29	73	0	-	-	-	-	27.9	41.4	-	17.2	65	8
				Open surgery	31	71	12.9	-	-	-	-	19.3	12.9	-	6.4	60	2
Wei et al. (2013) [18]	Retrospective observational	Juxtarenal	12	ChEVAR	37	-	-	-	-	-	-	-	-	-	-	-	-
				FEVAR	13	-	-	-	-	-	-	-	-	-	-	-	-
Lee et al. (2014) [19]	Retrospective observational	Juxtarenal	6	ChEVAR	15	76	26.6	93.3	100	-	6.6	33.3	-	-	-	66	-
				FEVAR	15	77	33.3	73.3	93.3	-	33.3	13.3	-	-	-	61	-
Barilla et al. (2014) [20]	Retrospective observational	Juxtarenal	60	Open surgery	50	78	6	16	75	56	22	44	54	8	20	-	-
				FEVAR	50	71	4	22	75	50	24	48	58	6	16	-	-
Barno et al. (2014) [21]	Retrospective observational	Juxta/pararenal	24	FEVAR	80	74	10	-	70	51	17.5	32.5	55	16.2	15	58	4
				ChEVAR	38	74	10.5	-	79	58	26.3	29	39.5	10.5	23.7	66	9
Shahverdyan et al. (2015) [22]	Retrospective observational	Juxtarenal	24	Open surgery	34	72	23.5	-	76.5	-	14.7	38.2	53	-	5.9	-	-
				FEVAR	35	72	14.3	-	85.7	-	5.7	20	45.7	-	11.4	-	-
Saratzis et al. (2015) [23]	Retrospective observational	Juxtarenal	20	FEVAR	58	75	12	81	63.8	67.2	31	-	31	8.6	-	52	-
				Open surgery	58	74	12	81	63.8	67.2	31	-	25.4	8.6	-	53	-
Maeda et al. (2015) [24]	Retrospective observational	Juxtarenal	33	FEVAR	81	71	14.8	72.8	74.1	40.7	24.7	23.4	54.3	24.7	22.2	58	-
				ChEVAR	34	77	11.7	58.8	82.3	50	17.6	20.6	26.5	20.6	23.5	55	-
Wooster et al. (2016) [25]	Retrospective observational	Juxtarenal	15	ChEVAR	37	77	10.8	59.4	81.1	48.6	18.9	21.6	27	18.9	21.6	56	-
				FEVAR	54	78	11.5	87	87	70.3	20.4	31.5	63	9.2	-	62	-
Caradu et al. (2017) [26]	Retrospective observational	Juxtarenal	24	FEVAR	39	72	12.8	79.5	82	66.6	15.4	38.5	53.8	17.9	-	68	-
				ChEVAR	90	71	2.2	70	80	61.1	12.2	26.6	-	10	14.4	58	-
					31	75	16.1	67.7	77.4	67.7	9.7	35.5	-	6.4	38.7	67	-

Table 1. Cont.

First Author (Year of Publication)	Study Design	AAA Type	Follow-Up Duration (Months)	Intervention	Sample Size	Mean AGE (years)	Female Gender (%)	Smoking (%)	HTN (%)	HLP (%)	Diabetes (%)	COPD (%)	CAD (%)	CVD (%)	CKD (%)	AAA Size (mm)	Previous Aortic Intervention
Fiorucci et al. (2018) [27]	Retrospective observational	Pararenal	50	FEVAR	92	75	9.8	-	84.8	32.6	11.9	41.3	57.6	10.8	18.5	-	-
				Open surgery	108	70	5.5	-	88.9	39.8	14.8	51.8	30.5	1	30.5	-	-
Chinsakchai et al. (2019) [28]	Retrospective observational	Juxtarenal	37	FEVAR	32	70	21.9	15.6	81.2	46.9	15.6	3.1	46.9	-	-	63	-
				Open surgery	20	72	15	15	85	15	20	15	30	-	-	55	-
				ChEVAR	23	76	34.8	4.3	65.2	30.4	8.7	8.7	30.4	-	-	68	-
Soler et al. (2019) [29]	Retrospective observational	Juxtarenal	27	Open surgery	134	69	7.4	86.5	67.9	61.2	14.2	33.6	40.3	-	20.9	59	5
				FEVAR	57	74	5.2	84.2	78.9	59.6	12.3	56.1	49.1	-	22.8	55	9
O'Donnell et al. (2020) [30]	Retrospective observational	Juxtarenal	36	Open surgery	1894	70	21	47	85	-	16	33	37	-	34	-	0
				FEVAR	822	73	20	34	86	-	19	38	45	-	42	-	6
Menegolo et al. (2021) [31]	Retrospective observational	Juxtarenal	43	ChEVAR	25	77	28	-	100	-	25	32	40	-	40	67	8
				Open surgery	61	71	3.3	-	82	-	14.7	9.8	29.5	-	22.9	65	0
Bootun et al. (2021) [32]	Retrospective observational	Juxtarenal	60	Open surgery	98	74	19	-	19.4	-	11.2	22.4	32.6	4.1	16.3	67	-
				FEVAR	64	76	4	-	6.2	-	9.4	25	45.3	20.3	18.7	76	-

AAA: abdominal aortic aneurysm;; FEVAR: fenestrated EVAR; ChEVAR: chimney EVAR; HTN: Hypertension; HLP: hyperlipidaemia; COPD: chronic obstructive pulmonary disease; CAD: coronary artery disease; CVD: cerebrovascular disease; CKD: chronic kidney disease.

Table 2. Procedural data of included studies.

First Author (Year of Publication)	AAA Type	Intervention	Sample Size	Stent Graft Manufacturer	Chimney/ Bridging Stent Graft Manufacturer	FEVAR/ChEVAR Configuration					Open Surgery								
						One Fenestration/One Chimney	Two Fenestrations/Two Chimneys	Three Fenestrations/One Chimneys	Four Fenestrations/One Chimneys	Mean Number of Fenestrations/Chimneys	Infrarenal Clamp	Interrenal Clamp	Suprarenal Clamp	Supraceliac Clamp	Mean Proximal Clamp Duration (min)	Operation Duration (min)	Blood Loss (ml)	ICU Stay (Days)	Hospital Stay (Days)
Donas et al. (2012) [17]	Juxtarenal AAA	Chimney EVAR	30	Medtronic	Advanta balloon expandable	22	5	3	0	1.4	-	-	-	-	-	90	-	-	3
		FEVAR	29	Cook Zenith		0	29	0	0	2	-	-	-	-	-	290	-	-	3
		Open surgery	31			-	-	-	-	-	-	-	-	-	23	-	-	-	7
Wei et al. (2013) [18]	Juxtarenal AAA	Chimney EVAR	37			-	-	-	-	-	-	-	-	-	-	-	-	-	-
		FEVAR	13			-	-	-	-	-	-	-	-	-	-	-	-	-	-
Lee et al. (2014) [19]	Juxtarenal AAA	Chimney EVAR	15	Medtronic/ Gore/Cook Zenith	iCAST and Viabahn	-	-	-	-	-	-	-	-	-	-	218	400	1	4
		FEVAR	15	Cook Zenith	iCAST	-	-	-	-	-	-	-	-	-	-	282	650	1	4
Barilla et al. (2014) [20]	Juxtarenal AAA	Open surgery	50			-	-	-	-	-	35	-	15	0	48	-	-	5	12
		FEVAR	50			2	48	0	0	1.9	-	-	-	-	-	-	-	3	12
Banno et al. (2014) [21]	Juxta/ pararenal AAA	FEVAR	60	Cook Zenith, Anaconda	BECSs. Advanta V12 Fluency	3	44	29	4	2.4	-	-	-	-	-	191	-	-	8
		Chimney EVAR	38		BECSs, Advanta V12 Fulency	20	14	4	0	1.6	-	-	-	-	-	183	-	-	2
Shahverdyan et al. (2015) [22]	Juxtarenal AAA	Open surgery	34			-	-	-	-	-	0	15	14	5	-	171	-	-	11
		FEVAR	35	Cook Zenith, Anaconda	Advanta V12	2	19	11	3	2.3	-	-	-	-	-	188	-	-	7
Saratzis et al. (2016) [23]	Juxtarenal AAA	FEVAR	58	Cook Zenith		3	23	27	5	2.6	-	-	-	-	-	-	-	-	6
		Open surgery	58			-	-	-	-	-	-	-	-	-	-	-	-	-	7
Maeda et al. (2016) [24]	Juxtarenal AAA	Open surgery	81	Gore Excluder		-	-	-	-	-	0	28	47	6	35	313	3120	-	15
		FEVAR	34	Cook Zenith	Advanta V12	-	-	-	-	-	-	-	-	-	-	282	550	-	8
		Chimney EVAR	37		Advanta V12	-	-	-	-	-	-	-	-	-	-	198	440	-	8
Woester et al. (2016) [25]	Juxtarenal AAA	Chimney EVAR	54	Medtronic, Core Excluder, Cook Zenith		27	21	4	2	1.6	-	-	-	-	-	233	634	2	6
		FEVAR	39	Cook Zenith		1	16	21	1	2.5	-	-	-	-	-	238	408	2	6

Table 2. Cont.

First Author (Year of Publication)	AAA Type	Intervention	Sample Size	Stent Graft Manufacturer	Chimney/Bridging Stent Graft Manufacturer	FEVAR/ChEVAR Configuration					Open Surgery					Operation Duration (min)	Blood Loss (ml)	ICU Stay (Days)	Hospital Stay (Days)
						One Fenestration/One Chimney	Two Fenestrations/Two Chimneys	Three Fenestrations/One Chimneys	Four Fenestrations/One Chimneys	Mean Number of Fenestrations/Chimneys	Infrarenal Clamp	Interrenal Clamp	Suprarenal Clamp	Supraceliac Clamp	Mean Proximal Clamp Duration (min)				
Caradu et al. (2017) [26]	Juxtarenal AAA	FEVAR	90	Cook Zenith, Anaconda	Advanta 12	0	72	14	4	2.2	-	-	-	-	-	182	-	1	7
		Chimney EVAR	31	Cook Zenith, Medtronic	Fluency	-	-	-	-	1.3	-	-	-	-	-	139	-	1	7
Fiorucci et al. (2018) [27]	Pararenal AAA	FEVAR	92	Cook Zenith	-	8	30	29	25	2.8	-	-	-	-	-	218	344	-	10
		Open surgery	108	-	-	-	-	-	-	-	-	-	-	-	-	237	758	-	9
Chinsakchai et al. (2019) [28]	Juxtarenal AAA	FEVAR	20	Cook Zenith	Advanta V12	-	-	-	-	2.4	3	9	10	10	-	242	-	1	8
		Chimney EVAR	23	-	Advanta V12, BeGraft, Viabahn	-	-	-	-	1.8	-	-	-	-	-	262	-	1	7
Soler et al. (2019) [29]	Juxtarenal AAA	Open surgery	134	-	-	-	-	-	-	-	0	10	91	33	23	270	-	1	9
		FEVAR	57	Cook Zenith	Blue Genesis, Advanta V12	3	25	22	7	2.6	-	-	-	-	-	-	-	1	11
O'Donnell et al. (2020) [30]	Juxtarenal AAA	Open surgery	1894	-	-	-	-	-	-	-	-	-	-	-	-	-	-	2	8
		FEVAR	822	-	-	-	-	-	-	-	-	-	-	-	-	-	-	-	-
Menegolo M et al. (2021) [31]	Juxtarenal AAA	Chimney EVAR	25	Medtronic, Gore Excluder, Cook Zenith	Advanta V12, Viabahn, Fluency	16	8	0	1	1.4	-	-	-	-	-	244	-	1	10
		Open surgery	61	-	-	-	-	-	-	-	0	28	21	12	22	214	-	3	8
Bootun et al. (2021) [32]	Juxtarenal AAA	Open surgery	98	-	-	-	-	-	-	-	0	43	55	0	24	-	1600	3	10
		FEVAR	64	-	-	4	22	23	15	2.7	-	-	-	-	-	-	-	1	6

AAA: abdominal aortic aneurysm; EVAR: endovascular aneurysm repair; FEVAR: fenestrated EVAR; ChEVAR: chimney EVAR.

3.2. Quality of Included Studies and Choice of Model

The overall quality of studies, as assessed by the ROBINS-I tool, was deemed "low", with 10 studies (62%) having being deemed as having either serious or critical risk of bias in one or more domains [17,18,20–22,24–27,31], and 6 (38%) assessed as having moderate risk of bias [19,23,28–30,32] (Figure 2). The GRADE quality of evidence for all outcomes is presented in Appendix SC and ranged from "very low" to "moderate".

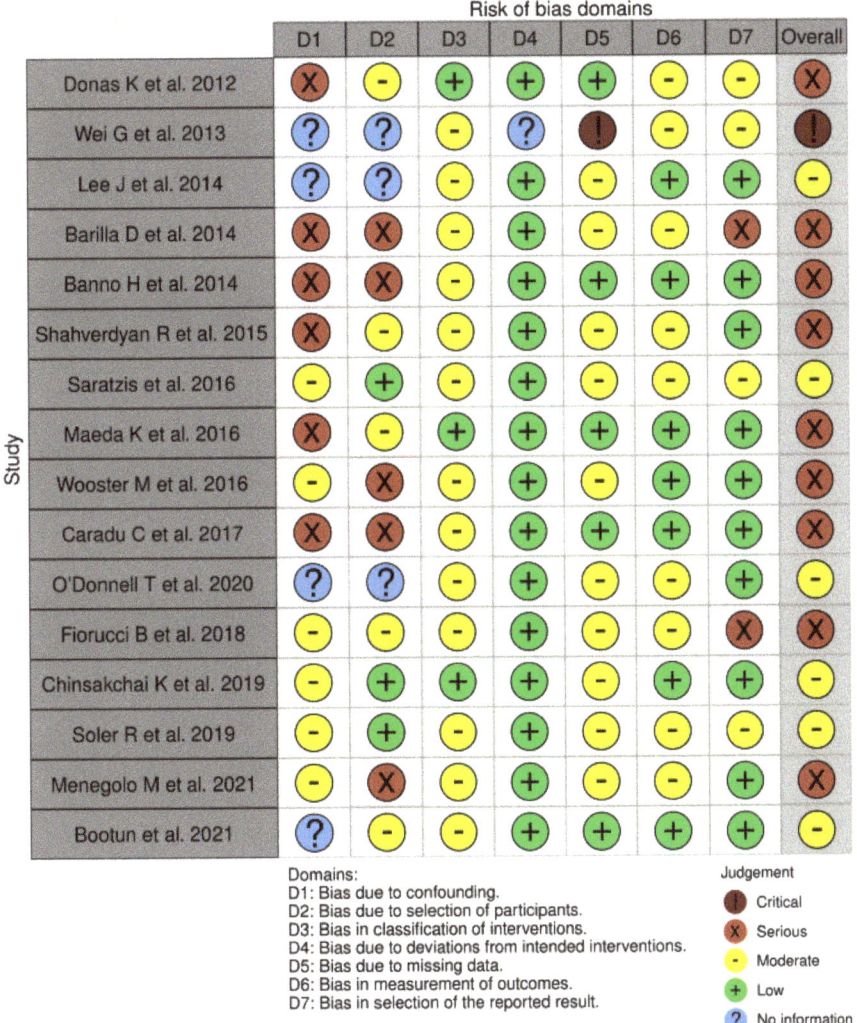

Figure 2. Risk of bias summary—judgments about each risk of bias item for each included study (for non-randomised studies using ROBINS-I tool) [17–32].

Values of the deviance information criteria (DIC) were similar in both models for all primary outcomes. However, lower values of residual deviance (Dres) were observed for the random-effects (RE) model compared with the fixed-effect model (FE) in all analyses. Seeing how both the values of Dres and the fact that studies were observational and heterogeneous were an indication for using the RE model, it was chosen in order for the estimate to be more conservative (Appendix SD).

3.3. Primary Outcomes

Fourteen studies reported on all-cause medium-term mortality. This NMA included 4229 patients, and 417 deaths were reported (9.8%) (Figure 3a). The unweighted pooled medium-term mortality rate was 8.1% for OS, 12.3% for FEVAR, and 14.3% for ChEVAR. The NMA results indicated that FEVAR (OR = 1.53, 95%CrI 1.03–2.11) was associated with higher medium-term mortality compared with OS (Table 3). The sensitivity analysis in which only studies with JAAA patients were included showed that FEVAR (OR = 1.65, 95%CrI 1.08–2.33) persisted to be associated with higher medium-term mortality when compared with OS (Appendixes SE and SF).

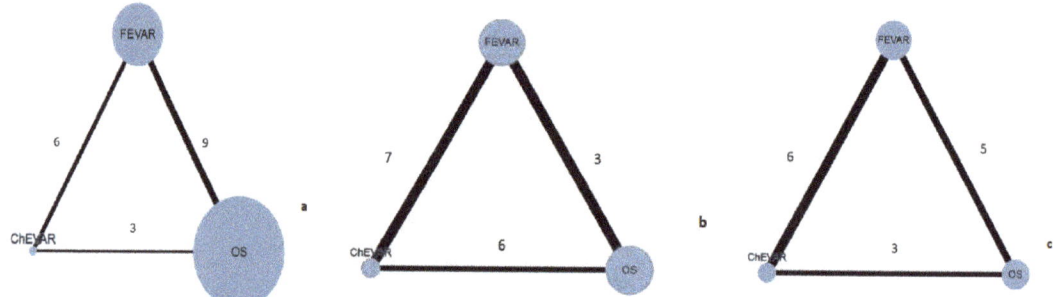

Figure 3. Network graph for mortality (**a**); aortic-related reintervention (**b**); and aortic-related mortality (**c**) (size of the node represents the sample size for the procedure, while the edge width represents the number of studies included in direct comparison).

Table 3. Network meta-analysis of major long-term outcomes in patients undergoing repair of JAAA/PAAA.

	FEVAR vs. OS	ChEVAR vs. OS	ChEVAR vs. FEVAR	Heterogeneity
Mortality	1.53 (1.03–2.11)	1.35 (0.74–2.40)	0.89 (0.50–1.58)	0.23 (0.01–0.71)
Aortic-related reintervention	8.32 (3.80–27.16)	5.95 (2.23–20.18)	0.72 (0.28–1.55)	0.63 (0.04–1.63)
Aortic-related mortality *	0.65 (0.06–5.67)	0.99 (0.07–9.76)	1.55 (0.20–11.06)	0.89 (0.04–1.93)

Legend: values are presented as OR (95% CrI), the treatment stated first is the reference treatment, OR < 1 favours the first treatment; OS—open surgery; FEVAR—fenestrated endovascular repair; ChEVAR—chimney endovascular repair; JAAA—juxtarenal abdominal aortic aneurysm; PAAA—pararenal abdominal aortic aneurysm. * The studies by Donas K et al. [17], and Wei G et al. [18], and Soler R et al. [29] were excluded from the quantitative analysis, as they had 0 outcomes in both groups.

Eleven studies reported on aortic-related reintervention as an outcome. A total of 1497 patients were included in this NMA, with 146 patients who underwent aortic-related reintervention (11.2%) (Figure 3b). The unweighted pooled aortic-related reintervention rate was 3.6% for OS, 17.1% for FEVAR, and 16.1% for ChEVAR. The NMA results showed that both FEVAR (OR = 8.32, 95%CrI 3.80–27.16) and ChEVAR (OR = 5.95, 95%CrI 2.23–20.18) were associated with a higher aortic-related reintervention rate than OS (Table 3), and this association persisted after sensitivity analysis including only JAAA (OR = 9.61, 95%CrI 3.44–44.22 for FEVAR; OR = 7.11, 95%CrI 2.06–32.67 for ChEVAR) (Appendixes SE and SF). There was no difference between FEVAR and ChEVAR in terms of aortic-related reintervention rates, not even after sensitivity analysis for JAAA (Table 3, Appendix SE).

Ten studies reported on aortic-related mortality. A total of 1150 patients were included in NMA, with 12 patients contributing to aortic-related mortality (1.1%) (Figure 3c). The unweighted pooled aortic-related mortality rate was 0.9% for OS, 0.8% for FEVAR, and 1.7% for ChEVAR. Results from NMA as well as from sensitivity analysis including only JAAA showed no difference between different treatment options in terms of aortic-related mortality (Table 3, Appendixes SE and SF).

3.4. Secondary Outcomes

Results from NMA showed that FEVAR (OR = 13.13, 95%CrI 2.70–105.2) and ChEVAR (OR = 16.82, 95%CrI 2.79–176.7) were associated with a higher rate of medium-term visceral branch occlusion/stenosis compared to OS; however, there was no difference between FEVAR and ChEVAR in terms of this complication. No difference was found between the three treatment options in terms of renal replacement therapy and MACEs. When comparing FEVAR and ChEVAR, no difference was found regarding the total number of endoleaks and more malignant ones such as type I/III (Table 4).

Table 4. Network meta-analysis of secondary long-term outcomes in patients undergoing repair of JAAA/PAAA.

	FEVAR vs. OS	ChEVAR vs. OS	ChEVAR vs. FEVAR	Heterogeneity
Long-term branch/bypass occlusion/stenosis	13.13 (2.701–105.2)	16.82 (2.79–176.7)	1.28 (0.34–5.11)	1.44 (0.39–1.97)
Renal replacement therapy	1.27 (0.13–13.87)	1.09 (0.02–48.97)	0.82 (0.02–32.71)	1.43 (0.13–1.98)
MACEs	1.57 (0.52–5.88)	6.96 (0.70–103.0)	4.39 (0.49–51.21)	0.49 (0.02–1.81)
Total endoleaks	/	/	1.14 (0.44–3.51)	0.84 (0.06–1.88)
Type I/III endoleaks	/	/	1.59 (0.52–5.43)	0.77 (0.05–1.88)

Legend: values are presented as OR (95% CrI), the treatment stated first is the reference treatment, OR < 1 favours the first treatment; OS—open surgery; FEVAR—fenestrated endovascular repair; ChEVAR—chimney endovascular repair; JAAA—juxtarenal abdominal aortic aneurysm; PAAA—pararenal abdominal aortic aneurysm.

4. Discussion

This NMA found only observational studies comparing medium-term outcomes of interventions for JAAA/PAAA, mostly of low quality. The results of this NMA showed that FEVAR had a higher mid-term mortality compared to OS. Both endovascular procedures had higher rates of aortic-related reintervention and side branch occlusion/stenosis compared to the OS group. When making a comparison between the endovascular techniques, no significant preferences for either FEVAR or ChEVAR were found for any of the outcomes.

In this meta-analysis, several attempts were made to ameliorate the limitations of the existing literature. Firstly, it is difficult to interpret the results of the existing meta-analyses due to anatomical heterogeneity of the patients [10,33]. We focused our attention on studies reporting outcomes for only JAAA/PAAA, thus excluding more complex AAAs such as suprarenal and ThAAAs. Secondly, meta-analyses usually focus their attention on two most commonly used treatment options, i.e., FEVAR vs. OS, neglecting ChEVAR as the treatment option that is often used in some centres as the first-line endovascular option for the treatment of JAAA/PAAA [33]. This has only limited value. Thirdly, most of the published meta-analyses included studies published earlier than 2010 [7,34]. This NMA included more updated publications, with 11/16 published after 2015. Fourthly, NMA has an advantage that it allows both direct and indirect comparison; thus, more data are incorporated in the final analysis, and a bigger scope of the picture is tackled, whereas a single pairwise sometimes offers a very fragmented picture due to its failure to incorporate indirect data in the comparison.

Current guidelines recommend that the choice of different techniques and options for the management of JAAA/PAAA in the elective setting should be considered based on patient status, anatomy, local routines, team expertise, and patient preference [4,5]. The findings of this NMA reconfirm the widely accepted observation that endovascular techniques are associated with a higher incidence of aortic-related reintervention and a higher incidence of branch stenosis/occlusion. Recommendation 96 in the ESVS guidelines states that "In complex endovascular repair of juxtarenal abdominal aortic aneurysm, endovascular repair with fenestrated stent grafts should be considered the preferred treatment option when feasible". Current guidelines favour the advantage of endovascular techniques (FEVAR and ChEVAR) over OS in terms of short-term outcomes [4,5].

According to recommendation 97 from the latest ESVS guidelines [4], FEVAR is preferred over ChEVAR in the elective setting, while recommendation 98 says that ChEVAR might be used in the emergent setting as a bailout procedure. However, this recommendation is based on expert opinion, and there are no high-quality data that might support these two recommendations. One of the major concerns with ChEVAR in the elective setting is that it is associated with a high rate of type Ia endoleak, especially with more than two chimneys [35]. Furthermore, gutters created between the main graft and chimneys may limit the durability of the technique.

This NMA showed one interesting finding that FEVAR patients had worse medium-term all-cause mortality compared to the OS group. A similar tendency was found for ChEVAR patients compared to OS, but this did not reach the level of statistical significance. Due to the non-randomised nature of all studies included in this NMA, it is possible that this reflects a confounding from the variations in baseline clinical characteristics between the groups, but it is an important finding and an indication for future RCTs regardless. It is also possible that a confounding due to indication is present, i.e., that surgeons tend to choose endovascular solutions for less fit patients, and therefore, these solutions have worse medium-term outcomes. A general observation from Table 1 is that patients from the endovascular group were older, with the presence of other cardiovascular risk factors. Although the inclusion criteria are somewhat different, focusing also on patients with adverse neck characteristics, a recently published NMA from Patel et al. [36] showed no differences in overall mid-term mortality between three groups of patients.

A significantly higher rate of mid-term reinterventions in both the FEVAR and ChEVAR group compared to OS was demonstrated in this NMA. A recent NMA [36] showed that only FEVAR patients had a higher mid-term reintervention rate. It must be noted that details about OS reintervention are often lacking. One good example is the rate of postincisial hernia repair, which was reported only in one study, and it is unclear whether it was counted as reintervention. Another contributing factor could be reintervention due to persistent type II endoleak (seven studies) in the FEVAR group without mentioning specific reasons. Additionally, FEVAR nowadays for JAAA repair usually has four vessel fenestrations, and this more proximal/extensive repair predisposes patients for mid-term complications [6]. Nevertheless, more frequent reinterventions coupled with the higher costs of endovascular devices could raise an additional concern. The results from Michel M. et al. [37] showed that FEVAR is more expensive and not a cost-effective option for JAAA/PAAA at 2 years. Since this study was performed, new devices from different companies have been developed, which will hopefully decrease the cost of these stent grafts in the future. It is, however, important to emphasise that the majority of reports failed to report data adequately, thus introducing difficulties in data interpretation. Unlike rigid reporting systems in RCTs and prospective observational trials, retrospective studies do not provide an insight into the variability of surgeon preferences and department policies. One of the explanations why the reintervention rate was higher in the endovascular groups could be the higher incidence of branch vessel stenosis/occlusion and the presence of the non-negligible overall unweighted pooled 6.6% rate of type I/III (malignant) endoleak for FEVAR/ChEVAR groups.

The branch vessel occlusion/stenosis rate was lower in OSR. However, the interpretation of results should be taken with caution since most of the patients had juxtarenal AAA, and only 11.5% of all patients undergoing OSR had renal artery bypass/reattachment, which makes comparison to FEVAR/ChEVAR difficult. Surprisingly, there was no difference between FEVAR and ChEVAR in terms of incidence of new onset endoleaks and branch vessel patency. Most of the trials used company-manufactured stent grafts from Zenith Cook (Cook Medical, Bloomington, IN, USA) for FEVAR and from Endurant (Medtronic, Minneapolis, MN, USA) for ChEVAR. In the meta-analysis of Katsargyris et al. [8], no difference was observed for target vessel patency and short-term mortality for the treatment of JAAA. Additionally, no difference was observed regarding new onset RRT. However, the absence of difference in terms of these outcomes could be due to the lack of papers with sufficient power to highlight any statistical difference.

One important factor that should not be neglected is the impact of centre volume on patient outcomes. As reported in a previous registry, centres with high (>14) volume of open JAAA repair demonstrated significant adjusted lower perioperative mortality (3.9%) compared to centres with low volume of open repair [38]. Possibly, a broad implementation of centralisation of treatment of JAAA/PAAA could further improve these results, especially in OS.

5. Limitations and Implications for Research

There are several concerns in this NMA. Our study included only observational studies and registries with significant differences in terms of baseline clinical characteristics. No RCTs have been performed comparing JAAA/PAAA repair. The GRADE rating for evidence was "low" for the majority of pairwise comparisons, reflecting the inherited bias. Data veracity is the Achilles' heel of all retrospective analyses. Such nuances were most apparent in big registries [22]. Another issue when analysing cohort studies as opposed to randomised controlled trials is confounding by indication. It is possible that frailer patients received endovascular treatment, while patients with better pre-operative conditions received OS. This confounding was impossible to account for in our analysis. Another cause of concern is the "learning curve bias" and the use of older generations of devices. We tried to avoid this issue by excluding studies that reported less than 10 patients per treatment arm and by only including studies that treated patients after 2010, but since the endovascular techniques have been further improved since then, it is possible that this bias is still present in our analysis. Furthermore, the role of physician-modified grafts and outside-of-use EVAR in the elective setting have not been investigated due to unstandardised use of these two techniques in the setting of JAAA/PAAA repair. There was a lack of standardisation of definitions and reporting of the anatomy. For example, some studies defined JAAA as a neck less than 10 mm, and others used the anticipated clamp site with no specific mention of whether the aneurysms had involved the renal artery ostia, i.e., PAAA. Although the analysis was focused on JAAA/PAAA, the majority of studies provide no detail on the AAA anatomy, such as neck length and other adverse features. Cost-effectiveness analysis and quality of life assessment were not performed and could be important outcomes that could help in the decision-making process between these patient groups.

6. Conclusions

The results of this NMA found an advantage for OS regarding aortic-related intervention and vessel branch/bypass stenosis/occlusion compared to FEVAR and ChEVAR after medium-term follow-up. This suggests that younger, low-surgical-risk patients might benefit from open surgery of JAAA/PAAA; however, this insight should be interpreted with caution due to the low quality of the included studies in the analysis and the possibility of confounding by indication, bearing in mind the observational design of the included studies. Further larger studies including experienced and high-volume AAA centres in patients with similar baseline patient characteristics are needed to adequately determine medium and long-term results of all three used treatment options.

Supplementary Materials: The following supporting information can be downloaded at: https://www.mdpi.com/article/10.3390/jcm11226779/s1, Appendix SA. Search strategy. Appendix SB. Extracted data from each study with a pre-specified proforma. Appendix SC (1). Summary of findings table showing comparison FEVAR vs open surgery for JAAA/PAAA treatment. Appendix SC (2). Summary of findings table showing comparison Chimney EVAR vs open surgery for JAAA/PAAA treatment. Appendix SC (3). Summary of findings table showing comparison Chimney EVAR vs FEVAR for JAAA/PAAA treatment. Appendix SD. Model comparison of fixed-effect vs. random-effects models for the primary outcomes. Appendix SE. Sensitivity analysis including studies which included only patients with juxtarenal abdominal aortic aneurysms. Appendix SF. The probability of each treatment being the best, second best, and worst for primary outcomes. Appendix SG. Definitions of JAA/PAAA patients in included studies.

Author Contributions: P.Z.: conceptualisation, methodology, software, formal analysis, data curation, writing—original draft preparation, writing—review and editing, visualization, project administration. A.J.: conceptualisation, methodology, software, formal analysis, data curation, writing—original draft preparation, writing—review and editing, visualization. P.T.: conceptualisation, methodology, data curation, writing—original draft preparation, writing—review and editing, visualization. L.D.: conceptualisation, resources, writing—original draft preparation, writing—review and editing, supervision, project administration. All authors have read and agreed to the published version of the manuscript.

Funding: This research received no external funding.

Institutional Review Board Statement: Not applicable.

Informed Consent Statement: Not applicable.

Conflicts of Interest: The authors declare no conflict of interest.

References

1. Gimenez-Gaibar, A.; Gonzalez-Canas, E.; Solanich-Valldaura, T.; Herranz-Pinilla, C.; Rioja-Artal, S.; Ferraz-Huguet, E. Could preoperative neck anatomy influence follow-up of EVAR? *Ann. Vasc. Surg.* **2017**, *43*, 127–133. [CrossRef] [PubMed]
2. Marone, E.M.; Freyrie, A.; Ruotolo, C.; Michelagnoli, S.; Antonello, M.; Speziale, F.; Veroux, P.; Gargiulo, M.; Gaggiano, A. Expert Opinion on Hostile Neck Definition in Endovascular Treatment of Abdominal Aortic Aneurysms (a Delphi Consensus). *Ann. Vasc. Surg.* **2019**, *62*, 173–182. [CrossRef]
3. Powell, J.; Sweeting, M.; Ulug, P.; Blankensteijn, J.; Lederle, F.; Becquemin, J.-P.; Greenhalgh, R.; Evar-1, D. Meta-analysis of individual-patient data from EVAR-1, DREAM, OVER and ACE trials comparing outcomes of endovascular or open repair for abdominal aortic aneurysm over 5 years. *Br. J. Surg.* **2017**, *104*, 166–178. [CrossRef] [PubMed]
4. Wanhainen, A.; Verzini, F.; Van Herzeele, I.; Allaire, E.; Bown, M.; Cohnert, T.; Dick, F.; van Herwaarden, J.; Karkos, C.; Koelemay, M.; et al. Editor's Choice—European Society for Vascular Surgery (ESVS) 2019 Clinical Practice Guidelines on the Management of Abdominal Aorto-iliac Artery Aneurysms. *Eur. J. Vasc. Endovasc. Surg.* **2019**, *57*, 8–93. [CrossRef] [PubMed]
5. Chaikof, E.L.; Dalman, R.L.; Eskandari, M.K.; Jackson, B.M.; Lee, W.A.; Mansour, M.A.; Mastracci, T.M.; Mell, M.; Murad, M.H.; Nguyen, L.L.; et al. The Society for Vascular Surgery practice guidelines on the care of patients with an abdominal aortic aneurysm. *J. Vasc. Surg.* **2018**, *67*, 2–77.e2. [CrossRef] [PubMed]
6. Oderich, G.S.; Forbes, T.L.; Chaer, R.; Davies, M.G.; Lindsay, T.F.; Mastracci, T.; Singh, M.J.; Timaran, C.; Woo, E.Y. Reporting standards for endovascular aortic repair of aneurysms involving the renal-mesenteric arteries. *J. Vasc. Surg.* **2020**, *73*, 4S–52S. [CrossRef]
7. Doonan, R.J.; Girsowicz, E.; Dubois, L.; Gill, H.L. A systematic review and meta-analysis of endovascular juxtarenal aortic aneurysm repair demonstrates lower perioperative mortality compared with open repair. *J. Vasc. Surg.* **2019**, *70*, 2054–2064. [CrossRef] [PubMed]
8. Katsargyris, A.; Oikonomou, K.; Klonaris, C.; Topfel, I.; Verhoeven, E. Comparison of outcomes with open, fenestrated, and chimney graft repair of juxtarenal aneurysms: Are we ready for a paradigm shift? *J. Endovasc. Ther.* **2013**, *20*, 159–169. [CrossRef]
9. Končar, I.B.; Jovanović, A.L.; Dučič, S.M. The role of fEVAR, chEVAR and open repair in treatment of juxtarenal aneurysms: A systematic review. *J. Cardiovasc. Surg.* **2020**, *61*, 24–36. [CrossRef]
10. Antoniou, G.A.; Juszczak, M.T.; Antoniou, S.A.; Katsargyris, A.; Haulon, S. Editor's Choice - Fenestrated or Branched Endovascular versus Open Repair for Complex Aortic Aneurysms: Meta-Analysis of Time to Event Propensity Score Matched Data. *Eur. J. Vasc. Endovasc. Surg.* **2021**, *61*, 228–237. [CrossRef]
11. Page, M.J.; McKenzie, J.E.; Bossuyt, P.M.; Boutron, I.; Hoffmann, T.C.; Mulrow, C.D.; Shamseer, L.; Tetzlaff, J.M.; Akl, E.A.; Brennan, S.E.; et al. The PRISMA 2020 statement: An updated guideline for reporting systematic reviews. *Int. J. Surg.* **2021**, *88*, 105906. [CrossRef] [PubMed]
12. Shea, B.J.; Reeves, B.C.; Wells, G.; Thuku, M.; Hamel, C.; Moran, J.; Moher, D.; Tugwell, P.; Welch, V.; Kristjansson, E.; et al. AMSTAR 2: A critical appraisal tool for systematic reviews that include randomised or non-randomised studies of healthcare interventions, or both. *BMJ* **2017**, *358*, j4008. [CrossRef] [PubMed]
13. Sterne, J.A.C.; Hernán, M.A.; Reeves, B.C.; Savović, J.; Berkman, N.D.; Viswanathan, M.; Henry, D.; Altman, D.G.; Ansari, M.T.; Boutron, I.; et al. ROBINS-I: A tool for assessing risk of bias in non-randomised studies of interventions. *BMJ* **2016**, *355*, i4919. [CrossRef] [PubMed]
14. Guyatt, G.H.; Oxman, A.D.; Kunz, R.; Atkins, D.; Brozek, J.; Vist, G.; Alderson, P.; Glasziou, P.; Falck-Ytter, Y.; Schünemann, H.J. GRADE guidelines: 2. Framing the question and deciding on important outcomes. *J. Clin. Epidemiology* **2011**, *64*, 395–400. [CrossRef]

15. McGuinness, L.A.; Higgins, J.P.T. Risk-of-bias VISualization (robvis): An R package and Shiny web app for visualizing risk-of-bias assessments. *Res. Synth. Methods.* **2021**, *12*, 55–61. [CrossRef]
16. Dias, S.; Ades, A.E.; Welton, N.J.; Jansen, J.P.; Sutton, A.J. *Network Meta-Analysis for Decision Making*; John Wiley & Sons Ltd.: Hoboken, NJ, USA, 2018. [CrossRef]
17. Donas, K.P.; Eisenack, M.; Panuccio, G.; Austermann, M.; Osada, N.; Torsello, G. The role of open and endovascular treatment with fenestrated and chimney endografts for patients with juxtarenal aortic aneurysms. *J. Vasc. Surg.* **2012**, *56*, 285–290. [CrossRef]
18. Wei, G. GW24-e3928 Endovascular chimney technique versus fenestrated endovascular aneurysm repair of juxtarenal abdominal aortic aneurysms. *Heart* **2013**, *99*, A257.3–A258. [CrossRef]
19. Lee, J.T.; Lee, G.K.; Chandra, V.; Dalman, R.L. Comparison of fenestrated endografts and the snorkel/chimney technique. *J. Vasc. Surg.* **2014**, *60*, 849–857. [CrossRef]
20. Barilla', D.; Sobocinski, J.; Stilo, F.; Maurel, B.; Spinelli, F.; Haulon, S. Juxtarenal aortic aneurysm with hostile neck anatomy: Midterm results of minilaparotomy versus f-EVAR. *Int Angiol* **2014**, *33*.
21. Banno, H.; Cochennec, F.; Marzelle, J.; Becquemin, J.-P. Comparison of fenestrated endovascular aneurysm repair and chimney graft techniques for pararenal aortic aneurysm. *J. Vasc. Surg.* **2014**, *60*, 31–39. [CrossRef]
22. Shahverdyan, R.; Majd, M.; Thul, R.; Braun, N.; Gawenda, M.; Brunkwall, J. F-EVAR does not Impair Renal Function more than Open Surgery for Juxtarenal Aortic Aneurysms: Single Centre Results. *Eur. J. Vasc. Endovasc. Surg.* **2015**, *50*, 432–441. [CrossRef] [PubMed]
23. Saratzis, A.; Bath, M.F.; Harrison, S.C.; Sayers, R.D.; Bown, M.J. Impact of Fenestrated Endovascular Abdominal Aortic Aneurysm Repair on Renal Function. *J. Endovasc. Ther.* **2015**, *22*, 889–896. [CrossRef] [PubMed]
24. Maeda, K.; Ohki, T.; Kanaoka, Y.; Baba, T.; Kaneko, K.; Shukuzawa, K. Comparison between Open and Endovascular Repair for the Treatment of Juxtarenal Abdominal Aortic Aneurysms: A Single-Center Experience with Midterm Results. *Ann. Vasc. Surg.* **2017**, *41*, 96–104. [CrossRef] [PubMed]
25. Wooster, M.; Tanious, A.; Patel, S.; Moudgill, N.; Back, M.; Shames, M. Concomitant Parallel Endografting and Fenestrated Experience in a Regional Aortic Center. *Ann. Vasc. Surg.* **2017**, *38*, 54–58. [CrossRef]
26. Caradu, C.; Morin, J.; Poirier, M.; Midy, D.; Ducasse, E. Monocentric Evaluation of Chimney Versus Fenestrated Endovascular Aortic Repair for Juxtarenal Abdominal Aortic Aneurysm. *Ann. Vasc. Surg.* **2017**, *40*, 28–38. [CrossRef]
27. Fiorucci, B.; Speziale, F.; Kölbel, T.; Tsilimparis, N.; Sirignano, P.; Capoccia, L.; Simonte, G.; Verzini, F. Short- and Midterm Outcomes of Open Repair and Fenestrated Endografting of Pararenal Aortic Aneurysms in a Concurrent Propensity-Adjusted Comparison. *J. Endovasc. Ther.* **2018**, *26*, 105–112. [CrossRef]
28. Chinsakchai, K.; Prapassaro, T.; Salisatkorn, W.; Hongku, K.; Moll, F.L.; Ruangsetakit, C.; Wongwanit, C.; Puangpunngam, N.; Hahtapornsawan, S.; Sermsathanasawadi, N.; et al. Outcomes of Open Repair, Fenestrated Stent Grafting, and Chimney Grafting in Juxtarenal Abdominal Aortic Aneurysm: Is It Time for a Randomized Trial? *Ann. Vasc. Surg.* **2019**, *56*, 114–123. [CrossRef]
29. Soler, R.; Bartoli, M.; Faries, C.; Mancini, J.; Sarlon-Bartoli, G.; Haulon, S.; Magnan, P.E. Fenestrated endovascular aneurysm repair and open surgical repair for the treatment of juxtarenal aortic aneurysms. *J. Vasc. Surg.* **2019**, *70*, 683–690. [CrossRef]
30. O'Donnell, T.F.X.; Boitano, L.T.; Deery, S.E.; Schermerhorn, M.L.; Schanzer, A.; Beck, A.W.; Green, R.M.; Takayama, H.; Patel, V.I. Open Versus Fenestrated Endovascular Repair of Complex Abdominal Aortic Aneurysms. *Ann. Surg.* **2020**, *271*, 969–977. [CrossRef]
31. Menegolo, M.; Xodo, A.; Penzo, M.; Piazza, M.; Squizzato, F.; Colacchio, E.C.; Grego, F.; Antonello, M. Open repair versus EVAR with parallel grafts in patients with juxtarenal abdominal aortic aneurysm excluded from fenestrated endografting. *J. Cardiovasc. Surg.* **2021**, *62*. [CrossRef]
32. Bootun, R.; Carey, F.; Al-Thaher, A.; Al-Alwani, Z.; Crawford, M.; Delbridge, M.; Ali, T.; Al-Jundi, W. Comparison between open repair with suprarenal clamping and fenestrated endovascular repair for unruptured juxtarenal aortic aneurysms. *J. Cardiovasc. Surg.* **2021**. [CrossRef] [PubMed]
33. O'Donnell, T.F.; Patel, V.I.; Deery, S.E.; Li, C.; Swerdlow, N.J.; Liang, P.; Beck, A.W.; Schermerhorn, M.L. The state of complex endovascular abdominal aortic aneurysm repairs in the vascular quality initiative. *J. Vasc. Surg.* **2019**, *70*, 369–380. [CrossRef] [PubMed]
34. Orr, N.T.; Davenport, D.L.; Minion, D.J.; Xenos, E.S. Comparison of perioperative outcomes in endovascular versus open repair for juxtarenal and pararenal aortic aneurysms: A propensity-matched analysis. *Vascular* **2016**, *25*, 339–345. [CrossRef] [PubMed]
35. Donas, K.P.; Lee, J.T.; Lachat, M.; Torsello, G.; Veith, F.J. Collected world experience about the performance of the snorkel/chimney endovascular technique in the treatment of complex aortic pathologies: The PERICLES registry. *J. Vasc. Surg.* **2015**, *262*, 546–553. [CrossRef]
36. Patel, S.R.; Ormesher, D.C.; Griffin, R.; Jackson, R.J.; Lip, G.Y.H.; Vallabhaneni, S.R.; UK-COMPASS Trial. Editor's Choice-Comparison of Open, Standard, and Complex Endovascular Aortic Repair Treatments for Juxtarenal/Short Neck Aneurysms: A Systematic Review and Network Meta-Analysis. *Eur. J. Vasc. Endovasc. Surg.* **2022**, *63*, 696–706. [CrossRef]
37. Michel, M.; Becquemin, J.P.; Marzelle, J.; Quelen, C.; Durand-Zaleski, I. Editor's Choice e A study of the cost-effectiveness of fenestrated/ branched EVAR compared with open surgery for patients with complex aortic aneurysms at 2 years. *Eur. J. Vasc Endovasc. Surg* **2018**, *56*, 15–428. [CrossRef]
38. O'Donnell, T.; Boitano, L.; Deery, S.; Lancaster, R.; Siracuse, J.; Schermerhorn, M. Hospital Volume Matters: The Volume-Outcome Relationship in Open Juxtarenal AAA Repair. *J. Vasc. Surg.* **2019**, *69*, 1323–1324. [CrossRef]

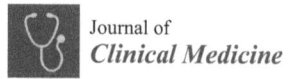

Article

Feasibility and Safety of Percutaneous Axillary Artery Access in a Prospective Series of 100 Complex Aortic and Aortoiliac Interventions

Tim Wittig [1,2,†], Arsen Sabanov [3,†], Andrej Schmidt [1], Dierk Scheinert [1], Sabine Steiner [1,2,*] and Daniela Branzan [2,3]

1. Department of Angiology, University Hospital Leipzig, 04103 Leipzig, Germany
2. Helmholtz Institute for Metabolic, Obesity and Vascular Research (HI-MAG) of the Helmholtz Center Munich at the University of Leipzig and University Hospital Leipzig, 04103 Leipzig, Germany
3. Department of Vascular Surgery, University Hospital Leipzig, 04103 Leipzig, Germany
* Correspondence: sabine.steiner@medizin.uni-leipzig.de; Tel.: +49-341-9718770; Fax: +49-341-9718779
† These authors contributed equally to this work.

Abstract: We aimed to review the feasibility and safe use of the percutaneous axillary artery (AxA, 100 patients) approach for endovascular repair (ER) of thoraco-abdominal aortic aneurysms (TAAA, 90 patients) using fenestrated, branched, and chimney stent grafts and other complex endovascular procedures (10 patients) necessitating AxA access. Percutaneous puncture of the AxA in its third segment was performed using sheaths sized between 6 to 14F. For closing puncture sites greater than 8F, two Perclose ProGlide percutaneous vascular closure devices (PVCDs) (Abbott Vascular, Santa Clara, CA, USA) were deployed in the pre-close technique. The median maximum diameter of the AxA in the third segment was 7.27 mm (range 4.50–10.80). Device success, defined as successful hemostasis by PVCD, was reported in 92 patients (92.0%). As recently reported results in the first 40 patients suggested that adverse events, including vessel stenosis or occlusion, occurred only in cases with a diameter of the AxA < 5 mm, in all subsequent 60 cases AxA access was restricted to a vessel diameter ≥ 5 mm. In this late group, no hemodynamic impairment of the AxA occurred except in six early cases below this diameter threshold, all of which could be repaired by endovascular measures. Overall mortality at 30 days was 8%. In conclusion, percutaneous approach of the AxA in its third segment is feasible and represents a safe alternative access to open access for complex endovascular aorto-iliac procedures. Complications are rare, especially if the maximum diameter of the access vessel (AxA) is ≥5 mm.

Keywords: aortic aneurysm; endovascular intervention; complex endovascular aneurysm repair; upper extremity access; percutaneous closure device

1. Introduction

Endovascular aortic repair has become a preferred strategy for the treatment of thoraco-abdominal aortic aneurysm (TAAA) because of the substantially lower peri-operative risk compared to open surgery [1]. However, in many cases, delivery of bridging and visceral stents necessitates an upper extremity access (UEA), which might also be required to stabilize the graft during the procedure via a through and through wire or in other aortoiliac interventions, such as delivery of iliac branch devices (IBD). UAE can be performed by a variety of techniques using open cut-down or percutaneous access, and four sites are usually suggested for access to the upper extremities: the distal brachial artery on the inside of the elbow, the brachial artery on the medial humerus, the proximal brachial artery just below the axillary grove, and the infraclavicular approach via the axillary fossa [2]. Compared to the brachial or radial approach, the axillary artery (AxA) can be used for large sheath sizes > 7F and successfully accommodation of sheath sizes up to 18F via the AxA have been reported in patients undergoing transcatheter aortic valve replacement [3].

So far, there are no clear guidelines for the best approach, but it depends on the clinical circumstances as well as operator's experience and preferences. Previous series providing results for both open and percutaneous access to upper extremity arteries reported overall low complication rates, but only a small number of percutaneous approaches were considered [2,4–6]. In case of percutaneous UAE, several approaches to closure have also been proposed, including manual compression and the use of closure devices.

We recently reported a preliminary series comprising 40 patients undergoing percutaneous axillary artery (AxA) access in the third segment with subsequent closure using the the Perclose ProGlide percutaneous vascular closure device (PVCD) (Abbott Vascular, Santa Clara, CA, USA) [7]. Importantly, results suggested that adverse events, including vessel stenosis or occlusion, occurred only in cases with a diameter of the AxA < 5 mm, and thus in all subsequent 60 cases AxA access was restricted to patients with a vessel diameter $\geq$ 5 mm. Here we report now the results of the full series of 100 patients undergoing percutaneous AxA access.

2. Material and Methods

2.1. Study Design and Patient Selection

This single-center cohort study enrolled 100 consecutive patients between September 2013 and November 2020 who required upper extremity access for endovascular aortoiliac procedures, primarily for TAAA with fenestrated, branched, and chimney stent grafts. In all patients, a percutaneous axillary approach with a 6–14F sheath was established in the third segment of the vessel under ultrasound guidance. Based on an interim analysis of the first 40 patients, complications at the puncture site were only seen when the maximum diameter of the axillary artery was <5 mm [7]. In all subsequent patients, percutaneous axillary access was only performed if the maximum diameter was $\geq$5 mm based on CT scan measurements. Eight patients were excluded from the study due to AxA diameter < 5 mm. There were no other exclusion criteria for percutaneous AxA access. The patients excluded for percutaneous AxA access were alternatively treated using a bilateral percutaneous brachial access. The Institutional Review Board of University of Leipzig approved the analysis of this data set obtained from a prospectively maintained aortic database.

2.2. Interventional Details and Postoperative Management

All interventions were performed under general anesthesia in a hybrid operating room equipped with a Philips Allura Xper FD 20 X-ray imaging system (Philips Healthcare, Amsterdam, The Netherlands) except for one patient who was locally anesthetized. Details on the branched and fenestrated stent graft implantation technique has been described previously [6,7]. Duplex ultrasound and computed tomography angiography (CTA) scans were evaluated before the procedure to assess the patency of the AxA, its size, and the presence of disease. An AxA with an anterior wall free of calcification and with a minimum diameter of 4.5 mm for the first 40 patients and with a minimum diameter of 5.0 mm for the subsequent 60 patients was considered suitable for large bore vascular access. Under ultrasound guidance, the operator aimed to puncture the anterior wall of the AxA in its third segment. Puncture was performed between the lateral border of the pectoralis minor muscle and the inferior border of the teres major muscle to minimize the risk of pneumothorax and to have the option for manual compression of the vessel against the humeral head using an 18 G needle and standard J wire. Care was taken to avoid injury to the brachial plexus and axillary vein. Access via the left AxA was preferred to avoid manipulation of the aortic arch. After 5F sheath insertion, a baseline control angiogram was performed to confirm correct positioning before proceeding with subsequent interventional steps. Five thousand international units of heparin were administered intravenously and then adjusted in order to achieve an activated clotting time of 250 s. A 5 mm skin incision was made at the axillary puncture site and the subcutaneous tissue was circumferentially stretched to facilitate insertion of the PVCDs. Two Perclose ProGlide PVCDs (Abbott Vascular, Santa Clara, CA, USA) were positioned in a typical 90 degree-angle fashion followed by sheath exchanges to achieve the size required for the planned endovascular aortoiliac procedure.

In those 90 patients treated for TAAA, a femoro-axillary through and through wire was established using a 300 cm long Lunderquist Guidewire (Cook Medical Inc, Bloomington, IN, USA) for percutaneous insertion of the aortic component of the thoracoabdominal stent graft. In order to ensure early restoration of blood flow to the pelvis and to the lower limbs, the right femoral access was closed, and the left femoral access was downsized by exchanging the stent graft sheath with a 9F 11 cm long introducer. Hemostasis of femoral access was achieved by pulling the long suture of the PVCDs. As the next step, stenting of the of the visceral target vessels was performed via the axillary approach.

At the end of the procedure, the axillary sheath was removed before final left femoral access removal and the sutures of the PVCDs were tied down over a safety J wire in place, while applying manual compression on the AxA over the humeral head. Adequate hemostasis was monitored clinically and angiographically. No additional external hemostatic agents were used.

A representative example of percutaneous AxA access and closure is presented in Figure 1A–C.

In patients with inadequate hemostasis, an additional PVCD was initially used, and if bleeding persisted, a covered self-expanding stent (Viabahn, W.L. Gore & Associates, Flagstaff, AZ, USA) was inserted into the AxA via the femoral approach after controlling proximal bleeding with semi-compliant balloon occlusion. In case of flow limiting dissection or occlusion, antegrade treatment of the injured vessel was performed by implantation of a self-expanding stent. The choice of the stent was at the discretion of the operator.

All patients under general anesthesia were transferred to an intensive care unit (ICU) for monitoring using a standardized post-operative management protocol and, if necessary, for further treatment. As part of clinical routine, all patients received a CT scan of the aorta as well as a duplex ultrasound of all puncture sites to identify access site complications before discharge.

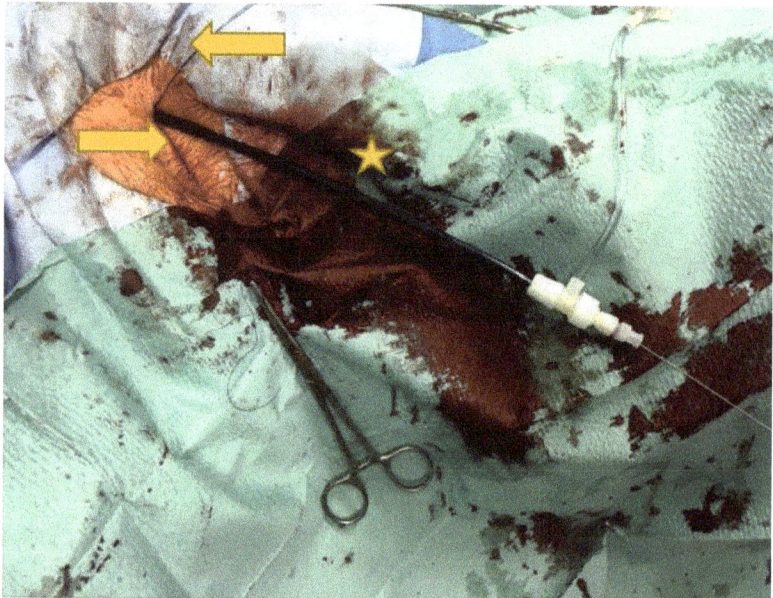

(A)

Figure 1. Cont.

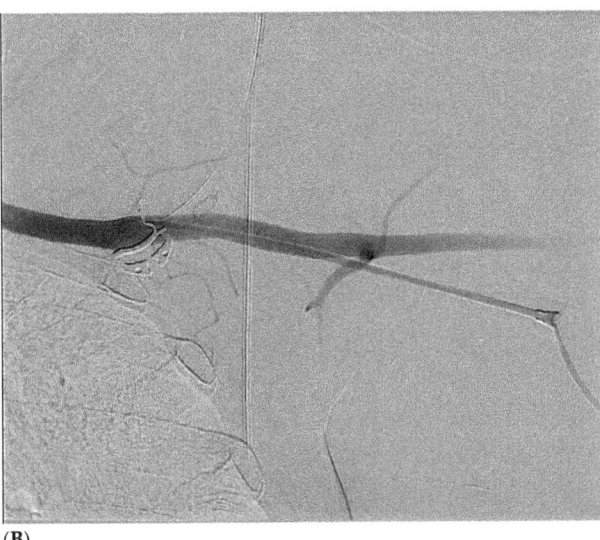

(B)

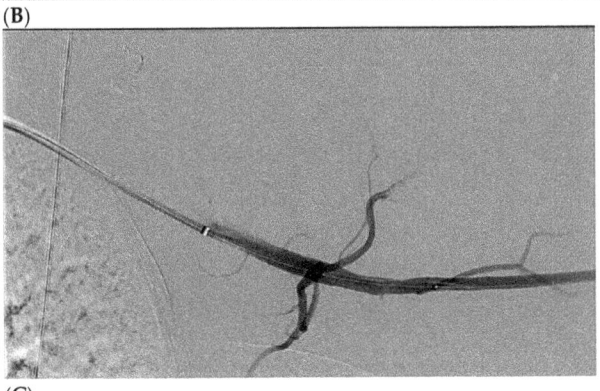

(C)

Figure 1. (A): Left axillary region. Puncture was made in the third segment of the AxA. The picture shows a 12F sheath (yellow star), which was introduced into the AxA. In addition, the two preloaded Perclose ProGlide PVCDs (Abbott Vascular, Santa Clara, CA, USA) (yellow arrows) can be seen. **(B)**: Baseline angiography of the axillary artery (AxA) after ultrasound guided puncture in the third segment of the vessel. Consistent with the results of a previous CT scan, no relevant atherosclerotic changes were detected in this vessel segment, and the vessel diameter was >5 mm. The patient required pre-planned treatment for chronic thoraco-abdominal aortic aneurysm. **(C)**: After successful fenestrated endovascular aortic repair (FEVAR) with fenestrations for the left and right renal artery, coeliac trunc, and superior mesenteric artery, closure of the axillary puncture site was performed using two Perclose ProGlide PVCDs (Abbott Vascular, Santa Clara, CA, USA). The control angiogram via the left femoral access showed no complications at the AxA puncture site.

2.3. Outcome Definitions

Device success was defined as successful puncture site closure using PVCD and no evidence of persistent bleeding or relevant hemodynamic impairment necessitating endovascular or open surgical repair. Procedural success was defined as establishing hemostasis and flow of the AxA using any endovascular method and freedom from major cerebrovascular and peripheral neurological complications by 48 h after the procedure. In addition, complications were recorded based on definitions from the Society for Vascular

Surgery's reporting standards for endovascular aortic aneurysm repair [8] and 30-day mortality was analyzed.

2.4. Statistical Analysis

All data were obtained from a prospectively maintained aortic database within our vascular center, in which imaging studies were evaluated using three-dimensional image analysis techniques (3Mensio Medical Imaging BV, Bilthoven, The Netherlands). Descriptive statistics were performed using SPSS version 20.0 (IBM, Armonk, NY, USA). Categorical variables are presented as number and percentages and continuous variables as mean ± SD or median values (range).

3. Results

3.1. Patient and Procedural Characteristics

Detailed patient demographics and characteristics of the AxA are presented in Tables 1 and 2.

Table 1. Patient characteristics.

Variables	No.	%
Sex		
Male	75	75.0
Female	25	25.0
Age, years		
Mean ± SD	73.8 ± 8.2	
Median (range)	76.0 (54–87)	
History of hypertension	98	98.0
COPD	24	24.0
Active smoking	51	51.0
CHD	30	30.0
Diabetes mellitus	28	28.0
Chronic renal insufficiency *	68	68.0
Hyperlipidaemia	88	88.0
BMI (kg/m^2)		
Mean ± SD	26.6 ± 4.6	
Median (range)	25.8 (20.0–42.4)	
PCI-pre-OP	10	10.0
CABG pre-OP	5	5.0
Creatinine pre-OP (µmol/L)		
Mean ± SD	125.3 ± 113.2	
Median (range)	95.5 (42.0–763.0)	
ASA Score		
ASA II	22	22.0
ASA III	77	77.0
ASA IV	1	1.0
Antiplatelets	81	81.0
Anticoagulant	21	21.0

Continuous data are presented as means ± SD; categorical data are given as counts (percentage). COPD = chronic obstructive pulmonary disease; CHD = coronary heart disease; BMI = body mass index; PCI = percutaneous coronary intervention; CABG = coronary artery bypass graft; ASA = American Society of Anesthesiologists; SD = standard deviation. * Defined as estimated glomerular filtration rate < 60 mL/min/1.73 m^2.

Included patients had a mean age of 73.8 ± 8.2 years and three quarters were male. Most procedures were performed for TAAA (90.0%). The mean aneurysm diameter of the TAAA cases was 65.7 mm (SD: 14.4 mm). Further characteristics of the treated TAAA are listed in Table 3. Endovascular TAAA treatment was pre-planned in 72 patients, while 18 patients presented as vascular emergencies: from those, 9 patients had an acute aortic rupture, 3 patients had a symptomatic penetrating aortic ulcer and 6 patients presented with acute, non-controllable pain.

Table 2. Characteristics of the AxA.

AxA Description Pre-OP		
Diameter AxA (mm)		
Mean ± SD	7.26 ± 1.29	
Median (range)	7.27 (4.50–10.80)	
Calcification > 50% circumference	0	0
Stenosis > 50%	0	0
Previous percutaneous access	0	0
Pacemaker on the punctured side	4	4.0
Dialysis AVF on the punctured side	5	5.0
Side of puncture AxA		
Left	93	93.0
Right	7	7.0

Continuous data are presented as means ± SD; categorical data are given as counts (percentage). AxA = axillary artery; AVF = arteriovenous fistula; SD = standard deviation.

Table 3. Characteristics of thoraco-abdominal aortic aneurysms.

Aneurysms Characteristics	No.	%
Acute	18	18.0
Rupture	9	9.0
Penetrating aortic ulcer	3	3.0
Pain	6	6.0
Chronic	72	72.0
Crawford Classification		
Type II	32	32.0
Type III	33	33.0
Type IV	25	25.0
Maximum aortic diameter, mm		
Mean ± SD	65.7 ± 14.4	
Median (range)	66.0 (25–102)	
Previous repair of the aorta	42	42.0
TEVAR	20	20.0
EVAR	22	22.0
TAAA		
Atherosclerotic	82	82.0
Dissection	8	8.0
Previous coil of segmental arteries	55	55.0

Continuous data are presented as means ± SD; categorical data are given as counts (percentage). TAAA = Thoraco-abdominal aortic aneurysms; SD = standard deviation; TEVAR = Thoracic endovascular aortic repair; EVAR = Endovascular aortic repair.

Most patients were treated by branched endovascular aortic repair (BEVAR; 45%), followed by fenestrated endovascular aortic repair (FEVAR; 30%), chimney endovascular aortic repair (ChEVAR; 9%), and fenestrated-branched endovascular aortic repair (FBEVAR; 6%). The remaining 10% were mixed cases with different indications: a coil embolization of the superior gluteal artery because of endoleak Type II was performed twice via UEA. In two cases, an axillary approach was needed for bi-iliac extension after endovascular aortic repair (EVAR) and in four cases for delivery of iliac branch devices. One case each required UEA access for endovascular repair of renal artery bleeding and subclavian artery aneurysm (Table 4).

Based on CT scan measurements, the median diameter of the AxA in its third segment was 7.27 mm (range: 4.50–10.80). Most procedures were performed with a 12F introducer (60%), followed by 7F (18%), 8F (15%) and 9F (5%). Just in two single cases, a 6 and 14F introducer was used. None of the patients had significant calcification of the anterior wall of the vessel as examined in CTA. Except for one case, all patients were treated under general anesthesia. The mean operating time was 191.0 min (SD: 69.0) (Table 4).

Table 4. Endovascular treatment characteristics.

Treatment Characteristics	No.	%
FEVAR (with no. of fenestrations)	30	30.0
2	5	5.0
4	25	25.0
BEVAR (with no. of branches)	45	45.0
2	3	3.0
3	7	7.0
4	34	34.0
5	1	1.0
FBEVAR (with no. of fenestrations)	6	6.0
4	5	5.0
5	1	1.0
ChEVAR (with no. of fenestrations)	9	9.0
3	3	3.0
4	5	5.0
5	1	1.0
Other	10	10.0
General anesthesia	99	99.0
Operative time (minutes)		
Mean ± SD	191.0 ± 69.0	
Median (range)	193 (53–480)	
Fluoroscopy time (minutes)		
Mean ± SD	50.3 ± 22.7	
Median (range)	49 (16–142)	
Radiation dose (Gycm^2)		
Mean ± SD	1567.6 ± 2156.2	
Median (range)	429.7 (52.0–8635.6)	
ID of introducer (French)		
6F	1	1.0
7F	18	18.0
8F	15	15.0
9F	5	5.0
12F	60	60.0
14F	1	1.0
Median (range)	12 (6–14)	

Continuous data are presented as means ± SD; categorical data are given as counts (percentage). FEVAR = fenestrated endovascular aortic repair. BEVAR = branched endovascular aortic repair; FBEVAR = fenestrated-branched endovascular aortic repair; ChEVAR = chimney endovascular aortic repair; SD = standard deviation.

3.2. Acute Procedural Outcomes

Device success was reached in 92 of the 100 patients (92.0%) using the two Perclose ProGlide PVCDs (Abbott Vascular, Santa Clara, CA, USA) inserted after puncture. Eight patients (8.0%) required additional procedures performed immediately during the index procedure via transfemoral access to either successfully close the puncture site (two patients) or restore adequate flow (six patients). Two bleedings occurred in the area of the puncture site despite use of closure devices, necessitating deployment of self-expanding covered stents. One of those patients exhibited a vessel diameter below 5 mm. In three patients, AxA occlusion occurred instantly after use of two PVCDs and was resolved in two cases by transfemoral implantation of 6 mm diameter self-expanding uncovered nitinol stents and by a 6 mm self-expanding covered stent in another patient. Furthermore, three patients experienced a high-grade stenosis at the percutaneous approach of the AxA, which was successfully repaired by implantation of self-expanding uncovered stents with a diameter of 6 mm. A total of six patients (6%) suffered stenosis or occlusion of the AxA at the puncture site. In all six cases with the above complications, the maximum diameter of the AxA was <5 mm. No cases required conversion to open surgical repair of the AxA.

Procedural success was achieved in 100% of the patients as there were no subsequent major vascular complications at the UEA access site requiring late reintervention or open surgery. No patient developed acute arm ischemia or deep arm vein thrombosis. Nine minor vessel complications (9.0%) were detected, including three pseudo-aneurysms and six hematomas, which all could be treated conservatively. No peripheral nerve injuries or brachial plexus damage were noted. Ischemia of the spinal cord occurred to varying degrees in 11 patients (11%) after the procedure. Seven patients also suffered a stroke (7%) and five of those events were considered peri-procedural based on neurologic assessment and CT scan. In three cases, symptoms completely resolved over the next few days and patients were asymptomatic at the time of discharge. Two patients with middle cerebral artery infarction had to be transferred to a neurological rehabilitation facility due to persisting hemiparesis and aphasia. The median ICU stay was 2 days and the median hospital stay 12 days (Table 5).

Table 5. In-hospital outcomes.

Variables	No.	%
Primary hemostasis AxA	92	92.0
Stenosis/occlusion AxA	6	6.0
Bleeding	2	2.0
Uncovered stent	5	5.0
Covered stent	3	3.0
Surgical repair	0	0
Hematoma	6	6.0
PSA	3	3.0
Arm ischemia	0	0
Peripheral nerve injury	0	0
DVT	0	0
Stroke	7	7.0
SCI	11	11.0
Death within 30 days	8	8.0
ICU stay (days)		
Median (range)	2 (0–34)	
Hospital stay (days)		
Median (range)	12 (1–95)	

Continuous data are presented as means ± SD; categorical data are given as counts (percentage). SD = standard deviation; AxA = axillary artery; PSA = pseudoaneurysm; DVT = deep vein thrombosis; SCI = spinal cord ischemia.

3.3. All-Cause Death through 30 Days

The thirty-day survival rate was 92%, but all deaths occurred during hospitalization. In four patients who died, the reason of death was aneurysm related. Three patients died within 24 h after endovascular treatment of ruptured TAAA and one because of a retrograde type A aortic dissection. Three patients developed multiorgan failure after the procedure, which could not be resolved despite intensive care measures. One patient became infected with SARS-CoV-2 virus after the endovascular procedure and died of COVID-related pneumonia with global respiratory insufficiency at day 30.

4. Discussion

As the complexity of endovascular aortic repairs has increased over time, the need for UEA has increased, particularly for bridging and visceral stent delivery, graft stabilization via a through and through wire, or complex aortoiliac procedures, such as IBD delivery. AxA access is often preferred over the brachial artery as the vessel can accommodate large sheath sizes up to 18F and is rarely atherosclerotic. To date, most surgeons prefer surgical exposure of the AxA, but the potential advantages of percutaneous access are shorter operation time and less vascular trauma with a lower risk of wound healing problems. However, only limited data are available on the safety of such an approach.

Our study aimed to characterize the feasibility and safety of percutaneous axillary artery access in its third segment in a series of 100 complex aortic and aortoiliac interventions with closure of the puncture site by percutaneous closure systems. While there are no specific vascular closure devices for the AxA, the use of two Proglide—deployed at the beginning of the procedure before sheath upsizing—has been suggested as a promising approach. The AxA can be divided into three segments based on anatomic structures [3]. Due to its deep submuscular location, the second segment is considered unsuitable for direct puncture. Its close location to the ribcage with the risk of pneumothorax in the context of puncture, as well as the lack of an adequate posterior bony structure for compression, are reasons against puncturing the first segment, and thus we decided to prefer the third segment of the AxA. Using this location, we report an overall 92% device success rate, which was even higher when we changed our practice after a preliminary analysis of the first 40 patients [7] excluding vessels below a 5 mm diameter threshold. Subsequently, no relevant stenosis or occlusion of the AxA was detected in the final control angiogram after puncture site closure. Bleeding events were rare (two cases), which also could be resolved using endovascular techniques. In no case was open surgical repair of the AxA required. Overall, our complication rate (e.g., occlusion/stenosis, bleeding, and hematoma) is comparable to similar studies in the field [3,8,9], but focusing on the excellent results of our late cohort, where we excluded vessel diameter < 5 mm, we actually report fewer complications. Importantly, we achieved these excellent results by using the third segment of the AxA, where the puncture risk can be considered lower due to the anatomical conditions, while most prior data were obtained after puncture of the first AxA segment. Bertoglio et al. investigated safety and effectiveness of UEA with percutaneous closure of the axillary artery (AxA) during endovascular treatment of TAA with fenestrated and branched endografts in 59 patients. They also used, for closing of the puncture site, the double ProGlide technique. In contrast to our study, the puncture of the AxA was carried out in the first segment using sheath sizes between 10 and 16F. The closure success rate was 90% with no open conversion required. A total of 5 out of 59 patients received a bare or covered stent implantation for either flow-limiting dissection or persistent bleeding. After a follow-up period of 6 months, there were no late complications, and all access vessels were patent [10]. Agrusa et al. investigated the safety and feasibility of a percutaneous AxA access also in the third segment in 46 patients with TAAA using two Perclose ProGlide devices (Abbott Vascular, Santa Clara, CA, USA) before inserting a large sheath. Technical success was achieved in 41 of 46 patients (89%) and 5 patients required endovascular covered stent implantation to control persistent access site bleeding. No surgical intervention was required in this cohort either [9].

Furthermore, Schaefer et al. reported percutaneous closure of AxA access in the first segment during transaxillary transcatheter aortic valve replacement in 100 patients and demonstrated the feasibility and safety of this approach as the rate of minor vascular complications was acceptable. Covered stent implantation was necessary in 11% of the cases [3].

Prior data from cardiac interventions also suggest that a percutaneous AxA access offers a similar safety compared to open cut-down. A systematic review studying patients undergoing transcatheter aortic valve replacement or mechanical circulatory support with large-bore axillary arterial access showed similar major vascular complications (2.8% vs. 2.3%) but less major bleeding (2.7% vs. 17.9%) using a percutaneous versus a surgical approach [11].

Limitation

The limitations of the study include the sample size of this single center, non-controlled study, which did not allow for adjusted analysis. Further, effect sizes tend to be overestimated in non-controlled studies. Proving the feasibility and safety of the percutaneous axillary access would require a randomized controlled trial versus open surgery and other UEA sites. Long-term data would be needed to adequately assess the consequences after bailout stenting in case of occlusion/stenosis or bleeding complications with covered and uncovered stents.

5. Conclusions

Percutaneous puncture of the AxA in its third segment for insertion of large sheaths up to 14F in the percutaneous endovascular treatment of complex aortic and aortoiliac interventions seems to be safe, especially in arterial segments with a diameter > 5 mm. Complication management can also be performed with endovascular techniques.

Author Contributions: Conceptualization: T.W., A.S. (Arsen Sabanov), S.S., A.S. (Andrej Schmidt) and D.B.; Methodology: T.W., A.S. (Arsen Sabanov), A.S. (Andrej Schmidt), D.S., S.S. and D.B.; Formal Analysis: T.W., A.S. (Arsen Sabanov), S.S. and D.B.; Investigation: A.S. (Andrej Schmidt) and D.B.; Data Curation: T.W. and A.S. (Arsen Sabanov); Writing—Original Draft Preparation: T.W. and A.S. (Arsen Sabanov); Writing—Review and Editing: A.S. (Andrej Schmidt), D.S., S.S. and D.B.; Visualization: T.W., A.S. (Arsen Sabanov), S.S. and D.B.; Supervision: A.S. (Andrej Schmidt), D.S., S.S. and D.B. All authors have read and agreed to the published version of the manuscript.

Funding: Funded by the Open Access Publishing Fund of Leipzig University supported by the German Research Foundation within the program Open Access Publication Funding.

Institutional Review Board Statement: The study conformed to the principles outlined in the Declaration of Helsinki and received approval (EK Votum 319/15-ek) from the institutional ethics committee.

Informed Consent Statement: Informed consent was obtained from all subjects involved in the study.

Data Availability Statement: The data presented in this study are available on request from the corresponding author. The data are not publicly available due to data privacy.

Conflicts of Interest: The author(s) declared the following relationships in connection with the article: Tim Wittig: None. Arsen Sabanov: None. Daniela Branzan: Consultant for Artivion, Bentley Innomed, Cook Medical, Cydar Medical, and Endologix. Andrej Schmidt: Consultant for Abbott, Boston Scientific, Cook Medical, Cordis, CR Bard, ReFlow Medical, and Upstream Peripheral Technologies. Dierk Scheinert: Consultant or advisory board member for Abbott, Biotronik, Boston Scientific, Cook Medical, Cordis, CR Bard, Gardia Medical, Medtronic/Covidien, TriReme Medical, Trivascular, and Upstream Peripheral Technologies. Sabine Steiner: Consultant for Boston Scientific and Cook Medical. Research funding: C.R. Bard.

Abbreviations

AxA	axillary artery
ER	endovascular repair
PVCD	percutaneous vascular closure devices
TAAA	thoraco-abdominal aortic aneurysms
UEA	upper extremity access
IBD	iliac branch devices
CTA	computer tomography angiography
BEVAR	branched endovascular aortic repair
FEVAR	fenestrated endovascular aortic repair
ChEVAR	chimney endovascular aortic repair
FBEVAR	fenestrated-branched endovascular aortic repair
EVAR	endovascular aortic repair
ICU	intensive care unit

References

1. Tenorio, E.R.; Dias-Neto, M.F.; Lima, G.B.B.; Estrera, A.L.; Oderich, G.S. Endovascular repair for thoracoabdominal aortic aneurysms: Current status and future challenges. *Ann. Cardiothorac. Surg.* **2021**, *10*, 744–767. [CrossRef] [PubMed]
2. Meertens, M.M.; van Herwaarden, J.A.; de Vries, J.P.P.; Verhagen, H.J.; van der Laan, M.J.; Reijnen, M.M.; Schurink, G.W.; Mees, B.M. Multicenter experience of upper extremity access in complex endovascular aortic aneurysm repair. *J. Vasc. Surg.* **2022**, *76*, 1150–1159. [CrossRef] [PubMed]
3. Schäfer, U.; Deuschl, F.; Schofer, N.; Frerker, C.; Schmidt, T.; Kuck, K.; Kreidel, F.; Schirmer, J.; Mizote, I.; Reichenspurner, H.; et al. Safety and efficacy of the percutaneous transaxillary access for transcatheter aortic valve implantation using various transcatheter heart valves in 100 consecutive patients. *Int. J. Cardiol.* **2017**, *232*, 247–254. [CrossRef] [PubMed]

4. Puippe, G.D.; Kobe, A.; Rancic, Z.; Pfiffner, R.; Lachat, M.; Pfammatter, T. Safety of percutaneous axillary artery access with a suture-mediated closing device for parallel endograft aortic procedures—A retrospective pilot study. *Vasa* **2018**, *47*, 311–317. [CrossRef] [PubMed]
5. Wooster, M.; Powell, A.; Back, M.; Illig, K.; Shames, M. Axillary Artery Access as an Adjunct for Complex Endovascular Aortic Repair. *Ann. Vasc. Surg.* **2015**, *29*, 1543–1547. [CrossRef] [PubMed]
6. Knowles, M.; Nation, D.A.; Timaran, D.E.; Gomez, L.F.; Baig, M.S.; Valentine, R.J.; Timaran, C.H. Upper extremity access for fenestrated endovascular aortic aneurysm repair is not associated with increased morbidity. *J. Vasc. Surg.* **2015**, *61*, 80–87. [CrossRef] [PubMed]
7. Branzan, D.; Steiner, S.; Haensig, M.; Scheinert, D.; Schmidt, A. Percutaneous Axillary Artery Access for Endovascular Treatment of Complex Thoraco-abdominal Aortic Aneurysms. *Eur. J. Vasc. Endovasc. Surg.* **2019**, *58*, 344–349. [CrossRef] [PubMed]
8. Chaikof, E.L.; Blankensteijn, J.D.; Harris, P.L.; White, G.H.; Zarins, C.K.; Bernhard, V.M.; Matsumura, J.S.; May, J.; Veith, F.J.; Fillinger, M.F.; et al. Reporting standards for endovascular aortic aneurysm repair. *J. Vasc. Surg.* **2002**, *35*, 1048–1060. [CrossRef] [PubMed]
9. Agrusa, C.J.; Connolly, P.H.; Ellozy, S.H.; Schneider, D.B. Safety and Effectiveness of Percutaneous Axillary Artery Access for Complex Aortic Interventions. *Ann. Vasc. Surg.* **2019**, *61*, 326–333. [CrossRef] [PubMed]
10. Bertoglio, L.; Grandi, A.; Melloni, A.; Kahlberg, A.; Melissano, G.; Chiesa, R. Percutaneous AXillary Artery (PAXA) Access at the First Segment During Fenestrated and Branched Endovascular Aortic Procedures. *Eur. J. Vasc. Endovasc. Surg.* **2020**, *59*, 929–938. [CrossRef] [PubMed]
11. Southmayd, G.; Hoque, A.; Kaki, A.; Tayal, R.; Rab, S.T. Percutaneous large-bore axillary access is a safe alternative to surgical approach: A systematic review. *Catheter. Cardiovasc. Interv.* **2020**, *96*, 1481–1488. [CrossRef] [PubMed]

Disclaimer/Publisher's Note: The statements, opinions and data contained in all publications are solely those of the individual author(s) and contributor(s) and not of MDPI and/or the editor(s). MDPI and/or the editor(s) disclaim responsibility for any injury to people or property resulting from any ideas, methods, instructions or products referred to in the content.

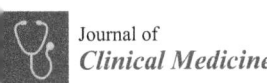

Article

Incidence and Outcomes of Abdominal Aortic Aneurysm Repair in New Zealand from 2001 to 2021

Sinead Gormley [1,2], Oliver Bernau [2], William Xu [2], Peter Sandiford [3,4] and Manar Khashram [1,2,*]

1. Department of Vascular & Endovascular Surgery, Waikato Hospital, Hamilton 3204, New Zealand
2. Faculty of Medical & Health Sciences, University of Auckland, Auckland 1010, New Zealand
3. Planning Funding and Outcomes Unit, Auckland and Waitemata District Health Boards, Auckland 1010, New Zealand
4. School of Population Health, University of Auckland, Auckland 1010, New Zealand
* Correspondence: manar.khashram@gmail.com

Abstract: Purpose: The burden of abdominal aortic aneurysms (AAA) has changed in the last 20 years but is still considered to be a major cause of cardiovascular mortality. The introduction of endovascular aortic repair (EVAR) and improved peri-operative care has resulted in a steady improvement in both outcomes and long-term survival. The objective of this study was to identify the burden of AAA disease by analysing AAA-related hospitalisations and deaths. Methodology: All AAA-related hospitalisations in NZ from January 2001 to December 2021 were identified from the National Minimum Dataset, and mortality data were obtained from the NZ Mortality Collection dataset from January 2001 to December 2018. Data was analysed for patient characteristics including deprivation index, repair methods and 30-day outcomes. Results: From 2001 to 2021, 14,436 patients with an intact AAA were identified with a mean age of 75.1 years (SD 9.7 years), and 4100 (28%) were females. From 2001 to 2018, there were 5000 ruptured AAA with a mean age of 77.8 (SD 9.4), and 1676 (33%) were females. The rate of hospitalisations related to AAA has decreased from 43.7 per 100,000 in 2001 to 15.4 per 100,000 in 2018. There was a higher proportion of rupture AAA in patients living in more deprived areas. The use of EVAR for intact AAA repair has increased from 18.1% in 2001 to 64.3% in 2021. The proportion of octogenarians undergoing intact AAA repair has increased from 16.2% in 2001 to 28.4% in 2021. The 30-day mortality for intact AAA repair has declined from 5.8% in 2001 to 1.7% in 2021; however, it has remained unchanged for ruptured AAA repair at 31.6% across the same period. Conclusions: This study highlights that the incidence of AAA has declined in the last two decades. The mortality has improved for patients who had a planned repair. Understanding the contemporary burden of AAA is paramount to improve access to health, reduce variation in outcomes and promote surgical quality improvement.

Keywords: abdominal aortic aneurysm; incidence; epidemiology; EVAR; ruptured AAA; New Zealand

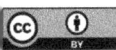

1. Introduction

The epidemiology and management of Abdominal Aortic Aneurysm (AAA) has changed in the last 20 years [1]. Some of these include a decline in prevalence, improvement in life expectancy and the introduction of Endovascular Aneurysm Repair (EVAR), along with the improvements in pre-operative work up and peri-operative care and the establishment of AAA screening programmes in some countries. The introduction of EVAR has made it possible to offer AAA repair to patients that previously might not have been candidates for open aneurysm repair (OAR). As a result, the proportion of AAA repairs using EVAR has increased [2], and the survival of both intact and ruptured AAA has improved.

The approach to population level screening is highly variable between different countries. New Zealand (NZ) has not established a policy for national AAA screening and mostly relies on background detection from medical imaging despite demonstrated cost-effectiveness [3]. In the United Kingdom [4] and Sweden [5], population screening programmes have contributed to the changes seen in the contemporary management and outcomes of AAA, such as the reduced incidence of ruptured aneurysms.

The incidence of hospitalisations and mortality of AAA in NZ has been previously reported from the years 1994–2009 [6]. However, the rate of decline, the changes in AAA management and patient outcomes have not been reported. The objective of this study was to report the incidence and outcomes of AAA in NZ.

2. Materials and Methods

2.1. Study Design

This was a retrospective observational cohort study and was prepared according to the Strengthening the Reporting of Observational Studies in Epidemiology (STROBE) guidelines [7]. Ethics approval was granted by the New Zealand Health and Disability Ethics Committees (Re13/STH/190/AM01).

2.2. Study Protocol and Data Collection

There were three datasets that contributed to the study population. The Analytics Services Team from the New Zealand Ministry of Health provided admission data from the National Minimum Dataset (NMDS) for all publicly and privately funded hospitalisations with any diagnosis or procedure relating to AAA (Appendix A, Table A1), with a discharge date from 1 January 2001 to 31 December 2021. Operative data from January 2010 onwards were cross referenced against the Australasian Vascular Audit (AVA) [8–10]. All deaths registered in NZ are recorded on the National Mortality collection dataset, and this database was interrogated to retrieve all deaths with a primary diagnosis of aortic aneurysm (ICD-10-AM codes I71.3 and I71.4) from January 2001 to December 2018. This permitted defining aneurysm-related mortality for patients who died because of a AAA-specific cause. In addition, two further groups were created for patients who died with a ruptured AAA in the community or those presented to the emergency department who died prior to hospital admission, and for the patients who were admitted to hospital with a ruptured AAA but did not have a repair.

AAA-related hospitalisations and repairs were analysed from 2001 to 2021, and AAA-related deaths were analysed from 2001 to 2018, as there is an approximately three-year lag time. Data collected from the NMDS included baseline characteristics, diagnoses and procedures performed. Only patients with a AAA diagnosis (I71.3, I71.4) were analysed. Data are presented on a patient-level basis using the index presentation. For patients with multiple hospitalisations across the study period, the index presentation was defined as the first occurrence of an aneurysm-related procedure or rupture, or the initial presentation with a AAA diagnosis if neither procedure nor rupture was found. There was no look back period during the study period. A pre-hospital death was defined as a death occurring in the community or whilst in the emergency department prior to admission. Aneurysm-related mortality was defined as any death occurring within 30 days of aneurysm treatment or date of rupture, or any death with a primary cause relating to AAA.

2.3. Ethnicity Definition

The New Zealand Ministry of Health ethnicity data protocols dictate the use of prioritisation of ethnicities. This means that if a patient identifies with more than one ethnicity, specific protocols are put in place to determine which ethnic group a patient will be included in for the purposes of statistical analysis. This is designed to ensure indigenous communities are counted and prioritised. It also works to ensure other ethnic minorities are enabled with the largest possible inclusion of membership to enable appropriate statistical analysis to be undertaken. New Zealand national ethnicity standards encourage all primary, secondary and tertiary health institutions to have patients complete a form in which they can self-identify with the ethnic group or groups that best describe their ethnic affiliations [11].

2.4. New Zealand Index of Deprivation (NZDep)

The New Zealand Index of Deprivation (NZDep) is a measure obtained from census data and is linked to geographical location rather than individuals [12]. The NZDep was calculated based on nine domains: access to transport, access to communication, living space, income, recipient of benefit, single-parent family, home ownership, qualifications and employment. NZDep groups deprivation scores into deciles, with 1 being the least deprived areas and 10 being the most deprived areas [13].

2.5. AAA-Related Hospitalisations

Age- and sex-specific rates per 100,000 population per year were calculated from the NZ population at each respective year. The World Health Organisation (WHO) standard population was used to age standardise the rates. All cases identified were assumed to be new cases and each case was identified once only.

2.6. Statistical Analysis

Data were presented as frequency (percentage) for categorical data and mean ± standard deviation (SD) or median (interquartile range). The Chi-squared test was used to compare categorial data and Student's *t*-test (two-tailed) was used for continuous variables. Age standardisation was completed using standard populations modelled after the NZ World Health Organisation standard population as per the methods of Robson et al. [14]. Age standardisation was completed with the dsr package, and 95% confidence intervals were calculated using well-documented methods. Statistical analyses were completed in R version 3.6.1 (R foundation for statistical computing, Vienna, Austria) [15].

3. Results

3.1. Patient Demographics

From January 2001 to December 2021, 14,436 patients were diagnosed with an intact AAA or registered as having died from an intact AAA-related death in NZ. The mean age was 75.1 years (SD 9.7 years), and 4100 (28%) were females. From January 2001 to December 2018, 5000 patients presented or died with a diagnosed ruptured AAA (rAAA). The mean age was 77.8 years (SD 9.4 years), and 1676 (33%) were females. For both intact and ruptured AAA groups, NZ Europeans made up over 80% of each patient cohort. There was a higher proportion of ruptured and intact AAA in those living in more deprived areas, with 4009 (22.7%) of patients living in deprivation deciles 9 to 10 versus 1993 (11.3%) in deciles 1 to 2. Patient characteristics are described for intact and ruptured AAA index presentations stratified by sex in Table 1. AAA prevalence grouped by age and sex are described in Figure 1. Crude estimated incidence of AAAs per 100,000 person-years stratified by gender and age are described in Table 2.

Table 1. Patient characteristics for intact and ruptured AAA index presentations stratified by sex. Intact AAA data from 2001 to 2021 and ruptured AAA data from 2001 to 2018.

	Intact (*n* = 14,436)			Ruptured (*n* = 5000)		
	Male	Female	*p*-Value	Male	Female	*p*-Value
Number	10,336	4100		3324	1676	
Age, mean (SD)	74.5	76.8	<0.001	76.5	80.6	<0.001
Ethnicity						
NZ/Other European	8794 (85.1%)	3319 (81%)	<0.001	2853 (85.8%)	1402 (83.7%)	<0.001
Māori	614 (5.9%)	480 (11.7%)		232 (7.0%)	176 (10.5%)	

Table 1. Cont.

	Intact (n = 14,436)			Ruptured (n = 5000)		
	Male	Female	p-Value	Male	Female	p-Value
Pacific	240 (2.3%)	84 (2.0%)		75 (2.3%)	40 (2.4%)	
Asian, African, Hispanic	295 (2.9%)	100 (2.4%)		80 (2.4%)	40 (2.4%)	
Not specified	393 (3.8%)	117 (2.9%)		84 (2.5%)	18 (1.1%)	
Deprivation index						
1–2	1371 (13.3%)	452 (11%)	<0.001	308 (9.3%)	122 (7.3%)	<0.001
3–4	1687 (16.3%)	601 (14.7%)		410 (12.3%)	199 (11.9%)	
5–6	2129 (20.6%)	867 (21.1%)		520 (15.6%)	235 (14%)	
7–8	2557 (24.7%)	1060 (25.9%)		631 (19%)	304 (18.1%)	
9–10	2349 (22.7%)	1058 (25.8%)		665 (20%)	342 (20.4%)	
Not available	243 (2.4%)	62 (1.5%)		790 (23.8%)	474 (28.3%)	
Intervention						
OAR	3411 (33%)	1028 (25.1%)	<0.001	1190 (35.8%)	321 (19.2%)	<0.001
EVAR	3150 (30.5%)	832 (20.3%)		76 (2.3%)	18 (1.1%)	
Not operated	3775 (36.5%)	2240 (54.6%)	<0.001	2058 (61.9%)	1337 (79.8%)	<0.001

Table 2. Crude estimated incidence of AAAs/100,000 person-years using NZ census statistics stratified by gender and age.

Category	Cases	Crude Overall Incidence (95% CI)
Gender		
Female	5905	12.44 (12.13–12.76)
Male	13929	30.34 (29.84–30.85)
Age Group		
44 Years and Under	300	0.04 (0.04–0.05)
45–49 Years	210	0.27 (0.23–0.31)
50–54 Years	432	0.59 (0.53–0.64)
55–59 Years	1016	1.52 (1.43–1.62)
60–64 Years	2424	4.22 (4.06–4.39)
65–69 Years	4530	9.49 (9.22–9.77)
70–74 Years	7038	18.44 (18.01–18.88)
75–79 Years	8788	30.46 (29.38–31.1)
80–84 Years	8024	39.8 (38.93–40.68)
85–89 Years	4780	40.98 (39.83–42.16)
90 Years and Over	2126	35.66 (34.16–37.2)

For the period 2001–2018, a total of 3874 AAA-related deaths were documented. There were 3601/3874 (93.0%) deaths from ruptured AAA and 273/3874 (7.0%) from intact AAA. The overall mortality for rAAA patients that underwent EVAR was 17/94 (18.1%). The overall mortality for rAAA patients that underwent OAR was 495/1511 (32.8%). Overall, there was a decline in AAA-related deaths per year across the study period, with 249 per year from 2001 to 2005 and 179 per year from 2014 to 2018.

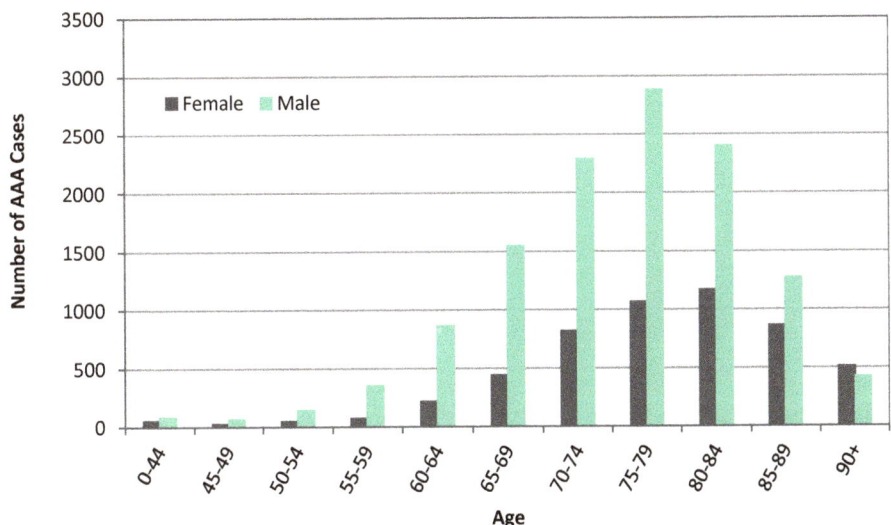

Figure 1. AAA prevalence grouped by age and sex, 2001–2018.

3.2. AAA Presentation and Repair

From 2001 to 2018, there was a 64.0% decrease in AAA presentations in males, from 61.5 to 22.1 per 100,000 per year. This was also observed in female presentations. There has been a decline in the incidence of intact AAA presentations and AAA repair from 24.8 per 100,000 in 2001 to 12.6 per 100,000 in 2021 and 11.9 per 100,000 in 2001 to 7.5 per 100,000 in 2021, respectively. There was a greater decline in the incidence of AAA hospitalisations in Maori females versus Maori males between 2001 and 2018. In 2018, there was 21.3 per 100,000 presentations in Maori females versus 28.3 per 100,000 in Maori males (Figure 2).

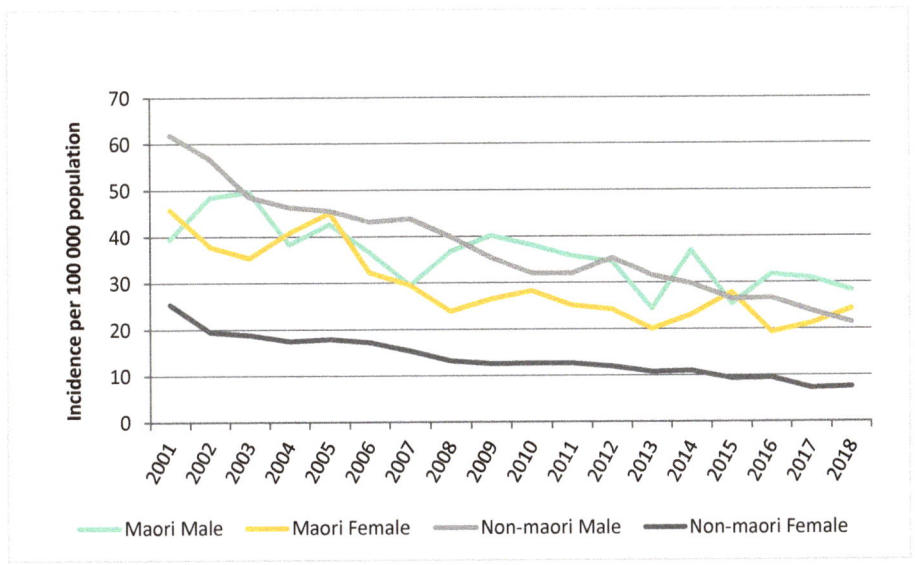

Figure 2. AAA hospitalisation age standardized to NZ population changes.

For ruptured AAA, the incidence decreased from 9.7 in 2001 to 4.7 per 100,000 in 2018. Similarly, repairs of ruptured AAA reduced from 4.0 per 100,000 in 2001 to 1.4 per 100,000 in 2018 (Figure 3).

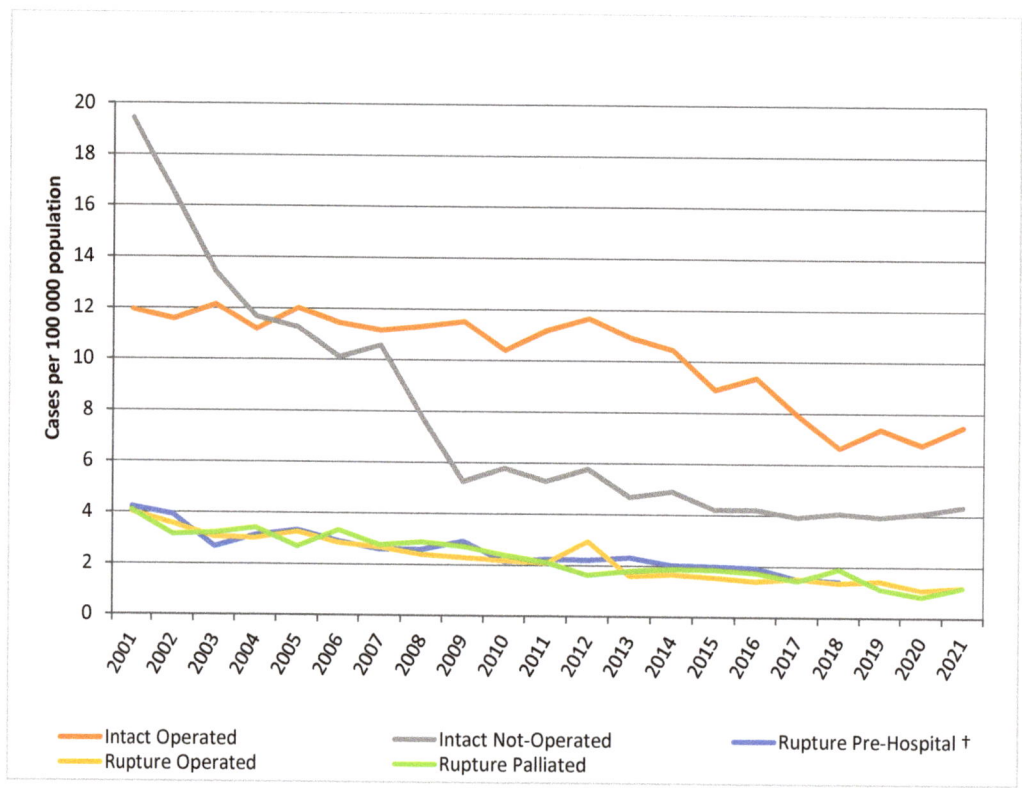

Figure 3. Trends in AAA presentation and management. † Pre-hospital rupture data available only from 2001 to 2018.

3.3. Trends of AAA Repair and Presentation

From 2001 to 2021, considering the AAA repairs performed, a total of 8421 (82.4%) were on intact AAA and 1802 (17.6%) were on ruptured AAA. The average annual number of intact AAA repairs remained fairly constant during the study period until 2015 after which it declined steadily.

From 2001 to 2018, considering those with a diagnosis of ruptured aneurysm, 1605 (32.1%) had a repair, 1673 (33.5%) were palliated or denied surgical intervention (treated conservatively) in the hospital and 1722 (34.4%) died prior to hospitalisation. Over the period 2001–2018, there was a decrease in the rate of patients with ruptured AAA dying pre-hospital from 4.2 per 100,000 population to 1.4 per 100,000 (Figure 3).

3.4. AAA Repair in Octogenarians

We observed a significant shift in AAA presentation to the older population driven by both the increased use of EVAR and the increasing number of octogenarians. The proportion of octogenarians undergoing intact AAA repair has increased from 16.2% in 2001 to 28.4% in 2021 (Figure 4). We also observed a decline in 30-day post-operative mortality in this age group following AAA repair, from 6.8% in 2001 to 0.9% in 2021.

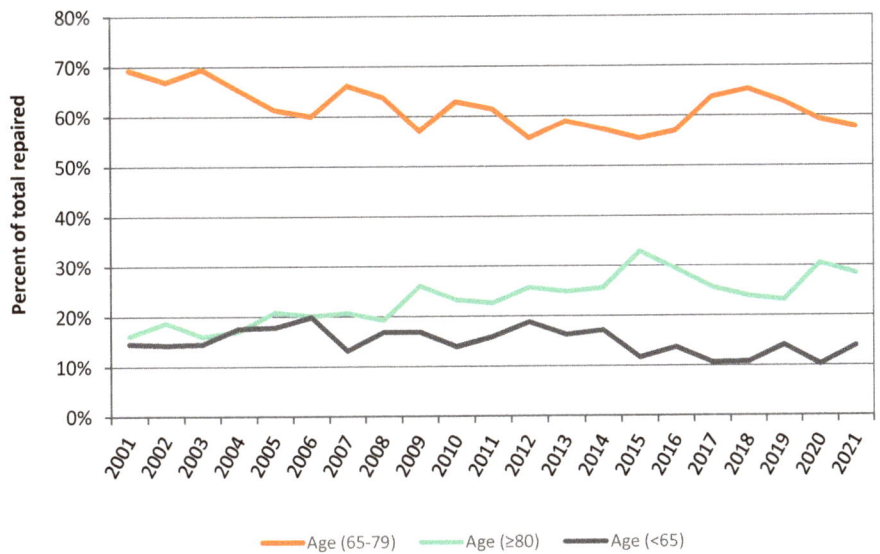

Figure 4. Proportion of intact AAA repaired by age.

3.5. Incidence of Ruptured AAA Stratified by Sex

From 2001 to 2018, there was a total of 5000 ruptured AAA presentations, of which 3324 (66.5%) were males and 1605 (32.1%) underwent repair. A greater number of males underwent surgery for ruptured AAA (1266 (78.9%) males). The proportion of males with a non-operative ruptured AAA decreased. The number of females with a ruptured AAA turned down for repair declined by 50% (Figure 5).

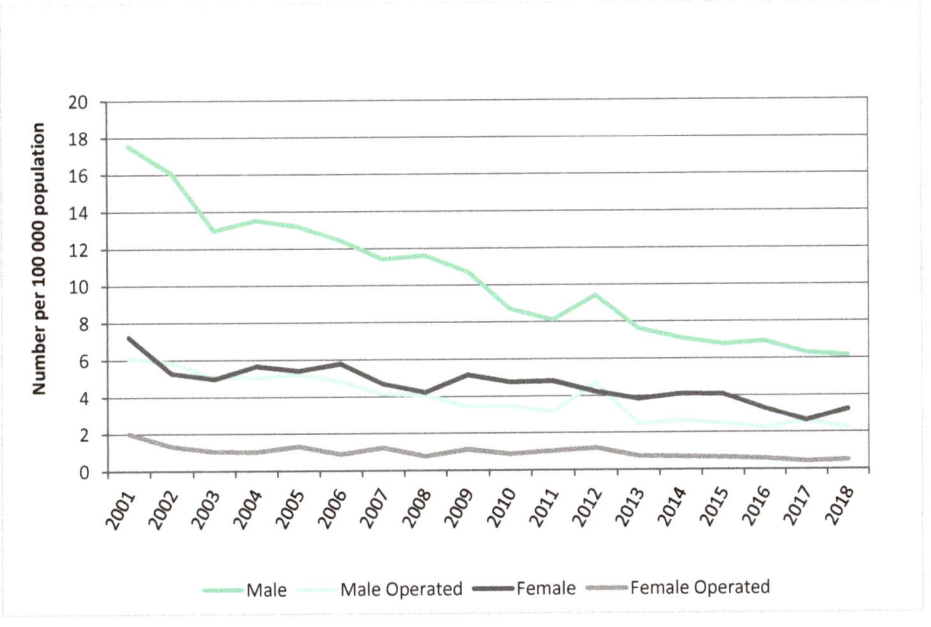

Figure 5. Trends or ruptured AAA incidence and repair between sexes.

3.6. Methods of AAA Repair and Trends in Operative Mortality

EVAR has gradually replaced OAR for patients requiring an intact AAA repair (4439 (52.7%) OAR cases vs. 3982 (47.2%) EVAR cases). There was an increase in the use of EVAR in all age groups for intact AAA repair from 18.1% in 2001 to 64.3% in 2021. There was a decline in 30-day mortality for patients undergoing intact AAA repair from 5.8% in 2001 to 1.7% in 2021. This coincided with the rise of EVAR usage from 18.1% in 2001 to 64.3% in 2021 (Figure 6).

For patients undergoing ruptured AAA repair, there was no change in outcomes with a mean 30-day mortality of 31.6%. There was an increase in EVAR usage for ruptured AAA from 0.8% in 2001 to 28.8% in 2021. (Figure 7). The 30-day mortality for patients who had an EVAR for a ruptured AAA (rEVAR) decreased from 34.1% to 28.8%. There was a decline in 30-day mortality for OAR from 5.4% in 2001–2005 to 4.2% in 2016–2020 (Figure 8).

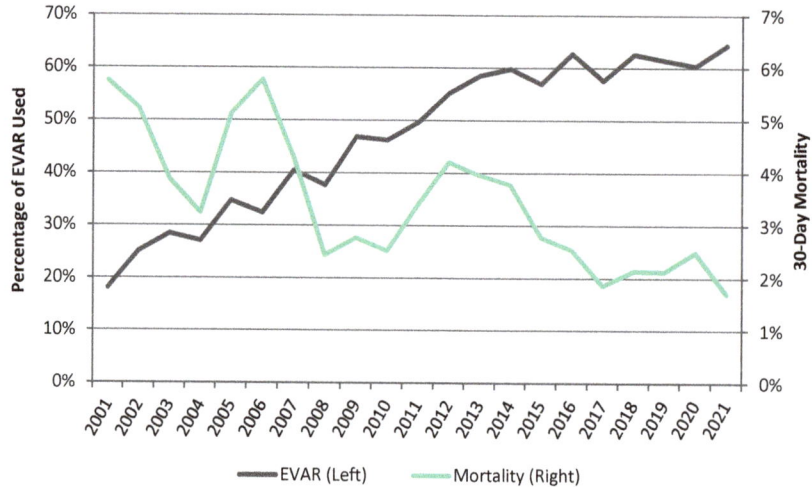

Figure 6. Intact AAA 30-day post-operative mortality and proportion of EVAR usage.

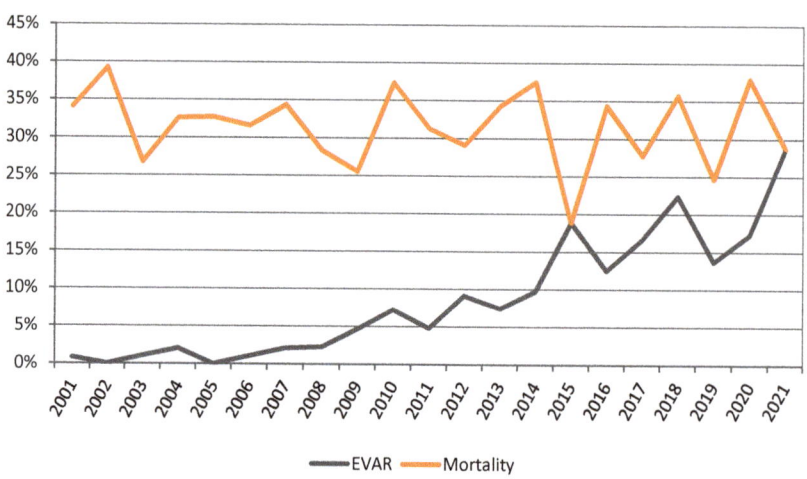

Figure 7. Ruptured AAA 30-day mortality versus proportion of EVAR used.

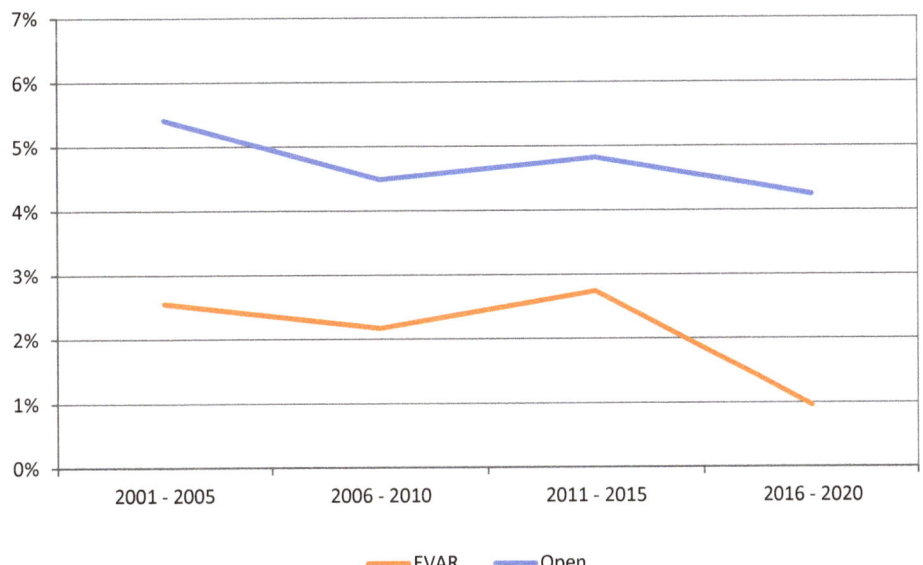

Figure 8. Intact AAA 30-day mortality by repair type.

3.7. Effect of Centralisation on Intact AAA Repair

Since centralisation of vascular surgical services has been implemented in NZ, there has been a steady increase in intact AAA repairs performed by tertiary centres since 2012, as demonstrated in the Figure 9. This increased from 79.2% in 2001 to 89.1% in 2021. As a result, AAA repairs are no longer performed in level three and four centres.

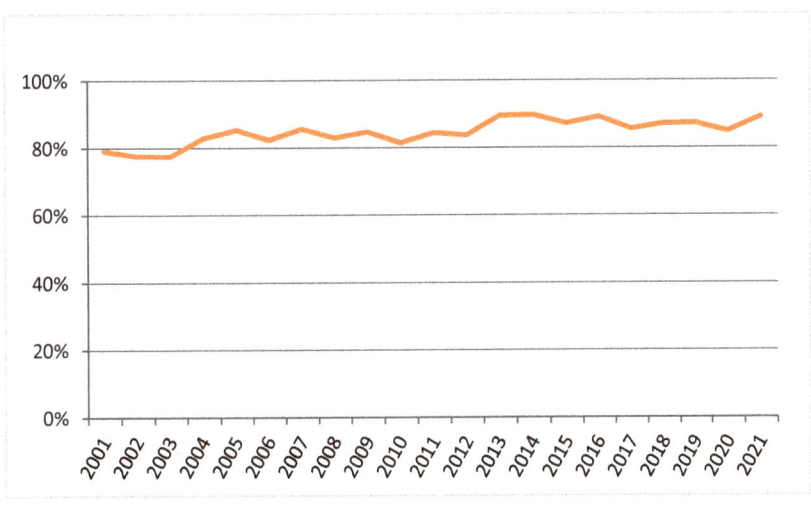

Figure 9. Trends of intact AAA repair performed by tertiary vascular centres.

4. Discussion

The salient findings observed in this study were firstly that the outcomes of intact AAA repair have improved during the last decade, with an overall reduction in 30-day mortality risk. Second, the overall counts of AAA repairs have remained fairly steady, but the age-standardized incidence has declined. However, the proportion of octogenarians undergoing intact AAA repair has increased with a significant reduction in mortality. Third, the incidence of ruptured aneurysms has not changed. In describing these findings, the disparity of sex on aneurysm presentations and outcomes has also become more apparent. These observations support that the burden of AAA disease in NZ that requires further investigation is likely to continue with the aging population and improved life expectancy.

This study differs from previous epidemiological studies of AAA in that we separated the AAA presentations into categories of acuity and repair [6,16]. By doing this, we noted that the largest decline in AAA presentations was in patients who had a had an intact AAA but did not have surgery. This group most likely presents patients being hospitalised for a non-AAA-related admission but who had an AAA present. In addition, we had access to patient unique identifiers; therefore, each hospitalisation was counted once, and the most clinically relevant AAA hospitalisation was identified.

4.1. Incidence of AAA

Sandiford and colleagues reported that AAA incidence, mortality, hospital admissions and hospital death rates between 1995 and 2008 in NZ have declined. In contrast to Sandiford's report, AAA presentations in this study were separated in order to provide some explanation for this decrease in age-standardized incidence [6]. In doing so, one of the major contributors to this decline appeared to be those patients who had an AAA diagnosis but did not have a repair. In 2001, there was 19.41 per 100,000 cases of intact AAA not repaired and in 2021 there was 4.94 cases per 100,000. In Sandiford's paper, AAA presentations were divided into ruptured and non-ruptured AAAs. In 2001, there was 5.29 per 100,000 cases of ruptured AAAs and 25.99 per 100,000 cases of unruptured AAAs.

In the 1990s, studies reported an increase in the incidence of asymptomatic AAA [17]. Smoking is considered one of the most causative risk factors for developing an AAA, and the decline in smoking prevalence in developed countries over the past 30 years is considered an important reason for the decline in the disease burden of AAA [18]. Norman et al. reported a declining rate of hospitalisation for both ruptured and non-ruptured AAA with a 38% decline in AAA mortality in men from 1999 to 2006 in Australia [19], and similarly, Sandiford et al. reported a 53% reduction in mortality from 1991 to 2007 in NZ [6]. In our study, we noted a decline in AAA incidence to be most prominent between 2005 and 2007.

The overall hospital presentations with ruptured and intact aneurysms have declined. As hospital admissions for AAA have decreased, the operative intervention for AAA has also declined due to the reduction in open aortic repair despite the increase in EVAR utilisation. Similar operative trends have also been observed in the UK National Vascular Registry and in the Swedish Vascular Registry [20,21]. These trends could be explained by the substantial changes that have influenced AAA management over the last two decades including the establishment of EVAR, the implementation of cardiovascular risk factor management, the introduction of statins and increased public health awareness on the importance of lowering blood pressure and smoking cessation. In addition, advances in perioperative medicine and quality improvement initiatives, such as centralisation of vascular surgery services, may have influenced these trends.

4.2. Effect of Social Deprivation and Ethnicity on Incidence of AAA

There is a higher proportion of intact and rupture AAA in patients living in more deprived areas in New Zealand. Socio-economic status (SES) and ethnicity have been reported as markers influencing the likelihood of increased mortality. A New Zealand study investigated how these factors impacted patient survival after AAA repair over a 14.5 year period and observed that patients living in areas of higher social deprivation had a higher risk of short- and medium-term mortality after AAA repair in a universal health setting [22]. The greatest proportion of Maori undergoing AAA repair lived in the most deprived areas, deciles 9–10. NZ Europeans were more likely to present to the hospital electively, live in less deprived areas and had the highest proportion undergoing an aneurysm repair at a private institution. In contrast the other ethnic groups, they had a higher proportion of patients presenting acutely with AAA rupture.

In a previous study to determine the prevalence of AAA in New Zealand, a group of patients undergoing computed tomography colonography had their infrarenal aorta measured [23]. The data suggest that the background detection of AAA might be lower in non-NZ Europeans, which might explain the higher rate of acute AAA hospital presentations. In addition, Maori men have a lower life expectancy in the general population than other men in New Zealand, resulting in an under-representation in those with AAA. The first population-based cross-sectional prevalence study to report the prevalence of AAA in NZ Maori or any other Polynesian group was published recently by Sandiford et al. Their study concluded that the prevalence of undiagnosed AAA in New Zealand Maori men is considerably higher than in screened populations of equivalent age in the United Kingdom and Sweden. The impact of ethnicity is likely to become more relevant given that the proportion of Maori patients has increased in the last 10 years and is likely to continue to do so. Our study has noted a change in population demographics over the last 20 years, and the proportion of non-NZ Europeans is increasing.

4.3. Mortality and Increase in EVAR Use

EVAR has resulted in a paradigm shift in the treatment of AAA worldwide and has gradually replaced open surgery [24]. In NZ, we have observed similar number of OAR and EVAR in the last 10 years. This can be partly explained by access to universal national healthcare and vascular surgeons' familiarity and skill set with both procedures. The decline in 30-day mortality following intact AAA repair has been observed elsewhere and has been predominantly related to the rise in EVAR usage [19,25]. Improvements in pre-operative, peri-operative and post-operative care along with centralisation of vascular services may have also contributed to the lower operative mortality. Previous studies have demonstrated that the mortality from AAA has declined in the last two decades in several countries, but this has not been consistent in all regions of the world [26,27]. A recent study analysed the death burden of aortic aneurysm and trends of four risk factors from 1990 to 2019 using the updated 2019 Global Burden of Disease study database and discovered that the global burden of death attributable to AAA began to increase after decreasing for two decades [28]. The study suggests that this trend will continue for the next decade and that high systolic blood pressure will replace smoking as the most important risk factor associated with aortic aneurysm death. A meta-analysis has shown that the risk of rupture in AAA patients with comorbid hypertension was 1.66 times higher than that in patients without comorbid hypertension [29].

4.4. Octogenarians

Predictions estimate that the population aged over 80 will increase fivefold by 2040. The repair of intact and ruptured AAA has increased in the older population with octogenarians constituting a significant fraction of intact AAA repairs performed in several countries [30]. In Sweden, the incidence of AAA repair in octogenarians has nearly tripled from 13% to 36% per 100,000 population >80 years in Sweden over the periods 1994–1999 to 2010–2014 [5]. Similarly in our study, AAA repair in octogenarians has almost doubled from 16.2% in 2001 to 28.4% in 2021. In a study by Park et al. among octogenarians treated for an intact AAA, 80% were treated by EVAR and patients older than 80 accounted for 25% of the total EVAR cohort [31].

This shift in AAA presentation to the older population has been driven by the increased use of EVAR and an increasing number of active octogenarians. A recent meta-analysis by Sweeting et al. of the Ruptured Aneurysm Trialists research group demonstrated that the 1-year mortality rate for an octogenarian with a ruptured AAA were 35% (95% CI = 18–56) following EVAR and 54% (95% CI = 47–60) following OAR compared to the overall population, with 38.6% treated by EVAR and 42.8% treated by OAR [32]. Compared to younger patients, EVAR in octogenarians is associated with a significantly higher but still acceptable peri-operative and midterm mortality rate. In our study, the 30-day mortality of octogenarians undergoing intact AAA repair decreased from 6.8% in 2001 to 0.9% in 2021. A multi-centre retrospective study was carried out in the Netherlands investigating the outcomes of ruptured AAA in octogenarians [33]. After one year, half of the octogenarians operated on for a ruptured AAA were alive, with >80% living at home.

4.5. Ruptured AAA Outcomes

AAA-related mortality is estimated at 150,000–200,000 deaths per year worldwide, which is equivalent to various types of cancer [34]. On average, since 2001, in New Zealand, approximately 215 people per year are recorded as dying of ruptured AAA, of which 80.9% are the result of ruptured AAA without undergoing any form of repair, and the remaining are a consequence of undergoing AAA procedures predominately for ruptured aneurysms.

As a substantial proportion of patients with rAAA die before hospitalisation, most studies do include prehospital deaths. Our study demonstrated that the overall mortality of rAAA was 72%, which is similar to a Norwegian study that found the incidence to be 68% [35]. In addition, the mortality for patients undergoing EVAR for rAAA (rEVAR) is static, from 34.1% in 2001 to 28.8% in 2021. During the same period, we observed a significant increase in EVAR utilisation from < 1% to 28.8%. Historically, the mortality rate for patients with ruptured aneurysms who undergo open surgery is 41% to 49% [36]. Centres that report outcomes for all rAAAs after the introduction of rEVAR have published mortality rates varying between 24% and 46%, and our results are keeping in line with these other studies [37].

4.6. Effect of Centralisation of Aortic Pathology in NZ

The volume outcome relationship in aortic aneurysm surgery has been well-studied, demonstrating that higher volume centres produce the best patient outcomes, which has subsequently led to a drive for centralisation of aortic and complex endovascular surgery [38,39]. A meta-analysis of the literature in 2007, comprising 421,299 elective aneurysm repairs, reported a weighted odds ratio of 0.66 in favour of higher volume centres [40]. An example of the benefits of the centralisation of vascular surgical services has been observed in the United Kingdom (UK) [41]. Twenty years ago, outcomes from aortic aneurysm surgery in the UK were among the worse in the Western world. Patients in lower volume centres had a higher mortality rate and poorer access to endovascular treatment than those treated in a higher volume centre. This subsequently led to a national quality improvement programme in AAA surgery in the last decade, which has resulted in a significant improvement in outcomes of AAA repair. In NZ, the model of care that is supported for vascular services is a regional model. Services are organised around Level 5 and/or 6 specialist vascular centres that provide a comprehensive range of vascular and endovascular services for adults and include the following hospitals: Auckland City Hospital, Waikato Hospital, Wellington Hospital, Christchurch Hospital, Middlemore Hospital and Dunedin Hospital. There has been no formal centralisation of vascular surgical services implemented, but as evident from these data, there has been a steady increase in intact AAA repairs performed in tertiary centres in the last decades. Vascular surgery only separated from general surgery training in NZ between 1995 and 1997 with the establishment of the establishment of the Board of Vascular Surgery of the Royal Australasian College of Surgeons (RACS) In 2002, the Australian and New Zealand Society for Vascular Surgery (ANZSVS) became the official administrator of vascular surgery in ANZ in association with RACS [42].

4.7. Limitations

This study has several limitations. As with all administrative databases, the data used in this study are subject to coding errors. Patients who were not hospitalised with a diagnosis of AAA or died without diagnosis despite having a AAA, might have been missed in our data capture. We are also unable to report the number of intact AAAs treated conservatively as surgical decision making was not recorded in our data. The AVA was implemented at the end of 2010, so we only have records of procedures performed in in private hospitals over the last 12 years.

In addition, our database contains no information regarding why EVAR was chosen over OAR or conservative management. Administrative data were used rather than patient-level data, so the patient risk profile, AAA diameter and extent of AAA anatomy were not recorded. Death status was based on mortality records that include only those deaths that occurred within New Zealand. Any deaths occurring outside New Zealand would not be captured, and this may have resulted in some degree of under reporting. We are unable to report mortality data from 2018 to 2021, as there is a three-year lag time with obtaining these data from the national mortality collection database.

5. Conclusions

This study highlights the epidemiological trends and survival outcomes of AAA management in NZ over 20 years and the challenges health services might encounter from the AAA burden. Important trends include the stabilisation of intact AAA repair, an increase in the number of octogenarians with AAA disease and the mortality rate of rAAA, which has remained static. Understanding the changing pattern of AAA burden is paramount to improve resource allocation and promote surgical quality improvement.

Author Contributions: Conceptualisation, S.G., P.S. and M.K. Methodology, S.G., O.B., W.X. and M.K.; Software, S.G., O.B. and W.X.; Validation S.G., O.B., W.X., P.S. and M.K.; Formal Analysis, S.G., O.B., W.X. and P.S.; Resources, M.K.; Data Curation S.G., O.B. and W.X.; Writing, S.G., O.B., P.S. and M.K.; Visualisation, S.G., O.B. and W.X.; Supervision, M.K.; Project administration, S.G. and M.K. All authors have read and agreed to the published version of the manuscript.

Funding: This research received no external funding.

Institutional Review Board Statement: Not applicable.

Informed Consent Statement: Not applicable.

Data Availability Statement: Ethics approval was granted by the New Zealand Health and Disability Ethics Committees (Re13/STH/190/AM01).

Acknowledgments: Analytical services at the New Zealand Ministry of Health Australia and New Zealand Society of Vascular Surgery (ANZSVS).

Conflicts of Interest: The authors declare no conflict of interest.

Appendix A

Table A1. Procedures.

9022800	Endoluminal repair of aneurysm
3318100	Repair of ruptured intra-abdominal aneurysm
3316300	Replacement of ruptured iliac artery aneurysm with graft
3316000	Replacement of ruptured infrarenal abdominal aortic aneurysm with bifurcation graft to femoral arteries
3315700	Replacement of ruptured infrarenal aortic aneurysm with bifurcation graft to iliac arteries
3315400	Replacement of ruptured infrarenal abdominal aortic aneurysm with tube graft
3315100	Replacement of ruptured suprarenal abdominal aortic aneurysm with graft
3314800	Replacement of ruptured thoraco-abdominal aneurysm with graft
3312700	Replacement of iliac artery aneurysm with graft, bilateral
3312400	Replacement of iliac artery aneurysm with graft, unilateral
3312100	Replacement of infrarenal abdominal aortic aneurysm with bifurcation graft to femoral arteries
3311800	Replacement of infrarenal abdominal aortic aneurysm with bifurcation graft to iliac arteries

Table A1. Cont.

3311500	Replacement of infrarenal abdominal aortic aneurysm with tube graft
3311200	Replacement of suprarenal abdominal aorta aneurysm with graft
3310900	Replacement of thoraco-abdominal aneurysm with graft
3308000	Repair of intra-abdominal aneurysm
3311600	Endovascular repair of aneurysm

References

1. Sampson, U.K.; Norman, P.E.; Fowkes, F.G.; Aboyans, V.; Song, Y.; Harrell, F.E., Jr.; Forouzanfar, M.H.; Naghavi, M.; Denenberg, J.O.; McDermott, M.M.; et al. Estimation of global and regional incidence and prevalence of abdominal aortic aneurysms 1990 to 2010. *Glob. Heart* **2014**, *9*, 159–170. [CrossRef] [PubMed]
2. Boyle, J.R.; Mao, J.; Beck, A.W.; Venermo, M.; Sedrakyan, A.; Behrendt, C.-A.; Szeberin, Z.; Eldrup, N.; Schermerhorn, M.; Beiles, B.; et al. Editor's Choice–Variation in Intact Abdominal Aortic Aneurysm Repair Outcomes by Country: Analysis of International Consortium of Vascular Registries 2010–2016. *Eur. J. Vasc. Endovasc. Surg.* **2021**, *62*, 16–24. [CrossRef] [PubMed]
3. Nair, N.; Kvizhinadze, G.; Jones, G.T.; Rush, R.; Khashram, M.; Roake, J.; Blakely, A. Health gains, costs and cost-effectiveness of a population-based screening programme for abdominal aortic aneurysms. *Br. J. Surg.* **2019**, *106*, 1043–1054. [CrossRef] [PubMed]
4. Sweeting, M.J.; Marshall, J.; Glover, M.; Nasim, A.; Bown, M.J. Evaluating the Cost-Effectiveness of Changes to the Surveillance Intervals in the UK Abdominal Aortic Aneurysm Screening Programme. *Value Health* **2021**, *24*, 369–376. [CrossRef] [PubMed]
5. Wanhainen, A.; Hultgren, R.; Linné, A.; Holst, J.; Gottsäter, A.; Langenskiöld, M.; Smidfelt, K.; Björck, M.; Svensjö, S. Outcome of the Swedish Nationwide Abdominal Aortic Aneurysm Screening Program. *Circulation* **2016**, *134*, 1141–1148. [CrossRef]
6. Sandiford, P.; Mosquera, D.; Bramley, D. Trends in incidence and mortality from abdominal aortic aneurysm in New Zealand. *Br. J. Surg.* **2011**, *98*, 645–651. [CrossRef]
7. von Elm, E.; Altman, D.G.; Egger, M.; Pocock, S.J.; Gøtzsche, P.C.; Vandenbroucke, J.P. Strengthening the Reporting of Observational Studies in Epidemiology (STROBE) statement: Guidelines for reporting observational studies. *BMJ* **2007**, *335*, 806–808. [CrossRef]
8. Beiles, C.B.; Bourke, B.M. Validation of Australian data in the Australasian Vascular Audit. *ANZ J. Surg.* **2014**, *84*, 624–627. [CrossRef]
9. Khashram, M.; Thomson, I.A.; Jones, G.T.; Roake, J.A. Abdominal aortic aneurysm repair in New Zealand: A validation of the Australasian Vascular Audit. *ANZ J. Surg.* **2017**, *87*, 394–398. [CrossRef]
10. Bernau, O.; Gormley, S.; Khashram, M. Validation of New Zealand Data in the Australasian Vascular Audit. *Eur. J. Vasc. Endovasc. Surg.* **2022**, *63*, 771–772. [CrossRef]
11. Khashram, M.; Pitama, S.; Williman, J.A.; Jones, G.T.; Roake, J.A. Survival Disparity Following Abdominal Aortic Aneurysm Repair Highlights Inequality in Ethnic and Socio-economic Status. *Eur. J. Vasc. Endovasc. Surg.* **2017**, *54*, 689–696. [CrossRef]
12. Salmond, C.; Crampton, P.; King, P.; Waldegrave, C. NZiDep: A New Zealand index of socioeconomic deprivation for individuals. *Soc. Sci. Med.* **2006**, *62*, 1474–1485. [CrossRef]
13. Jeffreys, M.; Sarfati, D.; Stevanovic, V.; Tobias, M.; Lewis, C.; Pearce, N.; Blakely, T. Socioeconomic inequalities in cancer survival in New Zealand: The role of extent of disease at diagnosis. *Cancer Epidemiol. Biomarkers Prev.* **2009**, *18*, 915–921. [CrossRef]
14. Robson, B.; Purdie, G.; Cram, F.; Simmonds, S. Age standardisation—An indigenous standard? *Emerg. Themes Epidemiol.* **2007**, *4*, 3. [CrossRef]
15. Team R.C. A language and environment for statistical computing. R Foundation for Statistical Computing: Vienna, Austria, 2015. Available online: http://www.R-project.org (accessed on 6 September 2022).
16. Sandiford, P.; Mosquera, D.; Bramley, D. Ethnic inequalities in incidence, survival and mortality from abdominal aortic aneurysm in New Zealand. *J. Epidemiol. Community Health* **2012**, *66*, 1097–1103. [CrossRef]
17. Eickhoff, J.H. Incidence of diagnosis, operation and death from abdominal aortic aneurysms in Danish hospitals: Results from a nation-wide survey, 1977–1990. *Eur. J. Surg. Acta Chir.* **1993**, *159*, 619–623.
18. Singh, K.; Bønaa, K.H.; Jacobsen, B.K.; Bjørk, L.; Solberg, S. Prevalence of and Risk Factors for Abdominal Aortic Aneurysms in a Population-based Study: The Tromsø Study. *Am. J. Epidemiol.* **2001**, *154*, 236–244. [CrossRef]
19. Norman, P.E.; Spilsbury, K.; Semmens, J.B. Falling rates of hospitalization and mortality from abdominal aortic aneurysms in Australia. *J. Vasc. Surg.* **2011**, *53*, 274–277. [CrossRef]
20. Lilja, F.; Mani, K.; Wanhainen, A. Editor's Choice—Trend-break in Abdominal Aortic Aneurysm Repair With Decreasing Surgical Workload. *Eur. J. Vasc. Endovasc. Surg.* **2017**, *53*, 811–819. [CrossRef]
21. Hanna, L.; Sounderajah, V.; Abdullah, A.A.; Marshall, D.C.; Salciccioli, J.D.; Shalhoub, J.; Gibbs, R.G.J. Trends in Thoracic Aortic Aneurysm Hospital Admissions, Interventions, and Mortality in England between 1998 and 2020: An Observational Study. *Eur. J. Vasc. Endovasc. Surg.* **2022**, *64*, 340–348. [CrossRef]
22. Han, Y.; Zhang, S.; Zhang, J.; Ji, C.; Eckstein, H.H. Outcomes of Endovascular Abdominal Aortic Aneurysm Repair in Octogenarians: Meta-analysis and Systematic Review. *Eur. J. Vasc. Endovasc. Surg.* **2017**, *54*, 454–463. [CrossRef] [PubMed]
23. Khashram, M.; Jones, G.T.; Roake, J.A. Prevalence of abdominal aortic aneurysm (AAA) in a population undergoing computed tomography colonography in Canterbury, New Zealand. *Eur. J. Vasc. Endovasc. Surg.* **2015**, *50*, 199–205. [CrossRef] [PubMed]

24. Karthikesalingam, A.; Holt, P.J.; Vidal-Diez, A.; Bahia, S.S.; Patterson, B.O.; Hinchliffe, R.J.; Thompson, M.M. The impact of endovascular aneurysm repair on mortality for elective abdominal aortic aneurysm repair in England and the United States. *J. Vasc. Surg.* **2016**, *64*, 321–327.e2. [CrossRef] [PubMed]
25. Choke, E.; Vijaynagar, B.; Thompson, J.; Nasim, A.; Bown, M.J.; Sayers, R.D. Changing epidemiology of abdominal aortic aneurysms in England and Wales: Older and more benign? *Circulation* **2012**, *125*, 1617–1625. [CrossRef]
26. Sidloff, D.; Stather, P.; Dattani, N.; Bown, M.; Thompson, J.; Sayers, R.; Choke, E. Aneurysm global epidemiology study: Public health measures can further reduce abdominal aortic aneurysm mortality. *Circulation* **2014**, *129*, 747–753. [CrossRef]
27. Mani, K.; Venermo, M.; Beiles, B.; Menyhei, G.; Altreuther, M.; Loftus, I.; Björck, M. Regional Differences in Case Mix and Peri-operative Outcome After Elective Abdominal Aortic Aneurysm Repair in the Vascunet Database. *Eur. J. Vasc. Endovasc. Surg.* **2015**, *49*, 646–652. [CrossRef]
28. Kobeissi, E.; Hibino, M.; Pan, H.; Aune, D. Blood pressure, hypertension and the risk of abdominal aortic aneurysms: A systematic review and meta-analysis of cohort studies. *Eur. J. Epidemiol.* **2019**, *34*, 547–555. [CrossRef]
29. Huang, X.; Wang, Z.; Shen, Z.; Lei, F.; Liu, Y.-M.; Chen, Z.; Qin, J.-J.; Liu, H.; Ji, Y.-X.; Zhang, P.; et al. Projection of global burden and risk factors for aortic aneurysm—Timely warning for greater emphasis on managing blood pressure. *Ann. Med.* **2022**, *54*, 553–564. [CrossRef]
30. Roosendaal, L.C.; Kramer, G.M.; Wiersema, A.M.; Wisselink, W.; Jongkind, V. Outcome of Ruptured Abdominal Aortic Aneurysm Repair in Octogenarians: A Systematic Review and Meta-Analysis. *Eur. J. Vasc. Endovasc. Surg.* **2020**, *59*, 16–22. [CrossRef]
31. Park, B.D.; Azefor, N.M.; Huang, C.C.; Ricotta, J.J. Elective endovascular aneurysm repair in the elderly: Trends and outcomes from the Nationwide Inpatient Sample. *Ann. Vasc. Surg.* **2014**, *28*, 798–807. [CrossRef]
32. Sweeting, M.J.; Ulug, P.; Powell, J.T.; Desgranges, P.; Balm, R. Ruptured Aneurysm Trials: The Importance of Longer-term Outcomes and Meta-analysis for 1-year Mortality. *Eur. J. Vasc. Endovasc. Surg.* **2015**, *50*, 297–302. [CrossRef]
33. Roosendaal, L.C.; Wiersema, A.M.; Yeung, K.K.; Ünlü, Ç.; Metz, R.; Wisselink, W.; Jongkind, V. Survival and Living Situation After Ruptured Abdominal Aneurysm Repair in Octogenarians. *Eur. J. Vasc. Endovasc. Surg.* **2021**, *61*, 375–381. [CrossRef]
34. Global, regional, and national age-sex-specific mortality for 282 causes of death in 195 countries and territories, 1980-2017: A systematic analysis for the Global Burden of Disease Study 2017. *Lancet* **2018**, *392*, 1736–1788. [CrossRef]
35. Visser, P.; Akkersdijk, G.J.; Blankensteijn, J.D. In-hospital operative mortality of ruptured abdominal aortic aneurysm: A population-based analysis of 5593 patients in The Netherlands over a 10-year period. *Eur. J. Vasc. Endovasc. Surg.* **2005**, *30*, 359–364. [CrossRef]
36. Bown, M.J.; Sutton, A.J.; Bell, P.R.; Sayers, R.D. A meta-analysis of 50 years of ruptured abdominal aortic aneurysm repair. *Br. J. Surg.* **2002**, *89*, 714–730. [CrossRef]
37. Larzon, T.; Lindgren, R.; Norgren, L. Endovascular treatment of ruptured abdominal aortic aneurysms: A shift of the paradigm? *J. Endovasc. Ther.* **2005**, *12*, 548–555. [CrossRef]
38. Holt, P.J.; Poloniecki, J.D.; Gerrard, D.; Loftus, I.M.; Thompson, M.M. Meta-analysis and systematic review of the relationship between volume and outcome in abdominal aortic aneurysm surgery. *Br. J. Surg.* **2007**, *94*, 395–403. [CrossRef]
39. Giles, K.A.; Hamdan, A.D.; Pomposelli, F.B.; Wyers, M.C.; Dahlberg, S.E.; Schermerhorn, M.L. Population-based outcomes following endovascular and open repair of ruptured abdominal aortic aneurysms. *J. Endovasc. Ther.* **2009**, *16*, 554–564. [CrossRef]
40. Young, E.L.; Holt, P.J.; Poloniecki, J.D.; Loftus, I.M.; Thompson, M.M. Meta-analysis and systematic review of the relationship between surgeon annual caseload and mortality for elective open abdominal aortic aneurysm repairs. *J. Vasc. Surg.* **2007**, *46*, 1287–1294. [CrossRef]
41. Loftus, I.M.; Boyle, J.R. A Decade of Centralisation of Vascular Services in the UK. *Eur. J. Vasc. Endovasc. Surg.* **2023**, *65*, 315–316. [CrossRef]
42. Mohan, I.V.; Khashram, M.; Fitridge, R. Vascular Surgery in Australia and New Zealand (Australasia). *Eur. J. Vasc. Endovasc. Surg.* **2021**, *62*, 338–339. [CrossRef] [PubMed]

Disclaimer/Publisher's Note: The statements, opinions and data contained in all publications are solely those of the individual author(s) and contributor(s) and not of MDPI and/or the editor(s). MDPI and/or the editor(s) disclaim responsibility for any injury to people or property resulting from any ideas, methods, instructions or products referred to in the content.

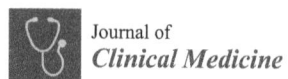

Systematic Review

A State-of-the-Art Review of Intra-Operative Imaging Modalities Used to Quality Assure Endovascular Aneurysm Repair

Petra Z. Bachrati [1,2], Guglielmo La Torre [1], Mohammed M. Chowdhury [1], Samuel J. Healy [1,2], Aminder A. Singh [1] and Jonathan R. Boyle [1,*]

1 Cambridge Vascular Unit, Cambridge University Hospitals NHS Foundation Trust, Cambridge CB2 0QQ, UK
2 School of Clinical Medicine, Cambridge University, Cambridge CB2 0SP, UK
* Correspondence: jonboyle@doctors.org.uk or jrb83@cam.ac.uk

Abstract: Endovascular aortic aneurysm repair (EVAR) is the preferred method for elective abdominal aortic aneurysm (AAA) repair. However, the success of this technique depends greatly on the technologies available. Intra-operative imaging is essential but can come with limitations. More complex interventions lead to longer operating times, fluoroscopy times, and greater contrast doses. A number of intra-operative imaging modalities to quality assure the success of EVAR have been developed. A systematic literature search was performed with separate searches conducted for each imaging modality in the study: computed tomography (CT), digital subtraction angiography (DSA), fusion, ultrasound, intra-operative positioning system (IOPS), and non-contrast imaging. CT was effective at detecting complications but commonly resulted in increased radiation and contrast dose. The effectiveness of DSA can be increased, and radiation exposure reduced, through the use of adjunctive technologies. We found that 2D-3D fusion was non-inferior to 3D-3D and led to reduced radiation and contrast dose. Non-contrast imaging occasionally led to higher doses of radiation. Ultrasound was particularly effective in the detection of type II endoleaks with reduced radiation and contrast use but was often operator dependent. Unfortunately, no papers made it past full text screening for IOPS. All of the imaging techniques discussed have advantages and disadvantages, and clinical context is relevant to guide imaging choice. Fusion and ultrasound in particular show promise for the future.

Keywords: endovascular aneurysm repair; imaging; computerised tomography; digital subtraction angiography; fusion; ultrasound

Citation: Bachrati, P.Z.; La Torre, G.; Chowdhury, M.M.; Healy, S.J.; Singh, A.A.; Boyle, J.R. A State-of-the-Art Review of Intra-Operative Imaging Modalities Used to Quality Assure Endovascular Aneurysm Repair. *J. Clin. Med.* **2023**, *12*, 3167. https://doi.org/10.3390/jcm12093167

Academic Editors: Martin Teraa and Constantijn E.V.B. Hazenberg

Received: 15 March 2023
Revised: 24 April 2023
Accepted: 24 April 2023
Published: 28 April 2023

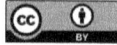

Copyright: © 2023 by the authors. Licensee MDPI, Basel, Switzerland. This article is an open access article distributed under the terms and conditions of the Creative Commons Attribution (CC BY) license (https://creativecommons.org/licenses/by/4.0/).

1. Introduction

Minimally invasive aortic surgery has been practised since the mid-1980s [1]. Since its inception, outcomes from endovascular aneurysm repair (EVAR) have been compared to open aortic repair. EVAR Trial 1, DREAM, and OVER did not demonstrate the mortality benefit of EVAR over open surgery beyond 30 days [2–5]. Despite new evidence regarding suboptimal long-term outcomes of decreasing survival benefit over time and almost double the reintervention rate compared to open aneurysm repair, it remains an attractive surgical intervention in those patients who are not physiologically capable to withstand open surgery [6,7]. What can be achieved with endovascular surgery, however, in large part depends on the technology used and accurate device deployment at the time of intervention. More complex repairs require longer fluoroscopy times, higher contrast doses, and greater exposure to ionising radiation to patients and interventionalists [8]. Imaging is fundamental to the correct approach and performance of EVAR and is categorised as pre-operative, peri-operative and post-operative. Pre-operatively, computed tomography angiogram (CTA) imaging plays a crucial role in the diagnosis and planning of the endovascular procedure. Intra-operatively, fluoroscopy and novel fusion imaging techniques aid the accurate deployment of stent grafts. Post-operatively, CTA and duplex imaging in surveillance allow for the detection of complications, with a particular focus on endoleaks [9]. The ESVS guidelines discuss the use of digital subtraction angiography (DSA) and intravascular ultrasound (IVUS) in the perioperative setting but conclude that these techniques are currently not widely available, difficult to perform, and add additional procedure time. These guidelines highlighted angiographic CT as a promising technique for the detection of complications, albeit with limited evidence presently [10]. Further, the introduction of fusion imaging has promised to revolutionise the EVAR technique by allowing a wider scope of intervention.

This review will aim to evaluate the role of CT, DSA, fusion, ultrasound, and non-contrast imaging for the detection of complications, radiation exposure, and contrast usage intra-operatively in EVAR.

2. Materials and Methods

A systematic literature search of PubMed, Scopus, Web of Science, and Cochrane Library was performed on 7 February 2022. Separate searches (Supplementary Table S1) were conducted for each of the imaging modalities in the present study; CT, DSA, fusion, ultrasound, intra-operative positioning system (IOPS), and non-contrast imaging. Title, abstract screening, and full text review were conducted independently by authors PZB and SJH. A third independent author verified findings (GLT). Data extraction was carried out by PZB and SJH, following a predetermined standardised method. The data collected included author, year of publication, DOI, image modality, type of endovascular intervention, study type, sample sizes, sex of participants, and information regarding detection of complications, radiation dose, and use of contrast. Following inclusion and exclusion criteria (Table 1), a total number of 32 studies were included in the review (Figure 1 PRISMA Diagram). Relevant complications of EVAR were defined predominately as endoleaks but included stent kinking or compression, thrombosis, or renal function decline. Risk of bias was calculated using the Newcastle-Ottawa Scale [11].

Table 1. Inclusion and Exclusion Criteria.

Inclusion Criteria	Exclusion Criteria
In English	Not in English
EVAR procedures	Not EVAR procedures
Intra-operative imaging	Involvement of iliac arteries in the aneurysm or not simple AAA (e.g., rupture or mycotic, etc.)
	Pre-operative or post-operative imaging only
Full text available	Clinical outcomes of imaging not discussed (e.g., purely technical papers, phantoms, etc.)
	Animal studies

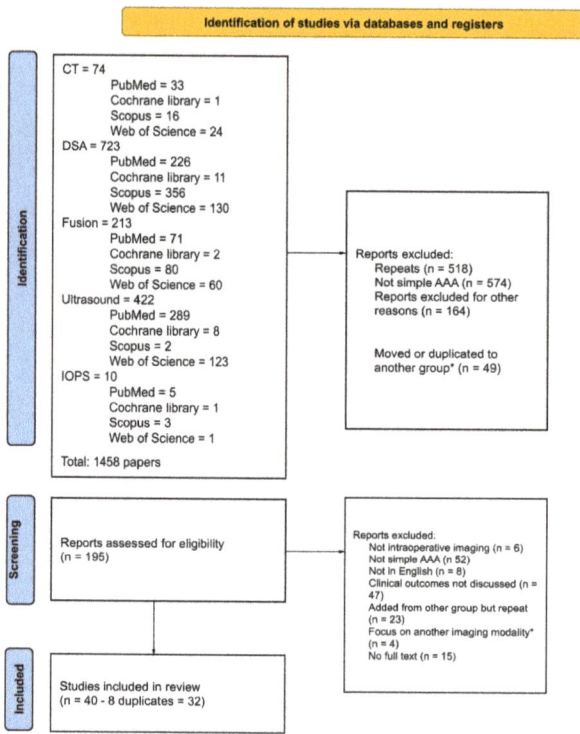

Figure 1. PRISMA Diagram. * those focusing on another imaging modality were moved or rarely duplicated to the relevant group and screened.

3. Results

The studies considered in this review were heterogeneous. Patient populations were pooled according to the imaging modality and study type where possible. Where this was not possible, the results were reported on a study-by-study basis. A summary of the included studies can be found in Table 2.

Table 2. Summary of included studies.

Author	Year	Imaging Modality	Aneurysm Type	Study Type	n	Summary of Technical Success & Complications	Contrast Usage	Radiation Dose
Biasi et al. [12]	2009	DynaCT vs DSA	Infrarenal	Prospective	392	DynaCT found 5 (6.25%) complications not seen on completion DSA with 3.8% having immediate intervention	No difference	Increased
Breininger et al. [13]	2019	2D3D	Non-specified EVAR	Retrospective	19	Successfully reconstructs Iliac displacement after stiffwire insertion from a 2D image	-	-
Bush et al. [14]	2002	Gadolinium-enhanced MRA, non-contrast CT, gadolinium or CO2 aortography, and IVUS	Infrarenal	Retrospective	297	Non-contrast technically successful in all patients	Reduced	-

Table 2. Cont.

Author	Year	Imaging Modality	Aneurysm Type	Study Type	n	Summary of Technical Success & Complications	Contrast Usage	Radiation Dose
Chao et al. [15]	2007	CO2-DSA vs. ICA-DSA	Infrarenal	Retrospective	100	No significant difference in technical success between groups	Reduced	Increased
de Ruiter et al. [16]	2016	DSA (mobile C-arm vs fixed C-arm/allura vs. fixed c-arm /AlluraClarity)	Infrarenal, complex	Retrospective	85	Image processing technology adjuncts can significantly help to reduce radiation exposure	-	Reduced
Dijkstra et al. [17]	2011	CBCT and 3D-3D fusion	Complex	Retrospective	82	Fusion technical success non inferior. No additional endoleaks found on MDCT.	Reduced	Reduced
Faries et al. [18]	2003	Standard angiography vs modified protocol	Non-specified AAA	Retrospective	391	Modified protocol detected more type II endoleaks but there was no significant difference in incidence of type II endoleaks by follow-up.	-	-
Gallitto et al. [19]	2020	3D2D fusion with intraop CO2-DSA	Complex	Prospective	45	CO2 angiography results in better renal function preservation	No contrast use	Increased
Garret, Jr. et al. [20]	2003	CT vs. IVUS	Infrarenal	Retrospective	78	IVUS resulted in changing stent graft size (n = 22). 4 patients treated with EVAR using IVUS after preop CT suggesting unsuitable.	-	-
Gennai et al. [21]	2021	Fusion but vessel cannulation with IVUS	Complex	Retrospective	10	IVUS was technically successful in all cases, identifying problems in 12% of bridging stents that were not detected by completion angiography.	Reduced	Reduced
Hertault et al. [22]	2018	3D2D with strict ALARA	Infrarenal	Prospective	85	-	Reduced	Reduced
Jansen et al. [23]	2021	3D2D	Complex	Retrospective	20	-	-	-
Kaladji et al. [24]	2015	3D2D without contrast	Infrarenal, thoracic	Prospective	6	EVAR graft deployment	No contrast use	-
Keschenau et al. [25]	2020	CEUS vs. DSA	Infrarenal, complex	Prospective	21	CEUS detected significantly more type II endoleaks than DSA. But only 5 of the 16 still persisted on pre-discharge CTA.	Reduced	Reduced
Kobeiter et al. [26]	2011	3D2D without ICM for registration	Thoracic	Retrospective	1	TEVAR deployment	No contrast use	-
Kopp et al. [27]	2010	CEUS vs. DSA	Infrarenal	Prospective	37	CEUS was effective at identifying proximal (82.4%) and distal (89.3%) landing zones and identified more endoleaks than angiography.	Reduced	Reduced
Koutouzi et al. [28]	2016	3D3D registration and 2D3D overlay	Infrarenal	Prospective	19	EVAR deployment	Reduced	Reduced
Lalys et al. [29]	2019	3D2D fusion	Infrarenal	Prospective	50	Assessment of displacement	-	-
Massoni et al. [30]	2021	CEUS vs. DSA	Infrarenal	Prospective	3	In two cases type Ia endoleak was missed by angiography but detected by CEUS	-	-
Massoni et al. [31]	2019	CEUS vs. DSA	Infrarenal	Prospective	60	Postdeployment CEUS detected more endoleaks than DSA	-	-
Maurel et al. [32]	2014	3D3D	Infrarenal, complex	Prospective	20	Stiffwire insertion causes significant displacement of main aortic branches	Reduced	Increased

Table 2. Cont.

Author	Year	Imaging Modality	Aneurysm Type	Study Type	n	Summary of Technical Success & Complications	Contrast Usage	Radiation Dose
McNally et al. [33]	2015	3D3D vs. fluoroscopy/DSA/IVUS	Complex	Retrospective	72	FEVAR deployment	Reduced	Reduced
Panuccio et al. [34]	2016	3D2D but with mathematical model	Infrarenal, complex	Prospective	25	Fully automated fusion imaging is possible although manual intervention may be needed in some cases	Reduced	Reduced
Rolls et al. [35]	2016	3D3D vs. standard fluoroscopic imaging	Complex	Prospective	42	Target vessel catheterisation and endoleak detection satisfactory. Fusion and team based approach reduced procedure time	-	Reduced
Schulz et al. [36]	2016	ceCBCT vs. cDSA	Infrarenal	Prospective	98	ceCBCT detected more endoleaks than CTA or DSA	Reduced	-
Schulz et al. [37]	2019	2D3D fusion vs. 3D3D fusion	Non-specified EVAR	Prospective	151	Fusion imaging is feasible, and non-inferior to 3D3D offering better radiation exposure and time demand	-	Reduced
Schwein et al. [38]	2018	3D-3D fusion and CTA-fluoroscopy	Complex	Retrospective	26	83% of ostia cannulated without angiogram	Reduced	Reduced
Stangenberg et al. [39]	2015	3D2D fusion using VesselNavigator	Infrarenal	Retrospective	75	Procedure time, fluoroscopy time and air kerma was lower with fusion	Reduced	Reduced
Steuwe et al. [40]	2016	CBCT vs MDCT	Infrarenal	Retrospective	66	CBCT reduces radiation dose compared to 3-phase MDCT required to assess technical success of EVAR	-	Reduced
Tenorio et al. [41]	2019	3D3D onlay CTA fusion and CBCT without digital zoom capability 2D2D onlay CTA fusion, high definition CBCT with subtraction capability and digital zoom.	Complex	Retrospective	386	Successful stent deployment and endoleak detection	Reduced	Reduced
Timaran et al. [42]	2021	Standard vs. dual fluoroscopy with live-image digital zooming	Complex	Prospective	151	No difference in technical success between the two groups	-	Reduced
Törnqvist et al. [43]	2015	CBCT vs. DSA	Infrarenal	Prospective	51	CBCT more effective at detecting stent graft compression and kinks. DSA detected more endoleaks than CBCT	-	-

3.1. Computerised Tomography

Intra-operative CT imaging during EVAR utilises an intravenous contrast agent, and there are different techniques in which images can be acquired. The recently developed cone beam CT (CBCT or dynaCT) involves converging beams and rotational flat panel detectors that allow accurate CT-like three-dimensional images to be produced. Multidetector CT (MDCT) uses multiple detectors to generate three-dimensional images [17].

3.1.1. Detection of Endoleaks

CT imaging allows the increased detection of endoleaks and technical complications intra-operatively and aids stent graft deployment. Törnqvist et al. [43] compared completion angiography and CBCT and suggested the need for multiple projections to compensate for the two-dimensional approach of angiography results in increased operating time and contrast use that may be offset using three-dimensional techniques such as CBCT. They concluded that CBCT is more effective at detecting stent graft compression and kinks, but angiography is better at detecting endoleaks, although the majority of these were type 2, which required no intervention. Schulz et al. [36] compared contrast-enhanced CBCT (ceCBCT) to completion DSA and post-operative CTA. All endoleaks found on DSA and CTA were also found on ceCBCT, but ceCBCT also detected intraluminal thrombus and limb stenoses, prompting intra-operative intervention in some cases. The authors suggest that completely replacing DSA and CTA with ceCBCT would result in a 38.8% reduction in the overall contrast used on the patient. Biasi et al. [12] compared dynaCT to completion DSA and found that 3.8% of the DSA group had a potentially preventable early re-intervention due to technical complications that were not identified during completion DSA. Patients undergoing an early reintervention for a secondary procedure had a statistically significantly higher mortality rate (14.3% vs. 3.3%). Their study showed no technical problems identified in pre-discharge surveillance imaging after dynaCT completion imaging, which was not the case with the completion DSA cohort, suggesting the superiority of dynaCT in assessing technical success. In contrast to previous studies, they did not find a statistically significant difference in contrast load between the DSA and the dynaCT groups, although there was an increase in radiation dose to the patient. Dijkstra et al. [17] evaluated patients undergoing fenestrated EVAR (FEVAR) and compared two protocols of imaging: pre-deployment CBCT fused with pre-operative multidetector CT (MDCT) to guide stent graft placement and post-deployment CBCT to assess technical success. For the post-deployment CBCT group, eight endoleaks were detected; all type I and type III endoleaks were resolved with adjunctive procedures, whilst the two type II endoleaks were left untreated. No endoleaks were found on pre-discharge MDCT that were not seen on CBCT. The contrast dose was significantly less for CBCT than MDCT, as was the radiation exposure.

3.1.2. Radiation Exposure

CT is associated with greater radiation exposure than DSA or other imaging techniques. Steuwe et al. [40] compared radiation exposure between intra-operative CBCT and post-operative follow-up MDCT and found that ceCBCT resulted in an average effective dose that was around 90–125% higher than a single venous phase MDCT image covering the same body area. However, with the actual MDCT protocol that was required to image the patients, intra-operative CBCT reduced the average effective dose by 60–65%. This difference was replicated in their phantom studies.

CBCT is found by these studies to be superior when compared to angiography and DSA in detecting technical complications, particularly better or non-inferior at detecting endoleaks. As a result, CBCT may allow intra-operative correction of endoleaks and graft kinks and reduce the rates of post-operative complications and subsequent secondary interventions. The increased contrast doses and radiation doses compared to DSA and angiography may be offset by the increased efficiency of CBCT, reducing the need for further imaging and therefore the total contrast and radiation dose of the patient.

3.2. Digital Subtraction Angiography

Digital subtraction angiography (DSA) uses a pre-contrast 'mask' image, which is then digitally subtracted from an image taken after contrast injection. The requirement of multiple images to be taken to obtain one image often results in higher radiation doses when compared to simple fluoroscopy [44].

3.2.1. Detection of Endoleaks

Faries et al. [18] compared standard completion angiograms with a modified angiographic protocol, which involved DSA continuously for 60 s after injection of 20 mL of iodinated contrast media in the pararenal aorta and within the graft. With the standard protocol, type II endoleaks were detected in 6% of patients vs. 41% with the modified protocol ($p < 0.001$). However, during follow-up, no significant difference was noted in the incidence of type II endoleaks.

3.2.2. Radiation Exposure

Timaran et al. [42] compared the radiation doses between standard magnification and dual fluoroscopy with live-image digital zooming during fenestrated-branched EVAR (F/B-EVAR). Procedures performed with the dual fluoroscopy with live image digital zooming resulted in significantly lower median patient and theatre staff radiation doses compared to standard electronic magnification, with no difference in the technical success, procedure time, or fluoroscopy time of the procedures. de Ruiter et al. [16] compared fixed C-arm fluoroscopy with mobile C-arm fluoroscopy and the addition of image processing technology in the form of the Allura ClarityIQ technology. They found that for non-complex EVAR procedures, there was no significant difference in fluoroscopy time between the groups. However, there was a significant difference in total radiation exposure between the fixed and mobile C-arm groups, with the mobile C-arm having reduced radiation, which was replicated for complex EVAR procedures.

The studies included here primarily focused on modifications to DSA protocols to improve on the limitations of DSA. The addition of technological adjuncts can reduce the radiation dose, whilst the modification of contrast injection and fluoroscopy timing was able to provide more information about endoleaks. These are often the limitations of DSA that are improved upon by other imaging modalities.

3.3. Fusion Imaging

Fusion imaging provides a patient-specific roadmap of blood vessels based on the fusion of intra-operative imaging with pre-operative imaging; this is most often a pre-operative CT angiogram. The intra-operative image may be DSA, fluoroscopy, or CBCT. Fusing the pre-operative CTA with intra-operative DSA or fluoroscopy provides a 2D-3D image, whereas fusion with intra-operative CBCT provides 3D-3D images [37]. This means that key operative landmarks can be continuously visualised throughout the operation without the need to continuously image, reducing patient exposure to excess radiation and contrast material.

3.3.1. Vascular Displacement after Stiff Wire

Fusion imaging helps to provide accurate measurements of stiff wire localisation and resultant vascular displacement. In particular, Breininger et al. [13] showed its accuracy by manually segmenting 2D images and fusing them with preoperative 3D CTA. Further work by Lalys et al. [29] set out to quantify vascular displacement after stiff wire insertion via a pre-op 3D reconstruction and 2D intra-operative fluoroscopic imaging. Significant displacement was picked up by the fusion imaging, with a mean error of 4.1 ± 2.4 mm at the level of the renal arteries. Similarly, Maurel et al. [32] aimed to quantify vascular displacement with the fusion of pre-operative CTA and perioperative ce-CBCT with fluoroscopic guidance. This fusion imaging modality was able to pick up a median vascular displacement of the MA of 6.7 mm with reduced overall use of contrast. They also found a strong correlation between body mass index (BMI) and the amount of radiation used by the ceCBCT. Similarly, Jansen et al. [23], used pre-operative CTA and intra-operative ceCBCT. This fusion modality was able to detect an average displacement of target vessels, encompassing coeliac, SMA, and renal arteries of 7.8 mm.

3.3.2. Image Registration

Koutouzi et al. [28] compared automatic vs. manual (based on the L1-L2 position) 3D-3D imaging registration. Of the manually registered scans, 7/19 showed sufficient accuracy in the alignment of the renal arteries when this was based on the L1-L2 position for EVAR. The remaining error with 3D-3D registration showed the ongoing need for pre-deployment DSA. Neither 2D-3D nor 3D-3D fusion was shown to successfully completely replace intra-operative angiograms. Panuccio et al. [34] also investigated the role of a fully automated co-registration fusion imaging engine of preoperative CTA and intra-operative fluoroscopy, which was successful in 92% of cases. Stangenberg et al. [39] showed that the utilisation of correct, up-to-date software decreased the necessary radiation dose, fluoroscopy time, and contrast agent dose.

3.3.3. 2D-3D vs. 3D-3D

Schulz et al. [37] compared 2D-3D (fluoroscopy and CBCT) vs. 3D-3D (CBCT and CBCT) fusion imaging. They showed the non-inferiority of 2D-3D compared to 3D-3D, but it had advantages in terms of radiation exposure and timeframe. Dijkstra et al. [17] compared the outcomes of intra-operative CBCT-MDCT fusion imaging with post-procedural CBCT and pre-discharge MDCT in FEVAR surgery. Fusion imaging resulted in overall lower contrast and skin doses. Schwein et al. [38] assessed the role of CTA-fluoroscopy fusion imaging in FEVAR. In total, 83% of blood vessels were successfully cannulated with the aid of fusion imaging alone without need for dedicated angiograms. These results show that 2D-3D fusion imaging may be precise enough to be more widely implemented but also offer lower radiation exposure and lower operative time.

3.3.4. Radiation Exposure

Tenorio et al. [41] found significant decreases in operator radiation exposure and effective dose in F-BEVAR with the use of fusion imaging. Furthermore, patients that had fusion imaging had significantly lower mortality (3% lower relative risk), incidences of major adverse events (24% lower relative risk), and need for secondary interventions (6% lower relative risk) at 30 days. McNally et al. [33] focussed on patients undergoing FEVAR or BEVAR. Fusion imaging provided a significant decrease in radiation exposure, fluoroscopy time, and contrast usage. The results were reproducible for three and four vessel stents. The estimated blood loss also decreased significantly. Results found by Rolls et al. [35] confirmed that fusion imaging significantly lowered exposure to ionising radiation and procedure time during FEVAR. Finally, Hertault et al. [22] confirmed that fusion imaging with a good collimator technique allows the achievement of very low radiation exposure doses.

3.3.5. Reduction of Iodinated Contrast

Kobeiter et al. [26] first reported the feasibility of CTA and low-dose CBCT fusion imaging without injection of iodinated contrast in FEVAR. Gallitto et al. [19] investigated the role of carbon dioxide angiography imaging vs. iodinated contrast imaging in the overall reduction of injected contrast medium during FEVAR. Carbon dioxide angiography led to overall lower doses of injected contrast media and similar detection rates of type 1, 2, and 3 endoleaks. The median hospitalisation in the carbon dioxide angiography group was significantly lower. Kaladji et al. [24] also set out to investigate the safety and usefulness of performing EVAR without pre- or intra-operative contrast. Six patients were enrolled due to low eGFR (median 17.5 mL/min/1.73 m^2). No intra-operative endoleak was noted on duplex scanning, and there were no changes in eGFR at 1 week or 1 month. The stent graft position was achieved satisfactorily.

3.4. Non-Contrast Imaging

Non-contrast imaging encompasses various techniques of intra-operative imaging during EVAR that attempt to reduce the use of iodinated contrast media (ICM). These imaging techniques include carbon dioxide DSA (CO_2-DSA), gadolinium-enhanced magnetic resonance angiography (MRA), and non-contrast CT. In CO_2-DSA, gaseous CO_2 is injected instead of contrast. The gas pushes away the blood column, allowing the visualisation of the affected vessel [45]. Gadolinium-enhanced MRA uses gadolinium, which is paramagnetic and can be detected through how it affects MR signals [46]. Both alternatives to ICM allow the enhancement of the target vessels during intra-operative imaging. In contrast, non-contrast CT simply does not use ICM.

Bush et al. [14] compared patients with either renal dysfunction or an ICM allergy and compared them to those who received ICM. Intra-operatively, intravascular ultrasound

(IVUS) was used to measure the aorta to ensure the correct deployment of stent grafts, and post-implantation aortography was used with gadolinium contrast media throughout the operation when necessary and at post-implantation to assess the successful deployment of the graft. There was no statistically significant increase in creatinine from baseline in any patient in the cohort. Chao et al. [15] analysed DSA with either iodinated contrast agents (ICA-DSA) or CO_2-DSA supplemented with ICA-DSA when needed. The CO_2-DSA group required longer fluoroscopy and operating times and experienced increased radiation exposure. Additionally, 13 of the 16 procedures required supplementation with ICA-DSA. There was no significant difference in the number of endoleaks detected or changes in renal function between groups. Both studies found their respective non-ICM-based imaging techniques to be technically successful in imaging during EVAR.

Studies looking at non-contrast imaging techniques primarily focussed on reduction of iodinated contrast use. Chao et al. [15] quoted literature values of 2 to 16% incidence of renal deterioration associated with EVAR, indicating the importance of reducing renal insults, including the use of iodinated contrast. This highlights that contrast dose reduction should be considered not only in patients with existing renal impairment but in all patients undergoing EVAR.

3.5. Ultrasound Imaging

Ultrasound imaging uses soundwaves to obtain images and carries no radiation risk. Contrast enhanced ultrasound (CEUS) produces images based on the interaction between the ultrasound waves, oscillations, and resonance of microbubbles [27]. Intravascular ultrasound (IVUS) is another ultrasound-based imaging technique used to obtain imaging for EVAR. Here, a rotational catheter with ultrasound-emitting capabilities is inserted intraluminally, allowing 360-degree images inside the vessel to be obtained [47]. This allows for precise measurements of vessel diameter and vessel wall composition [14].

3.5.1. Detection of Endoleaks

Massoni et al. [31] compared intra-operative CEUS with completion DSA in the early detection of endoleaks. The two imaging modalities agreed in 65% of cases, but CEUS detected more endoleaks (25 vs. 11). In a further study in 2021, Massoni et al. [30] looked specifically at the use of CEUS in the detection of type Ia endoleaks. In two cases, a type Ia endoleak was missed by angiography but detected on CEUS, resulting in an adjunctive procedure. In case 3, DSA detected an endoleak thought to be a type Ia, however, CEUS identified it as a type II from a lumbar artery, and as a result, no adjunctive procedure was performed. Keschenau et al. [25] also looked at the efficacy of CEUS in endoleak detection in patients undergoing F-BEVAR or infrarenal EVAR. Similar to Massoni et al. [31] in 2019, they found CEUS to detect significantly more type II endoleaks than completion angiography. However, many of those seen on CEUS were not seen on the pre-discharge CTA. In a later stage of their study, Keschenau et al. [25] carried out CEUS examinations at the same time as the pre-discharge CTA and found that of the four patients examined (who had type II endoleaks on the post-implantation CEUS), three had slow-flowing type II endoleaks that were detected by CEUS but not by CTA. The authors argued the value of CEUS as an investigation that reduces both contrast and radiation dose, and is superior in detecting type II endoleaks; however, it remains unclear whether this has clinical relevance.

3.5.2. Stent Deployment

Kopp et al. [27] used CEUS in their study to identify the proximal landing zone of the stent and to confirm complete aneurysm exclusion at the proximal and distal landing zone. They found CEUS to be successful in 14 out of 17 patients at identifying the infrarenal landing zone and successfully releasing the graft proximally. CEUS was also found to be successful at visualising the distal landing zone at the iliac bifurcation in 25 out of 28 iliac arteries. Additionally, CEUS identified significantly more endoleaks than angiography. Operative time was similar for both groups, but time for radiation exposure and contrast use was significantly lower in the CEUS group. In contrast, Gennai et al. [21] used IVUS as a post-deployment imaging technique to assess the success of BEVAR/FEVAR stent graft deployment in a retrospective study of 10 patients, with 33 target visceral vessels. IVUS was technically successful in all cases. An increase in the operating time with the addition of IVUS was noted; however, IVUS identified problems in 4 of the 33 bridging stents that were not identified by completion angiography. Given the 12% of bridging stent issues that were only detected by IVUS, the authors concluded that there was a benefit to using IVUS as an adjunctive imaging modality in B-FEVAR, especially given its lack of contrast use and radiation exposure.

3.5.3. Measuring Stent Graft Size

Garrett et al. [20] evaluated aorta measurements taken by CT and by IVUS. They also conducted these measurements on a phantom tube, comparing the CT, IVUS, and calliper measurements. No statistically significant difference was found between the imaging techniques for the phantom. However, 22 cases had a sufficient disagreement between the pre-operative CT and intra-operative IVUS to result in changing stent graft size. In four cases, patients were considered inappropriate for EVAR based on the CT measurements, but IVUS suggested they were candidates, and these patients had successful interventions. No type I endoleaks were noted. The authors argue that the flexible sheath of the IVUS behaves more like the stent graft and is thus able to show more accurately the fit of the proximal aortic neck.

Ultrasound-based imaging techniques significantly reduce contrast and radiation dose and may be superior in the detection of endoleaks. However, the clinical relevance of these endoleaks is questioned in these studies. Both CEUS and IVUS had value in helping guide deployment of the stent graft, ensuring correct positioning both in standard infrarenal EVAR and more complex interventions with branches or fenestrations.

3.6. Intra-Operative Positioning System

Intra-operative positioning system (IOPS) is a novel endovascular navigation system that does not use radiation or contrast, instead using electromagnetic sensors to provide 3D roadmaps to guide intervention [48]. Unfortunately, no papers passed through the full text search stage for IOPS.

3.7. Risk of Bias

The risk of bias was assessed using the Newcastle-Ottawa Scale, with a median score of 8 (IQR 6–8) for all included studies (Supplementary Table S2).

4. Discussion

This study reviewed intra-operative imaging techniques used to quality assure EVAR by identifying technical complications and endoleaks that can be corrected at the time of initial intervention to improve EVAR durability and reduce the need for reintervention. The overall data on these techniques are limited to a small series and are of poor quality.

Patients requiring aortic aneurysm repair often have multiple comorbidities. Pre-existing renal impairment or renal insults from intra-operative contrast use can complicate endovascular intervention. Further, following EVAR, surveillance imaging is required to assess for stent position, endoleaks, and other complications. This monitoring is primarily conducted with duplex ultrasound, but patients often receive a post-operative CT scan, which adds to the lifetime radiation burden. Safe patient care involves minimising renal insult and exposure to ionising radiation as far as possible. Operators and theatre staff are also regularly exposed to ionising radiation during these procedures. Where ALARA principles are not followed or where the use of protection is lax, there may be an increased risk of harm to the operator including cataracts, skin damage, or even cancer [49–51]. These risks can be stochastic, such as cancer where there is no threshold dose, or deterministic, such as cataracts, where there is a threshold dose above which effects are seen. Thus, efforts to reduce the use of ionising radiation during procedures are not just beneficial to the patient. If preventable complications are not detected intra-operatively, then regardless of efforts to reduce radiation exposure during the surgery, the patient will be further exposed during re-intervention.

This review found that CT was good for identification of complications, with CBCT most often used intra-operatively. Whilst contrast use and ionising radiation exposure tended towards higher than comparative imaging, authors argued this to be acceptable in the context of reducing the need for re-intervention. Studies involving DSA focussed on reduction of radiation exposure, and the different protocols studied succeeded in this. Fusion imaging found 2D-3D fusion to be non-inferior to 3D-3D. Fusion imaging was also found to be useful in measuring vascular displacement after the insertion of stiff guidewires. Ionising radiation exposure and contrast usage was lower for fusion imaging, to the benefit of both the patient and the operator. Studies looking at automatic registration found it to be variable, but it shows promise in the future with further developments. Data regarding fusion imaging, albeit heterogeneous, indicate its utility to reduce overall radiation dose to patients and staff. The latest European Society for Vascular Surgery (ESVS) guidelines on radiation safety are clear regarding the importance placed on the judicious use of ionising radiation, encouraging operators to follow the ALARA principle (as low as reasonably possible). The ALARA principle should be adhered to by using low-dose protocols and limiting fluoroscopy time and screening time [52]. To achieve this, the ESVS stresses the importance of utilising more advanced imaging techniques such as fusion imaging. Concurrently, our review found data supporting that fusion imaging may help achieve shorter operative time. We show that there are data available to support the wider implementation of fusion imaging to achieve ALARA radiation exposure. Unsurprisingly, non-contrast imaging provided lower doses of contrast to the patient, but depending on the imaging used, occasionally resulted in higher doses of radiation, for example, in CO_2-DSA. Ultrasound was found to be effective, particularly in the detection of type II endoleaks. It frequently resulted in interventions with reduced radiation and contrast use, indicating it to be both safe and effective. However, it is not widely used and may be less effective in patients with higher BMIs. Additionally, it is highly operator-dependent and costly; thus, widespread use may be limited by this. IVUS was found to be useful in device kinks and endoleak detection but is costly due to disposable IVUS catheters and is not widely used. Furthermore, Fibre Optic RealShape (FORS) could show real promise in the future. This modality utilises fibre optic laser technology to enable real-time device visualisation. So far, this is not a widely available technique although it has been used with some degree of success both pre-clinically and in the clinical setting [53,54]. This novel technique also promises to further reduce exposure to ionising radiation.

5. Conclusions

This review provides an overall synopsis of the intra-operative imaging modalities used to quality assure endovascular aortic surgery. All of the imaging modalities discussed have advantages and disadvantages and can be of use if utilised appropriately. Recent advances in intra-operative fusion and ultrasound imaging modalities seem to be particularly promising for future developments and may reduce radiation doses to patients and operators.

6. Limitations

The overall data quality of this study is poor and heterogenous, making it difficult to draw robust conclusions. There are limited data on long-term outcomes after intra-operative CT fusion or IVUS that suggest these intra-operative imaging techniques reduce re-intervention rates or long-term aortic aneurysm rupture. This may be the case, but at present, there is insufficient evidence to support this claim.

Supplementary Materials: The following supporting information can be downloaded at: https://www.mdpi.com/article/10.3390/jcm12093167/s1, Table S1: Search strategy; Table S2: Risk of bias.

Author Contributions: Conceptualisation, J.R.B.; Methodology, J.R.B., P.Z.B., S.J.H. and M.M.C.; Software, P.Z.B., S.J.H.; Validation, P.Z.B., S.J.H. and G.L.T.; Formal analysis, P.Z.B., G.L.T.; Investigation, P.Z.B., S.J.H. and G.L.T.; Resources, P.Z.B., S.J.H.; Data curation, P.Z.B., S.J.H.; Writing—original draft preparation, P.Z.B., S.J.H., G.L.T.; Writing—review and editing, M.M.C., A.A.S., G.L.T., J.R.B.; Supervision, M.M.C., A.A.S., J.R.B.; Project administration, J.R.B., M.M.C., A.A.S. All authors have read and agreed to the published version of the manuscript.

Funding: This research received no external funding.

Institutional Review Board Statement: Not applicable.

Informed Consent Statement: Not applicable.

Data Availability Statement: No new data were created or analyzed in this study. Data sharing is not applicable to this article.

Conflicts of Interest: The authors declare no conflict of interest.

References

1. Volodos, N.L.; Shekhanin, V.E.; Karpovich, I.P.; Troian, V.I.; Gur'ev Iu, A. A self-fixing synthetic blood vessel endoprosthesis. *Vestn Khir Im I I Grek* **1986**, *137*, 123–125.
2. United Kingdom EVAR Trial Investigators; Greenhalgh, R.M.; Brown, L.C.; Powell, J.T.; Thompson, S.G.; Epstein, D.; Sculpher, M.J. Endovascular versus Open Repair of Abdominal Aortic Aneurysm. *N. Engl. J. Med.* **2010**, *362*, 1863–1871. [CrossRef] [PubMed]
3. Prinssen, M.; Verhoeven, E.L.G.; Buth, J.; Cuypers, P.W.M.; van Sambeek, M.R.H.M.; Balm, R.; Buskens, E.; Grobbee, D.E.; Blankensteijn, J.D. A Randomized Trial Comparing Conventional and Endovascular Repair of Abdominal Aortic Aneurysms. *N. Engl. J. Med.* **2004**, *351*, 1607–1618. [CrossRef] [PubMed]
4. Lederle, F.A.; Kyriakides, T.C.; Stroupe, K.T.; Freischlag, J.A.; Padberg, F.T.; Matsumura, J.S.; Huo, Z.; Johnson, G.R. Open versus Endovascular Repair of Abdominal Aortic Aneurysm. *N. Engl. J. Med.* **2019**, *380*, 2126–2135. [CrossRef]
5. Patel, R.; Sweeting, M.J.; Powell, J.T.; Greenhalgh, R.M. Endovascular versus open repair of abdominal aortic aneurysm in 15-years' follow-up of the UK endovascular aneurysm repair trial 1 (EVAR trial 1): A randomised controlled trial. *Lancet* **2016**, *388*, 2366–2374. [CrossRef]
6. The Lancet. Open versus endovascular repair of aortic aneurysms. *Lancet* **2020**, *395*, 1090. [CrossRef]
7. National Institute for Health and Care Excellence. Abdominal aortic aneurysm: Diagnosis and management (NG156). NICE Guideline [NG156], 2020. Available online: https://www.nice.org.uk/guidance/ng156 (accessed on 8 January 2023).
8. Dua, A.; Eagleton, M.J. A Revolution of EVAR Imaging Technologies. *Endovascular Today*, 1 November 2019.
9. Belvroy, V.M.; Houben, I.B.; Trimarchi, S.; Patel, H.J.; Moll, F.L.; Van Herwaarden, J.A. Identifying and addressing the limitations of EVAR technology. *Expert. Rev. Med. Devices* **2018**, *15*, 541–554. [CrossRef]
10. Moll, F.L.; Powell, J.T.; Fraedrich, G.; Verzini, F.; Haulon, S.; Waltham, M.; van Herwaarden, J.A.; Holt, P.J.E.; van Keulen, J.W.; Rantner, B.; et al. Management of Abdominal Aortic Aneurysms Clinical Practice Guidelines of the European Society for Vascular Surgery. *Eur. J. Vasc. Endovasc. Surg.* **2011**, *41*, S1–S58. [CrossRef] [PubMed]
11. Stang, A. Critical evaluation of the Newcastle-Ottawa scale for the assessment of the quality of nonrandomized studies in meta-analyses. *Eur. J. Epidemiol.* **2010**, *25*, 603–605. [CrossRef]
12. Biasi, L.; Ali, T.; Hinchliffe, R.; Morgan, R.; Loftus, I.; Thompson, M. Intraoperative DynaCT detection and immediate correction of a type Ia endoleak following endovascular repair of abdominal aortic aneurysm. *Cardiovasc. Intervent. Radiol.* **2009**, *32*, 535–538. [CrossRef] [PubMed]
13. Breininger, K.; Hanika, M.; Weule, M.; Kowarschik, M.; Pfister, M.; Maier, A. Simultaneous reconstruction of multiple stiff wires from a single X-ray projection for endovascular aortic repair. *Int. J. Comput. Assist. Radiol. Surg.* **2019**, *14*, 1891–1899. [CrossRef]
14. Bush, R.L.; Lin, P.H.; Bianco, C.C.; Lumsden, A.B.; Gunnoud, A.B.; Terramani, T.T.; Brinkman, W.T.; Martin, L.G.; Weiss, V.J. Endovascular aortic aneurysm repair in patients with renal dysfunction or severe contrast allergy: Utility of imaging modalities without iodinated contrast. *Ann. Vasc. Surg.* **2002**, *16*, 537–544. [CrossRef]
15. Chao, A.; Major, K.; Kumar, S.R.; Patel, K.; Trujillo, I.; Hood, D.B.; Rowe, V.L.; Weaver, F.A. Carbon dioxide digital subtraction angiography-assisted endovascular aortic aneurysm repair in the azotemic patient. *J. Vasc. Surg.* **2007**, *45*, 451–458. [CrossRef] [PubMed]
16. de Ruiter, Q.M.; Moll, F.L.; Gijsberts, C.M.; van Herwaarden, J.A. AlluraClarity Radiation Dose-Reduction Technology in the Hybrid Operating Room During Endovascular Aneurysm Repair. *J. Endovasc. Ther.* **2016**, *23*, 130–138. [CrossRef] [PubMed]
17. Dijkstra, M.L.; Eagleton, M.J.; Greenberg, R.K.; Mastracci, T.; Hernandez, A. Intraoperative C-arm cone-beam computed tomography in fenestrated/branched aortic endografting. *J. Vasc. Surg.* **2011**, *53*, 583–590. [CrossRef] [PubMed]

18. Faries, P.L.; Briggs, V.L.; Bernheim, J.; Kent, K.C.; Hollier, L.H.; Marin, M.L. Increased recognition of type II endoleaks using a modified intraoperative angiographic protocol: Implications for intermittent endoleak and aneurysm expansion. *Ann. Vasc. Surg.* **2003**, *17*, 608–614. [CrossRef]
19. Gallitto, E.; Faggioli, G.; Vacirca, A.; Pini, R.; Mascoli, C.; Fenelli, C.; Logiacco, A.; Abualhin, M.; Gargiulo, M. The benefit of combined carbon dioxide automated angiography and fusion imaging in preserving perioperative renal function in fenestrated endografting. *J. Vasc. Surg.* **2020**, *72*, 1906–1916. [CrossRef]
20. Garrett, H.E.; Abdullah, A.H.; Hodgkiss, T.D.; Burgar, S.R. Intravascular ultrasound aids in the performance of endovascular repair of abdominal aortic aneurysm. *J. Vasc. Surg.* **2003**, *37*, 615–618. [CrossRef]
21. Gennai, S.; Leone, N.; Saitta, G.; Migliari, M.; Lauricella, A.; Farchioni, L.; Silingardi, R. Intravascular Ultrasound in Branched and Fenestrated Endovascular Aneurysm Repair: Initial Experience in a Single-Center Cohort Study. *J. Endovasc. Ther.* **2021**, *28*, 828–836. [CrossRef]
22. Hertault, A.; Rhee, R.; Antoniou, G.A.; Adam, D.; Tonda, H.; Rousseau, H.; Bianchini, A.; Haulon, S. Radiation Dose Reduction During EVAR: Results from a Prospective Multicentre Study (The REVAR Study). *Eur. J. Vasc. Endovasc. Surg.* **2018**, *56*, 426–433. [CrossRef]
23. Jansen, M.M.; van der Stelt, M.; Smorenburg, S.P.M.; Slump, C.H.; van Herwaarden, J.A.; Hazenberg, C. Target vessel displacement during fenestrated and branched endovascular aortic repair and its implications for the role of traditional computed tomography angiography roadmaps. *Quant. Imaging Med. Surg.* **2021**, *11*, 3945–3955. [CrossRef] [PubMed]
24. Kaladji, A.; Dumenil, A.; Mahé, G.; Castro, M.; Cardon, A.; Lucas, A.; Haigron, P. Safety and accuracy of endovascular aneurysm repair without pre-operative and intra-operative contrast agent. *Eur. J. Vasc. Endovasc. Surg.* **2015**, *49*, 255–261. [CrossRef] [PubMed]
25. Keschenau, P.R.; Alkassam, H.; Kotelis, D.; Jacobs, M.J.; Kalder, J. Intraoperative contrast-enhanced ultrasound examination for endoleak detection after complex and infrarenal endovascular aortic repair. *J. Vasc. Surg.* **2020**, *71*, 1200–1206. [CrossRef]
26. Kobeiter, H.; Nahum, J.; Becquemin, J.P. Zero-contrast thoracic endovascular aortic repair using image fusion. *Circulation* **2011**, *124*, e280–e282. [CrossRef]
27. Kopp, R.; Zürn, W.; Weidenhagen, R.; Meimarakis, G.; Clevert, D.A. First experience using intraoperative contrast-enhanced ultrasound during endovascular aneurysm repair for infrarenal aortic aneurysms. *J. Vasc. Surg.* **2010**, *51*, 1103–1110. [CrossRef]
28. Koutouzi, G.; Roos, H.; Henrikson, O.; Leonhardt, H.; Falkenberg, M. Orthogonal Rings, Fiducial Markers, and Overlay Accuracy When Image Fusion is Used for EVAR Guidance. *Eur. J. Vasc. Endovasc. Surg.* **2016**, *52*, 604–611. [CrossRef]
29. Lalys, F.; Barré, A.; Kafi, M.; Benziane, M.; Saudreau, B.; Dupont, C.; Kaladji, A. Identification of Parameters Influencing the Vascular Structure Displacement in Fusion Imaging during Endovascular Aneurysm Repair. *J. Vasc. Interv. Radiol.* **2019**, *30*, 1386–1392. [CrossRef]
30. Massoni, C.B.; Perini, P.; Fanelli, M.; Ucci, A.; Azzarone, M.; Rossi, G.; D'ospina, R.M.; Freyrie, A. The utility of intraoperative contrast-enhanced ultrasound for immediate treatment of type ia endoleak during evar: Initial experience. *Acta Biomed.* **2021**, *92*, e2021046. [CrossRef]
31. Massoni, C.B.; Perini, P.; Fanelli, M.; Ucci, A.; Rossi, G.; Azzarone, M.; Tecchio, T.; Freyrie, A. Intraoperative contrast-enhanced ultrasound for early diagnosis of endoleaks during endovascular abdominal aortic aneurysm repair. *J. Vasc. Surg.* **2019**, *70*, 1844–1850. [CrossRef]
32. Maurel, B.; Hertault, A.; Gonzalez, T.M.; Sobocinski, J.; Le Roux, M.; Delaplace, J.; Azzaoui, R.; Midulla, M.; Haulon, S. Evaluation of visceral artery displacement by endograft delivery system insertion. *J. Endovasc. Ther.* **2014**, *21*, 339–347. [CrossRef] [PubMed]
33. McNally, M.M.; Scali, S.T.; Feezor, R.J.; Neal, D.; Huber, T.S.; Beck, A.W. Three-dimensional fusion computed tomography decreases radiation exposure, procedure time, and contrast use during fenestrated endovascular aortic repair. *J. Vasc. Surg.* **2015**, *61*, 309–316. [CrossRef]
34. Panuccio, G.; Torsello, G.F.; Pfister, M.; Bisdas, T.; Bosiers, M.J.; Torsello, G.; Austermann, M. Computer-aided endovascular aortic repair using fully automated two- and three-dimensional fusion imaging. *J. Vasc. Surg.* **2016**, *64*, 1587–1594. [CrossRef] [PubMed]
35. Rolls, A.E.; Rosen, S.; Constantinou, J.; Davis, M.; Cole, J.; Desai, M.; Stoyanov, D.; Mastracci, T.M. Introduction of a Team Based Approach to Radiation Dose Reduction in the Enhancement of the Overall Radiation Safety Profile of FEVAR. *Eur. J. Vasc. Endovasc. Surg.* **2016**, *52*, 451–457. [CrossRef]
36. Schulz, C.J.; Schmitt, M.; Böckler, D.; Geisbüsch, P. Intraoperative contrast-enhanced cone beam computed tomography to assess technical success during endovascular aneurysm repair. *J. Vasc. Surg.* **2016**, *64*, 577–584. [CrossRef] [PubMed]
37. Schulz, C.J.; Böckler, D.; Krisam, J.; Geisbüsch, P. Two-dimensional-three-dimensional registration for fusion imaging is noninferior to three-dimensional- three-dimensional registration in infrarenal endovascular aneurysm repair. *J. Vasc. Surg.* **2019**, *70*, 2005–2013. [CrossRef]
38. Schwein, A.; Chinnadurai, P.; Behler, G.; Lumsden, A.B.; Bismuth, J.; Bechara, C.F. Computed tomography angiography-fluoroscopy image fusion allows visceral vessel cannulation without angiography during fenestrated endovascular aneurysm repair. *J. Vasc. Surg.* **2018**, *68*, 2–11. [CrossRef] [PubMed]
39. Stangenberg, L.; Shuja, F.; Carelsen, B.; Elenbaas, T.; Wyers, M.C.; Schermerhorn, M.L. A novel tool for three-dimensional roadmapping reduces radiation exposure and contrast agent dose in complex endovascular interventions. *J. Vasc. Surg.* **2015**, *62*, 448–455. [CrossRef] [PubMed]

40. Steuwe, A.; Geisbüsch, P.; Schulz, C.J.; Böckler, D.; Kauczor, H.U.; Stiller, W. Comparison of Radiation Exposure Associated With Intraoperative Cone-Beam Computed Tomography and Follow-up Multidetector Computed Tomography Angiography for Evaluating Endovascular Aneurysm Repairs. *J. Endovasc. Ther.* **2016**, *23*, 583–592. [CrossRef]
41. Tenorio, E.R.; Oderich, G.S.; Sandri, G.A.; Ozbek, P.; Kärkkäinen, J.M.; Macedo, T.A.; Vrtiska, T.; Cha, S. Impact of onlay fusion and cone beam computed tomography on radiation exposure and technical assessment of fenestrated-branched endovascular aortic repair. *J. Vasc. Surg.* **2019**, *69*, 1045–1058.e1043. [CrossRef]
42. Timaran, L.I.; Timaran, C.H.; Scott, C.K.; Soto-Gonzalez, M.; Timaran-Montenegro, D.E.; Guild, J.B.; Kirkwood, M.L. Dual fluoroscopy with live-image digital zooming significantly reduces patient and operating staff radiation during fenestrated-branched endovascular aortic aneurysm repair. *J. Vasc. Surg.* **2021**, *73*, 601–607. [CrossRef]
43. Törnqvist, P.; Dias, N.; Sonesson, B.; Kristmundsson, T.; Resch, T. Intra-operative cone beam computed tomography can help avoid reinterventions and reduce CT follow up after infrarenal EVAR. *Eur. J. Vasc. Endovasc. Surg.* **2015**, *49*, 390–395. [CrossRef] [PubMed]
44. Gyánó, M.; Berczeli, M.; Csobay-Novák, C.; Szöllősi, D.; Óriás, V.I.; Góg, I.; Kiss, J.P.; Veres, D.S.; Szigeti, K.; Osváth, S.; et al. Digital variance angiography allows about 70% decrease of DSA-related radiation exposure in lower limb X-ray angiography. *Sci. Rep.* **2021**, *11*, 21790. [CrossRef]
45. Rezaee, A.; Mehrabinejad, M.-M.; Bell, D.J.; Weerakkody, Y. Carbon dioxide angiography. Available online: https://radiopaedia.org/articles/53045 (accessed on 24 January 2023).
46. Bashir, U.; Bell, D.J.; Chieng, R.; Yap, J.; Francavilla, M.; Sharma, R.; MacManus, D.; Gaillard, F.; Gamage, P.J.; Murphy, A.; et al. Gadolinium Contrast Agents. Available online: https://radiopaedia.org/articles/18340 (accessed on 24 January 2023).
47. Shlofmitz, E.; Kerndt, C.C.; Parekh, A.; Khalid, N. Intravascular Ultrasound. In *StatPearls*; StatPearls Publishing: Treasure Island, FL, USA, 2022.
48. Muluk, S.C.; Elrakhawy, M.; Chess, B.; Rosales, C.; Goel, V. Successful endovascular treatment of severe chronic mesenteric ischemia facilitated by intraoperative positioning system image guidance. *J. Vasc. Surg. Cases Innov. Tech.* **2022**, *8*, 60–65. [CrossRef] [PubMed]
49. Vano, E.; Gonzalez, L.; Fernández, J.M.; Haskal, Z.J. Eye Lens Exposure to Radiation in Interventional Suites: Caution Is Warranted. *Radiology* **2008**, *248*, 945–953. [CrossRef] [PubMed]
50. Wan, R.C.; Chau, W.W.; Tso, C.Y.; Tang, N.; Chow, S.K.; Cheung, W.-H.; Wong, R.M. Occupational hazard of fluoroscopy: An invisible threat to orthopaedic surgeons. *J. Orthop. Trauma Rehabil.* **2021**, *28*, 22104917211035547. [CrossRef]
51. Mastrangelo, G.; Fedeli, U.; Fadda, E.; Giovanazzi, A.; Scoizzato, L.; Saia, B. Increased cancer risk among surgeons in an orthopaedic hospital. *Occup. Med.* **2005**, *55*, 498–500. [CrossRef]
52. Modarai, B.; Haulon, S.; Ainsbury, E.; Böckler, D.; Vano-Carruana, E.; Dawson, J.; Farber, M.; Van Herzeele, I.; Hertault, A.; van Herwaarden, J.; et al. Editor's Choice—European Society for Vascular Surgery (ESVS) 2023 Clinical Practice Guidelines on Radiation Safety. *Eur. J. Vasc. Endovasc. Surg.* **2023**, *65*, 171–222. [CrossRef]
53. Jansen, M.; Khandige, A.; Kobeiter, H.; Vonken, E.-J.; Hazenberg, C.; van Herwaarden, J. Three dimensional visualisation of endovascular guidewires and catheters based on laser light instead of fluoroscopy with fiber optic RealShape technology: Preclinical results. *Eur. J. Vasc. Endovasc. Sur.* **2020**, *60*, 135–143. [CrossRef]
54. Panuccio, G.; Schanzer, A.; Rohlffs, F.; Heidemann, F.; Wessels, B.; Schurink, G.W.; van Herwaarden, J.A.; Kölbel, T. Endovascular navigation with fiber optic RealShape technology. *J. Vasc. Surg.* **2023**, *77*, 3–8.e2. [CrossRef]

Disclaimer/Publisher's Note: The statements, opinions and data contained in all publications are solely those of the individual author(s) and contributor(s) and not of MDPI and/or the editor(s). MDPI and/or the editor(s) disclaim responsibility for any injury to people or property resulting from any ideas, methods, instructions or products referred to in the content.

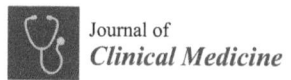

Article

Three-Dimensional Characterization of Aortic Root Motion by Vascular Deformation Mapping

Taeouk Kim [1,†], Nic S. Tjahjadi [2,†], Xuehuan He [3], JA van Herwaarden [4], Himanshu J. Patel [2], Nicholas S. Burris [3,*] and C. Alberto Figueroa [1,5,*]

1. Department of Biomedical Engineering, University of Michigan, Ann Arbor, MI 48109, USA; taeouk@umich.edu
2. Department of Cardiac Surgery, University of Michigan, Ann Arbor, MI 48109, USA; nicasiut@med.umich.edu (N.S.T.); hjpatel@med.umich.edu (H.J.P.)
3. Department of Radiology, University of Michigan, Ann Arbor, MI 48109, USA; xuhe@med.umich.edu
4. Department of Vascular Surgery, University Medical Center Utrecht, 3584 CX Utrecht, The Netherlands; j.a.vanherwaarden@umcutrecht.nl
5. Department of Surgery, University of Michigan, Ann Arbor, MI 48109, USA
* Correspondence: nburris@med.umich.edu (N.S.B.); figueroc@med.umich.edu (C.A.F.)
† These authors contributed equally to this work.

Abstract: The aorta is in constant motion due to the combination of cyclic loading and unloading with its mechanical coupling to the contractile left ventricle (LV) myocardium. This aortic root motion has been proposed as a marker for aortic disease progression. Aortic root motion extraction techniques have been mostly based on 2D image analysis and have thus lacked a rigorous description of the different components of aortic root motion (e.g., axial versus in-plane). In this study, we utilized a novel technique termed vascular deformation mapping (VDM(D)) to extract 3D aortic root motion from dynamic computed tomography angiography images. Aortic root displacement (axial and in-plane), area ratio and distensibility, axial tilt, aortic rotation, and LV/Ao angles were extracted and compared for four different subject groups: non-aneurysmal, TAA, Marfan, and repair. The repair group showed smaller aortic root displacement, aortic rotation, and distensibility than the other groups. The repair group was also the only group that showed a larger relative in-plane displacement than relative axial displacement. The Marfan group showed the largest heterogeneity in aortic root displacement, distensibility, and age. The non-aneurysmal group showed a negative correlation between age and distensibility, consistent with previous studies. Our results revealed a strong positive correlation between LV/Ao angle and relative axial displacement and a strong negative correlation between LV/Ao angle and relative in-plane displacement. VDM(D)-derived 3D aortic root motion can be used in future studies to define improved boundary conditions for aortic wall stress analysis.

Keywords: aortic root motion; VDM; 3D displacement; dynamic 3D CTA; age; LV/Ao angle

Citation: Kim, T.; Tjahjadi, N.S.; He, X.; van Herwaarden, J.A.; Patel, H.J.; Burris, N.S.; Figueroa, C.A. Three-Dimensional Characterization of Aortic Root Motion by Vascular Deformation Mapping. *J. Clin. Med.* **2023**, *12*, 4471. https://doi.org/10.3390/jcm12134471

Academic Editor: Giovanni Mosti

Received: 5 June 2023
Revised: 29 June 2023
Accepted: 2 July 2023
Published: 4 July 2023

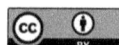

Copyright: © 2023 by the authors. Licensee MDPI, Basel, Switzerland. This article is an open access article distributed under the terms and conditions of the Creative Commons Attribution (CC BY) license (https://creativecommons.org/licenses/by/4.0/).

1. Introduction

Current guidelines for management of aortic diseases such as thoracic aortic aneurysms (TAA) and aortic dissection largely focus on maximal diameter as a primary metric of disease severity and risk [1,2]. Aortic diameter is an inherently static metric, typically performed in diastole [3]. However, the aorta is in constant motion due to the combination of cyclic loading and unloading with its mechanical coupling to the contractile left ventricle (LV) myocardium. Electrocardiogram (ECG)-gated computed tomography angiography (CTA) affords the opportunity to visualize motion of the thoracic aorta throughout the cardiac cycle and is capable of depicting such dynamic aortic root motion in a three-dimensional (3D) manner [4]. Abnormalities in aortic root motion have been proposed to be a potential risk factor for disease progression and complications in thoracic aortic disease [5–8].

Previous studies have characterized aortic root motion from dynamic imaging and have incorporated this data into methods to estimate wall stresses in the ascending thoracic aorta (ATAA). However, some studies have used idealized aortic models rather than patient-specific anatomy [5]. Furthermore, most techniques used to extract and quantify aortic root motion are based on 2D imaging and thus lack a comprehensive description of the multi-directional components of aortic root motion [5–9]. An accurate 3D assessment of cyclic motion of the ATAA could have significant implications for estimating mechanical properties of the aorta, informing computational simulations, endovascular device design, and, importantly, for refining diameter-based assessment of disease severity.

Vascular deformation mapping (VDM) is a validated medical image registration technique which allows for comprehensive assessment of the degree and extent of growth mapping of the aorta (VDM(G): VDM growth) [10–12] using longitudinal CTA data acquired at two different points during clinical surveillance. However, when applied to dynamic CTA data (i.e., time-resolved CTA), VDM allows for 3D assessment of the aortic deformation throughout the cardiac cycle (VDM(D): VDM dynamic).

The objective of this study is to utilize VDM(D) to accurately quantify aortic root motion in a 3D manner using patient-specific data in a cohort of patients with various manifestations of TAA disease (i.e., sporadic TAA and Marfan syndrome (MFS)) as well as non-aneurysmal controls.

2. Materials and Methods

2.1. Study Population

All procedures were approved by the local institutional review board with a waiver of informed consent obtained for this retrospective study and were Health Insurance Portability and Accountability Act-compliant. On the basis of available high-quality, retrospectively electrocardiogram-gated CTA data, electronic medical records search software was used to identify patients aged 18 years and older with a clinical diagnosis of thoracic aortic aneurysm (TAA) that was either sporadic or associated with MFS. For comparison, we also identified a cohort of patients with available retrospective CTA data that had non-aneurysmal thoracic aortic dimensions (i.e., maximal diameter < 40 mm) as well as a group of patients who had undergone prior open surgical repair of their aortic root and/or ascending aorta. Exclusion criteria were non-ECG-gated acquisition, suboptimal thoracic aortic enhancement (<250 Hounsfield units), image slice thickness > 2.5 mm, or significant motion/respiratory artifacts preventing accurate delineation of the aortic wall and thus accurate registration in VDM analysis. At random, 51 patients meeting these criteria were included in this study and were divided into four groups: non-aneurysmal, sporadic TAA (henceforth referred to as "TAA"), MFS (henceforth referred to as "Marfan"), and ascending graft repair (henceforth referred to as "repair"). Patient demographics and clinical characteristics were collected through medical chart review. Maximum diameter measurements of the thoracic aorta were collected from clinical radiology reports. Peak systolic and end-diastolic phases of the ECG-gated CTA imaging were selected and extracted using OsirixMD [13]. The angle between the aortic annulus and the mitral annulus (LV/Ao angle) was also measured using OsirixMD for each patient. Figure 1 depicts the definition of LV/Ao angle adopted in this study, namely the angle (φ) between two lines perpendicular to the aortic and mitral annuli, respectively.

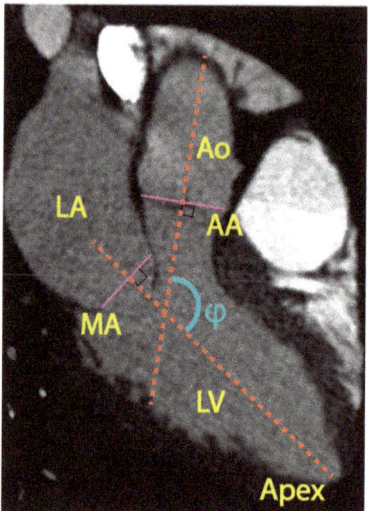

Figure 1. Definition of LV/Ao angle (φ) adopted in this study. LV: left ventricle, MA: mitral annulus, LA: left atrium, AA: aortic annulus, Ao: aorta. Purple lines indicate MA and AA. The LV/Ao angle (φ) is the angle between the lines perpendicular to the aortic and mitral annuli, respectively.

ECG-gated CTA examinations were performed on either 64- or 246-detector CTA scanners using helical (Lightspeed VCT or Discovery CT750HD; GE Healthcare) or axial (Revolution; GE Healthcare) acquisition modes. Dynamic CT imaging was acquired through the entire thoracic aorta, from lung apices to at least 2 cm below the celiac trunk.

2.2. VDM(D)

VDM employs b-spline deformable image registration techniques to quantify the 3D deformation of the aortic wall surface between two CTA images of a given subject. This approach has been previously applied to assess 3D aortic growth based on CTA images acquired at two time points spanning several years and has been validated in expert-rater and in silico phantom studies [10–12]. We refer to this growth assessment technique as VDM(G).

In this study, the VDM concept is expanded to study 3D aortic deformation between the diastolic and systolic phases extracted from the dynamic CTA images. Therefore, instead of assessing 3D growth over a long period of time, the method quantifies 3D deformation over the cardiac cycle. We refer to this technique as VDM(D). Figure 2 illustrates the VDM(D) workflow. First, the selected systolic and diastolic phase images are segmented using an in-house aortic segmentation neural network [14]. Next, rigid and deformable registrations were conducted to align the two segmentations. Registration accuracy was confirmed using a dual-channel plotting technique to assure alignment of the fixed diastolic and warped systolic configurations, as previously described [10]. Lastly, the 3D displacement field resulting from the deformable registration was used to perform a vertex-wise deformation of a triangulated mesh based on the diastolic configuration. The 3D displacement field between the diastolic and systolic aortic phases is amenable to performing engineering analysis of strains, stretches, and 3D motions of specific regions of the aorta, such as the aortic annulus.

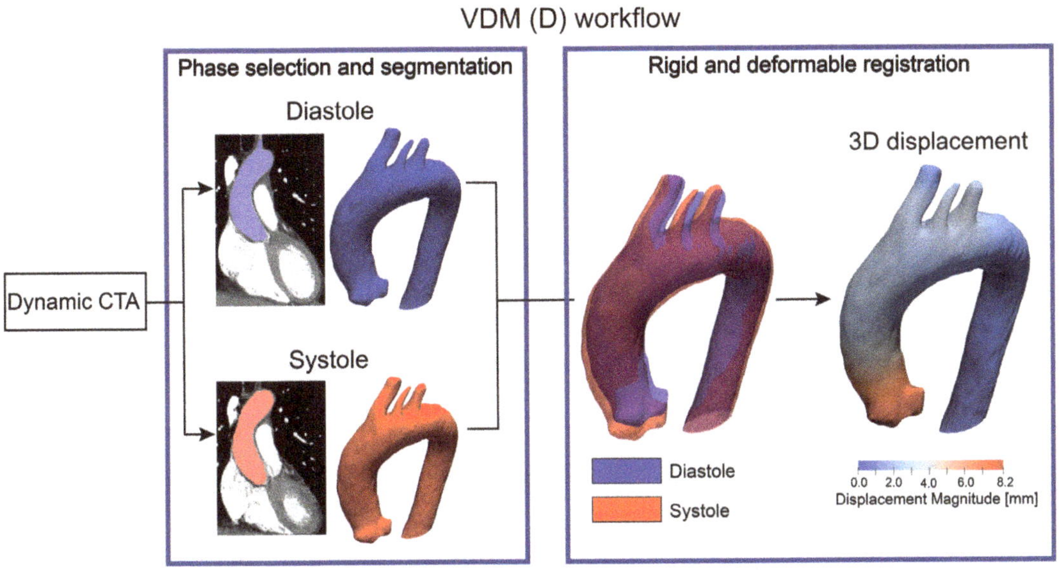

Figure 2. VDM(D) workflow.

2.3. Metrics Extracted from VDM(D)

2.3.1. Defining a Suitable Location to Study Aortic Root Motion

VDM(D) provides the 3D displacement from diastole to systole over the entire surface of the thoracic aorta. However, for the purposes of this study, we extracted and analyzed aortic root motion at the sinuses of Valsalva in a plane perpendicular to the aortic centerline. Specifically, the analysis plane was placed at the level of the coronary arteries (i.e., coronary ostia) as this location provides a distinct anatomic feature for deformable registration during VDM(D) (Figure 3a). A normal vector to this analysis plane was obtained via cross-product of in-plane unit vectors. The green and magenta arrows in Figure 3b show normal vectors to the analysis plane in diastole and systole, respectively.

2.3.2. Displacement

Figure 3a represents the total, axial, and in-plane displacement vectors in 3D space. The total displacement (black arrow) was obtained by averaging the 3D displacement field as given by VDM(D) over the entire analysis plane. The axial displacement (orange arrow) was defined as the projection of the total displacement vector in the direction of the diastolic normal vector (green arrow in panel b). Conversely, the in-plane displacement (purple arrow) was defined as the projection of the total displacement in the direction perpendicular to the diastolic normal vector. In addition, relative displacements in axial and in-plane directions can be defined as follows:

$$Relative\ axial(in\text{-}plane) dislacement = \frac{axial(in\text{-}plane) displacement\ [mm]}{total\ displacement\ [mm]} \quad (1)$$

2.3.3. Distensibility and Area Ratio

Distensibility is a metric that reflects aortic stiffness as it includes changes in both strain and pressure. Here, the ratio between diastolic and systolic analysis plane areas was obtained to calculate the distensibility (Figure 3c) using the following formula [15]:

$$Distensibility\left[10^{-3}\ mmHg^{-1}\right] = \frac{A_{sys} - A_{dia}}{A_{dia}} \times \frac{1}{PP} = (area\ ratio - 1) \times \frac{1}{PP} \quad (2)$$

where A_{sys} and A_{dia} refer to the systolic and diastolic annulus areas, respectively, and PP is the pulse pressure. Area ratio is A_{sys}/A_{dia}.

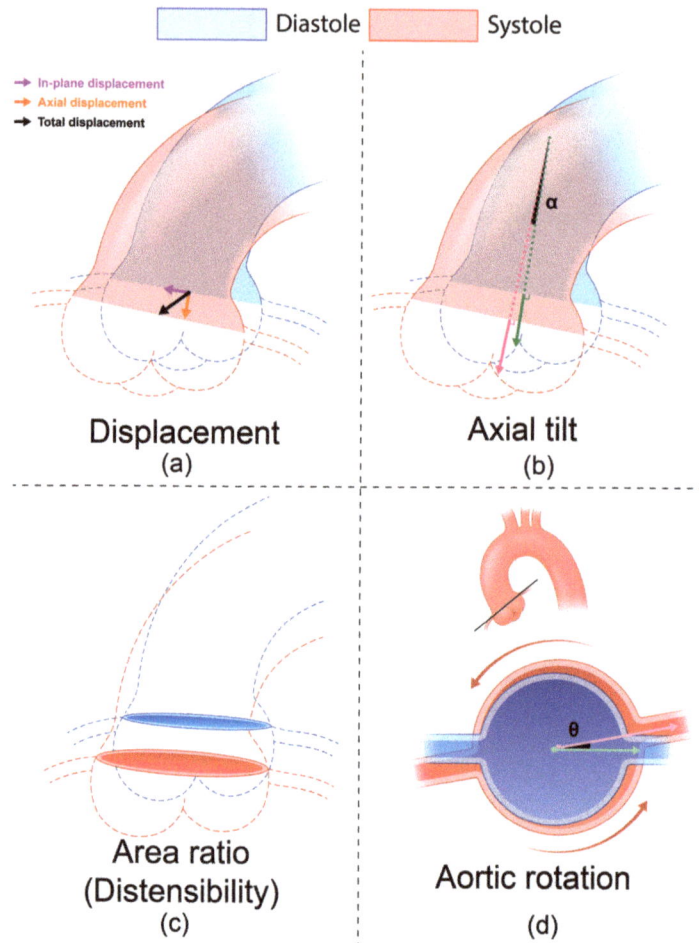

Figure 3. Four metrics of aortic root motion considered in this study, all calculated from 3D displacement extracted from VDM(D): (**a**) total, axial, and in-plane displacements, (**b**) axial tilt, (**c**) area ratio (distensibility), and (**d**) aortic rotation.

2.3.4. Axial Tilt and Aortic Rotation

The aortic root experiences a complex motion involving rotation and twisting around multiple axes due to its mechanical coupling with the contracting left ventricle. To characterize these complex rotations, in this paper we defined the following metrics.

Axial tilt α, defined as the angle between the diastolic (green arrow) and systolic (magenta arrow) normal vectors and their corresponding analysis plane areas (Figure 3b).

Aortic rotation θ, defined as the angle between two vectors from the centroid of the diastolic and systolic analysis plane areas and a reference point such as the initial point of the centerline of the left coronary artery (Figure 3d). Here, the green arrow represents the reference diastolic vector, and the magenta arrow represents the projection of the reference systolic vector onto the diastolic annulus plane. This aortic rotation θ represents the cyclic twisting motion of the aorta.

2.4. Statistical Analysis

Due to the small sample size of the different groups considered in this study (~10 subjects per group), we could not assume normal distribution behavior for each group. Therefore, a Kruskal–Wallis test was performed to compare different groups [16]. A p-value < 0.05 was considered significant. Correlations between variables were assessed using linear regression. Again, a p-value < 0.05 was considered a strong correlation. The 'kruskalwallis' and 'fitlm' MATLAB functions were used for the Kruskal–Wallis test and linear regression, respectively.

3. Results

3.1. Patient Demographics

The 51 subjects included in this study were divided into four groups, as follows: 13—non-aneurysmal; 15—TAA; 11—Marfan; and 12—repair. Patient demographics are shown in Table 1. Overall mean age was 55 ± 14.4 years old. Age distribution among the four groups is depicted in Figure 4 and Table 1. Age was significantly different between groups except between Marfan and non-aneurysmal groups, with the repair group demonstrating the highest mean age (Figure 4). Mean systolic/diastolic and pulse pressures were 127/71 mmHg and 56 mmHg, respectively, and did not differ across groups.

Table 1. Patient characteristics.

Characteristic ($n = 45$)	Non-Aneurysmal ($n = 13$)	TAA ($n = 15$)	Marfan ($n = 11$)	Repair ($n = 12$)	p-Value
Age (years)	48.6 ± 12.5	57.3 ± 9.5	43.1 ± 14.7	68.0 ± 9.0	<0.01
Female (n)	6	5	6	2	-
BP (systolic) (mmHg)	130 ± 22	125 ± 19	125 ± 17	129 ± 11	0.86
BP (diastolic) (mmHg)	77 ± 15	68 ± 8	69 ± 10	71 ± 10	0.21
Pulse pressure (mmHg)	53 ± 12	56 ± 19	56 ± 14	58 ± 16	0.86
HTN (n)	8	8	7	6	-
BAV (n)	0	6	1	0	-
AS (n)	0	5	0	0	-
AI (n)	0	3	0	0	-
CAD (n)	2	2	0	3	-
Hyperlipidemia (n)	2	7	2	5	-
Diameter (sinus) (mm)	32 ± 4	43 ± 5	43 ± 6	36 ± 5	<0.01
Diameter (STJ) (mm)	28 ± 3	43 ± 5	36 ± 6	32 ± 3	<0.01
Diameter (MAA) (mm)	30 ± 4	45 ± 4	33 ± 4	32 ± 3	<0.01
LV/Ao angle (degrees)	132.5 ± 9.5	134.4 ± 6.4	134.9 ± 7.4	126.4 ± 6.4	<0.01

Mean ± standard deviation. TAA = thoracic aortic aneurysm, BP = blood pressure, HTN = hypertension, BAV = bicuspid aortic valve, AS = aortic stenosis, AI = aortic insufficiency, CAD = coronary artery disease, STJ = sinotubular junction, MAA = mid-ascending aorta, LV/Ao angle = left-ventricular/aortic root angle.

TAA and Marfan groups demonstrated larger maximal sinus compared to the non-aneurysmal and repair groups (p-value < 0.001). Maximal diameter at the sinotubular junction (STJ) and mid-ascending aorta (MAA) was higher in the TAA group compared to the other groups (p-value < 0.001), concordant with the predilection for MAA dilation in sporadic TAA. LV/Ao angle was lowest in the repair group.

3.2. Aortic Root Motion Metrics

Figure 5 shows diastolic and systolic aortic geometries extracted from VDM(D) as well as the corresponding sinus contours at the analysis plane for representative subjects in each group (e.g., subject with motion patterns closest to the mean of the group). The 3D geometries and sinus contours demonstrate downward (axial) motion and contour expansion in systole across all groups and subjects. In addition, in-plane motion was apparent for all subjects but was lowest in the repair group. The non-aneurysmal and repair subjects show the largest and smallest axial displacements, respectively. The largest component of the aortic root motion in the repair subjects was in the in-plane direction.

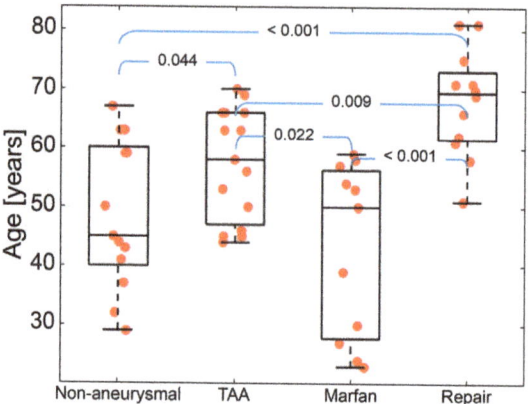

Figure 4. Age whiskers box plots for different groups; *p*-values are given at the top of the blue brackets.

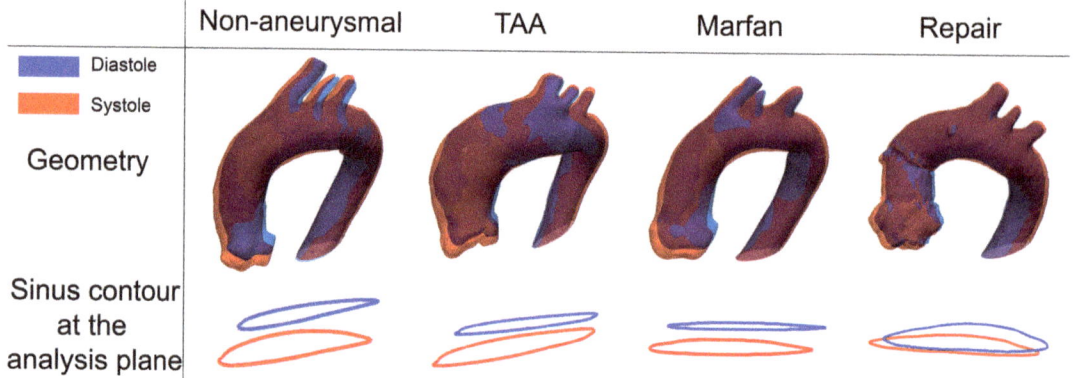

Figure 5. Diastolic (blue) and systolic (red) aortic geometries extracted from VDM(D) and the corresponding sinus contours at the analysis plane for representative subjects in each group.

Table 2 and Figure 6 summarize the results for the aortic root motion metrics across all patients and groups. On average, the repair group showed approximately 3.5 mm less total displacement than the other three groups; however, there was no significant difference between non-aneurysmal, TAA, and Marfan groups. The Marfan group showed the largest heterogeneity in total displacement (range: 1.77 to 10.03 mm). In contrast, the repair group demonstrated the narrowest range of total displacements (range: 1.93 to 4.99 mm, Figure 6a).

The axial and in-plane displacements show similar trends to the total displacement. The repair group showed significantly smaller axial and in-plane displacement than the other groups (Figure 6b,c). Table 2 also summarizes the relative axial and in-plane displacements (i.e., the directional component normalized by the total displacement). The repair group showed smaller relative axial displacement and larger relative in-plane displacement than the other three groups (p-value < 0.01). The non-aneurysmal group was the only group showing larger relative axial displacement (0.72) compared to relative in-plane displacement (0.66).

Table 2. Aortic root metrics for different subject groups.

	Non-Aneurysmal	TAA	Marfan	Repair
Sinus contour at the analysis plane (blue= diastolic, red= systolic)				
Displacement [mm] Total	7.34 ± 1.69	7.14 ± 2.30	7.01 ± 3.09	3.60 ± 1.00
Displacement [mm] Axial	5.20 ± 1.17	4.23 ± 2.27	4.84 ± 2.88	1.37 ± 1.14
Displacement [mm] In-plane	4.98 ± 1.93	5.33 ± 2.32	4.79 ± 2.08	3.13 ± 1.06
Relative axial displacement	0.72 ± 0.14	0.58 ± 0.27	0.63 ± 0.21	0.38 ± 0.26
Relative in-plane displacement	0.66 ± 0.14	0.68 ± 0.25	0.73 ± 0.17	0.88 ± 0.17
Axial tilt (degree)	3.06 ± 2.06	2.79 ± 1.65	2.96 ± 0.83	3.83 ± 2.08
Aortic rotation (degree)	1.93 ± 1.35	1.92 ± 0.97	1.70 ± 1.02	1.03 ± 0.43
Distensibility (10^{-3} mmHg^{-1})	2.21 ± 1.30	1.75 ± 0.37	1.34 ± 0.68	0.93 ± 0.26

Mean ± standard deviation. TAA = thoracic aortic aneurysm. Relative axial (in-plane) displacement = axial (in-plane) displacement/total displacement.

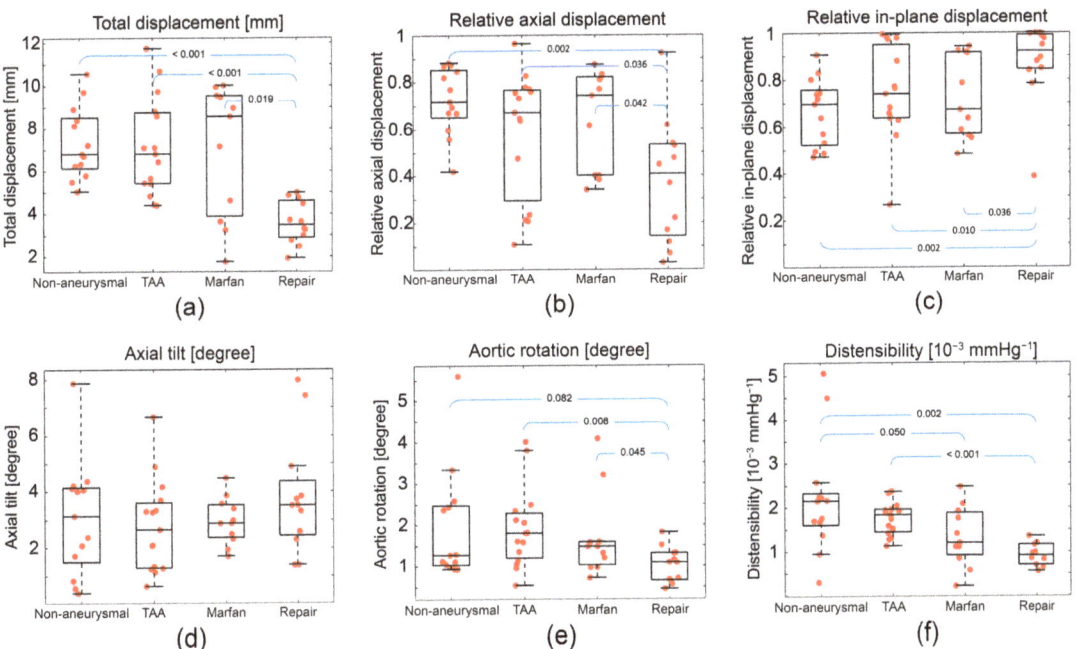

Figure 6. Whiskers box plots for the different subject groups: (**a**) total displacement, (**b**) axial displacement, (**c**) in-plane displacement, (**d**) axial tilt, (**e**) aortic rotation, and (**f**) distensibility; *p*-values are given at the top of the blue brackets.

There was no statistical difference in axial tilt between the four groups (Figure 6d). The repair group showed smaller aortic rotation values than the other groups (Figure 6e), but there was no statistical difference in rotation between non-aneurysmal, TAA, and Marfan groups. Figure 6f represents the distensibility results. The non-aneurysmal group showed higher median distensibility compared to the Marfan and repair groups; however, there was no statistical difference between non-aneurysmal and TAA groups. The TAA group displayed higher median distensibility compared to the repair group. The Marfan group showed the largest heterogeneity, with distensibility values ranging from 0.2 to 2.5×10^{-3} mmHg^{-1}. In contrast, the repair group shows the smallest heterogeneity in distensibility, ranging from 0.4 to 1.3×10^{-3} mmHg^{-1}.

3.3. Correlation with Age

Figure 7 summarizes the correlation between age and total displacement (panel a) and distensibility (panel b) for each group. Although each group showed a negative correlation between displacement and age, these correlations were weak–moderate and not statistically significant (Figure 7a). In contrast, there was a strong negative correlation between distensibility and age in the non-aneurysmal group but not in the other groups. In a subgroup of young patients (<40 years), distensibility was lower in Marfan compared to non-aneurysmal patients (1.73 vs. 4.04, p-value = 0.025).

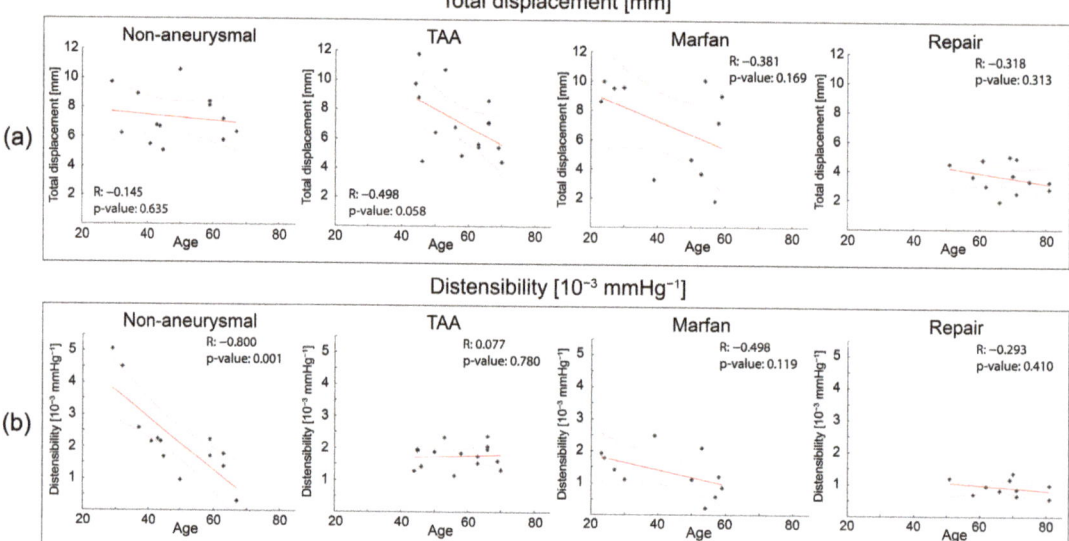

Figure 7. Scatter plots correlating (a) total displacement vs. age and (b) distensibility vs. age for the different subject groups. Solid and dotted red lines are fit and confidence bounds, respectively.

3.4. LV/Ao Angle Results

The LV/Ao angle (φ) represents the alignment between the aortic annulus and long-axis of the left ventricle (see Figure 1). The smaller this angle, the more perpendicularly oriented the heart and the aorta. Figure 8a summarizes the distribution of LV/Ao angles for each group. The repair group showed an approximately 5-degree smaller LV/Ao angle than the other groups. There was no statistical difference between non-aneurysmal, TAA, and Marfan groups. Combining the results in Figures 4 and 8a, we can appreciate that, in general, smaller LV/Ao angles are associated with older age.

Figure 8b,c illustrates the correlation between the LV/Ao angle and relative axial and in-plane displacements, respectively, for all subjects of all groups. Panel b shows that there was a strong positive correlation between LV/Ao angle and relative axial displacement. Conversely, Panel c shows a moderate negative correlation between LV/Ao angle and relative in-plane displacement.

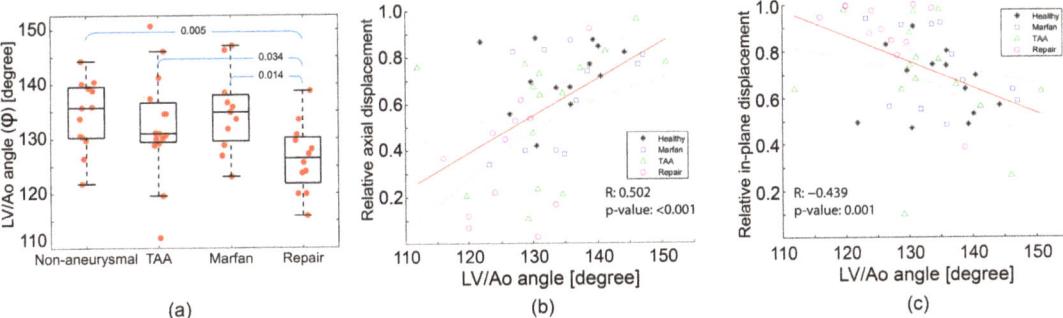

Figure 8. LV/Ao angle results. (**a**) Whiskers box plots of LV/Ao angle for each group; *p*-values are given at the top of the blue brackets. (**b**) Scatter plot correlating relative axial displacement and LV/Ao angle. (**c**) Scatter plot correlating relative in-plane displacement and LV/Ao angle. Solid and dotted red lines are fit and confidence bounds, respectively.

4. Discussion

High-level summary: In this study, 3D aortic root motion was characterized using dynamic CTA data and VDM(D) analysis. Aortic root motion metrics such as axial and in-plane displacements, area ratio/distensibility, axial tilt, aortic rotation, and LV/Ao angles were extracted and compared for four different subject groups: non-aneurysmal, TAA, Marfan, and repair. Our results revealed differences in aortic root motion metrics, most notably between the repair group and other groups with native ascending aortas. The repair group showed the smallest aortic root displacement, aortic rotation, and distensibility compared to other groups. There was no difference in axial tilt between groups. The repair group was also the only group that showed a larger relative in-plane displacement than relative axial displacement, likely explained by the lowest (i.e., more perpendicular) LV/Ao angle in this group. The Marfan group showed the largest heterogeneity in aortic root displacement, distensibility, and age, compatible with well-reported heterogeneity in this syndrome. We also showed that there were moderate–strong correlations between LV/Ao angle and relative axial and in-plane displacements.

This study adds several clinically relevant advances and insights. First, our proposed method is performed on ECG-gated dynamic CTA data acquired as part of routine clinical care. Thus, this is a technique that can be applied to routine clinical imaging without the need for non-standard or research imaging techniques. Second, given that stresses in the ascending aorta are in part determined by the downward pulling on the aortic root by the LV and that there is a large body of evidence connecting aortic stresses to disease progression and development of complications such as aortic dissection, the analytic tools to assess root motion may yield important insights into a patient's disease severity that may have implications for risk stratification. Additionally, our methods could be employed to better understand the biomechanical effects of stiff fabric or metallic endografts on aortic function. Clearly, making these inferences will require substantial additional research, but the immediate applicability of techniques to clinical data will greatly lessen barriers to these translational studies.

Repair group: Table 2 and Figure 6 show that the repair group presented smaller and more homogeneous displacements and rotations than the other groups. These findings are consistent with previous studies [17], indicative of the higher graft stiffness relative to the native aortic tissue [18,19]. Distensibility was also lowest in the repair group, an expected finding given the very stiff properties of synthetic fabric vascular grafts [20–22].

Marfan group: The Marfan group had the largest heterogeneity in displacement and distensibility (Figure 6) as well as in age (Figure 4). Such heterogeneity has been previously documented among patients with MFS [23]. While a pathogenic mutation in the fibrillin-1 gene is pathognomonic of MFS disease, it is well recognized that large degrees of phenotypic heterogeneity exist between patients, an observation that aligns with the variability we observed in root motion and mechanical metrics studied in this paper [24]. From a clinical perspective, methods to define the phenotypic severity of disease are greatly desirable, particularly at earlier stages of disease, to allow for improved estimates of risk and better-informed decisions surrounding prophylactic aortic repair. Given that aortic aneurysm is one of the defining manifestations of MFS disease and a leading cause of morbidity and mortality, novel methods that can better understand the severity of aortic disease may be impactful. A prior study using echocardiography to assess root distensibility in MFS demonstrated the same heterogeneity in these metrics that we observed [25]. However, this study did not examine the additional root motion metrics we considered in our work. Thus, while there is still much to learn about the clinical significance of such findings, we are encouraged by both replicating previous observations and identifying differences in root motion and distensibility metrics in a disease that is known to present highly variable manifestations between different affected individuals.

Distensibility: Our results revealed that the Marfan and repair groups had lower aortic root distensibility than the non-aneurysmal and TAA groups, in alignment with prior reports [21,26]. Interestingly, we observed no statistical difference between non-aneurysmal and TAA groups (Figure 6f), in contrast with prior studies that have reported higher aortic stiffness in TAA compared to non-aneurysmal aortas [27–29]. This discrepancy may be explained by several factors. First, the location where aortic motion is extracted in our study is at sinuses of Valsalva, which is different from the location of maximum aneurysm diameter in our TAA subjects, suggesting a potential gradient in distensibility (and therefore stiffness) from the aortic root to the aneurysm location in TAA subjects. Secondly, we may have simply failed to capture a statistical difference in these groups owing to relatively small group sizes and the confounding effects of age on aortic stiffness in the non-aneurysmal group.

LV/Ao angle: Previous studies have reported a negative correlation between age and LV/Ao angle [30,31]. Our results are consistent with these studies (see Appendix A, Figure A1). To better understand the correlation between LV/Ao angle and root motion metrics, we examined relative aortic displacements normalized to total displacement given that LV/Ao angle would be expected to affect the directional proportion of root motion more than its absolute degree (more reflective of the underlying aortic pathology). Further, normalizing the displacements allowed us to mitigate the relationship between age and aortic displacement and therefore to directly compare all subjects across groups.

Variation of metrics with age: Previous studies have reported clearly demonstrated increasing aortic stiffness with aging [32–34]. Therefore, the negative correlation between age and distensibility (inversely related to stiffness) in the non-aneurysmal group (Figure 7b) is consistent with prior results. However, the TAA, Marfan, and repair groups did not show significant correlations between distensibility and age. All three groups presented lower distensibility compared to the non-aneurysmal group. For instance, young (<40 years) Marfan subjects had lower distensibility compared to non-aneurysmal patients (1.73 vs. 4.04, p-value = 0.025). This suggests that the effects of aortic stiffening related to these patients' aneurysmal disease supersedes the effects of age-related aortic stiffening.

Figure 7a shows that there was no strong correlation between age and aortic root displacement. Only the TAA group suggested a pattern of larger total displacements for younger subjects. However, this TAA group is highly heterogenous with six bicuspid aortic valve, five aortic stenosis, and three aortic insufficiency patients. Unlike distensibility, which is dictated by aortic properties only, aortic root displacement results from the interactions between heart and aorta. Previous studies have reported that there is no significant correlation between age and LV ejection fraction [35,36]. Therefore, one could argue that aortic root motion is independent of age unless heart function is compromised.

Correlation with aortic diameter: Aortic diameter has been widely used as a clinical metric to assess aortic disease severity and progression [25,37,38]. However, numerous studies have demonstrated its poor predictive value [39–41]. Our results agree with such studies as we have observed no significant correlation between sinus diameter, distensibility, and aortic displacement (see Appendix A, Figure A2).

4.1. Displacement Extraction Comparison between 2D and 3D

Most studies thus far have characterized aortic root motion using 2D approaches [5,7–9,17,42,43]. However, extracting aortic root motion from 2D images without accounting for the full 3D motion of the aorta may provide a distorted assessment. Figure 9 illustrates diastolic (blue) and systolic (red) aortic geometries extracted from VDM(D) for a non-aneurysmal subject. The motion is observed under two different views. View 1 shows that there is an axial (downward) motion and almost no in-plane motion. However, view 2 shows that there are both axial and in-plane displacements. This is a simple demonstration of how a VDM(D) analysis of dynamic CTA data can more fully capture 3D motion of the root compared to 2D approaches.

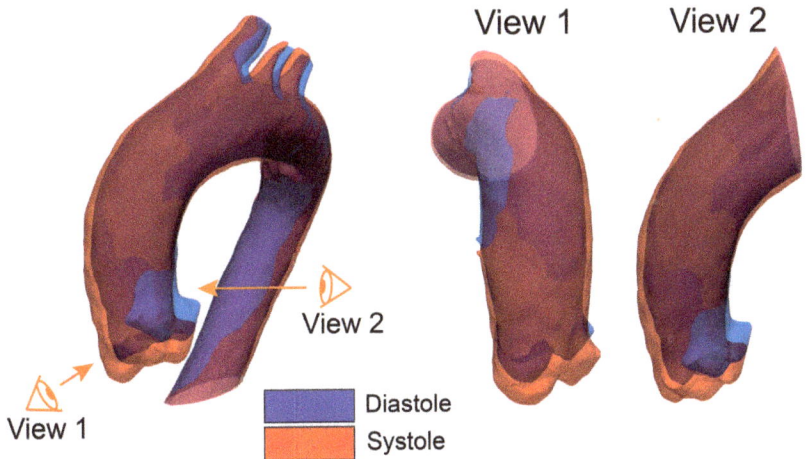

Figure 9. Diastolic (blue) and systolic (red) aortic geometries extracted from VDM(D) for a non-aneurysmal subject. Two different 2D views provide different characterizations of aortic root motion.

4.2. Implications for Aortic Wall Stress Analysis

Three-dimensional aortic root motion extracted from VDM(D) can be used to provide improved boundary conditions for aortic wall stress analysis [44,45]. Most previous computational studies of ascending aortic stress hold the inlet boundary as fixed (no root motion) [46–50]. Few studies have investigated the effect of aortic root motion on ascending aortic wall stress under simplified and unidirectional (e.g., axial) aortic root motion assumptions [5,7,51]. A recent study demonstrated that in-plane displacements contribute significantly to the stress level in the ascending aorta [8]. However, this study considered simplified, circumferentially uniform values of in-plane displacements extracted from 2D dimensional data. In reality, the aortic root has circumferentially variable in-plane and axial displacements which can be fully quantified by VDM(D). This 3D information could be used to define improved boundary conditions for aortic wall stress analysis.

4.3. Limitations

The small number of subjects per group is one limitation of this study which may result in a lack of strong correlations for some of the reported aortic root metrics in some of the subject groups. The composition of the TAA group was heterogenous as one third of the patients had BAV, one third had aortic stenosis, and one fifth had aortic insufficiency. These comorbidities may have an impact on aortic root motion. However, the primary objective of this study was to assess feasibility of VDM(D) rather than provide a comprehensive assessment of metrics across different patient groups and characteristics. Future studies will expand the sample size of the TAA group and thus enable us to define subgroups according to the presence or absence of valvular disease.

Additionally, the different patient groups had statistically significant differences in age. As expected, the TAA and repair groups were older than non-aneurysmal and Marfan groups (Figure 4). These trends therefore reflect the strong association between sporadic/degenerative TAA and age [52]. The Marfan group was youngest overall and had the largest variability in age (from mid-20s to nearly 60 years old), consistent with the well-known variability in phenotypes among Marfan patients [20]. Future studies using groups matched on age and other characteristics will be important to more fully understand the unique contribution of such factors on the described aortic root motion metrics.

Lastly, this study focused on establishing the feasibility of VDM(D) analysis using dynamic CTA data rather than comparing our method against other 2D root motion methods using cardiac MRI (CMR) or echocardiography. Such a comparative study, while interesting, would require prospective studies since it is highly unlikely that a patient would have analyzable images from all three modalities to allow assessment of inter-modality agreement.

5. Conclusions

VDM(D) analysis of dynamic CTA data enables a rigorous characterization of 3D aortic root motion. Directional aortic displacements, area ratio and distensibility, axial tilt, and aortic rotation can be extracted across a variety of TAA etiologies as well as in post-repair groups. Our results revealed differences in aortic root motion metrics, most notably between the repair group and other groups with native aortic tissue. The non-aneurysmal group showed a negative correlation between age and distensibility, consistent with widely reported age-related aortic stiffening. Additionally, our results demonstrated that the LV/Ao angle is an important determinant of the proportions of axial and in-plane displacements and should thus be included in future studies focused on dynamic assessment of the ascending aorta.

Author Contributions: Conceptualization, T.K., N.S.T., N.S.B. and C.A.F.; data curation, N.S.T. and N.S.B.; formal analysis, T.K., N.S.T., N.S.B. and C.A.F.; funding acquisition, H.J.P., N.S.B. and C.A.F.; investigation, T.K., N.S.T., N.S.B. and C.A.F.; methodology, T.K., N.S.T., N.S.B. and C.A.F.; project administration, N.S.B. and C.A.F.; resources, J.v.H., H.J.P., N.S.B. and C.A.F.; software, T.K. and X.H.; supervision, J.v.H., N.S.B. and C.A.F.; validation, H.J.P., N.S.B. and C.A.F.; visualization, T.K.; writing—original draft, T.K., N.S.T., N.S.B. and C.A.F.; writing—review and editing, T.K., N.S.T., X.H., J.v.H., H.J.P., N.S.B. and C.A.F. All authors have read and agreed to the published version of the manuscript.

Funding: This research was funded as follows. N.S.B: National Institutes of Health (SBIRR44 HL145953); H.J.P.: David Hamilton Fund, Phil Jenkins Breakthrough Fund, and Joe D. Morris Collegiate Professorship in Cardiac Surgery; C.A.F.: Edward B. Diethrich Professorship in Biomedical Engineering and Vascular Surgery, MI-AORTA at the Samuel and Jean Frankel Cardiovascular Center, University of Michigan.

Institutional Review Board Statement: All procedures were approved by the local institutional review board and were Health Insurance Portability and Accountability Act-compliant. A waiver of informed consent was obtained for this retrospective study.

Informed Consent Statement: Informed consent was waived for subjects involved in the study due to its retrospective nature.

Data Availability Statement: The data presented in this study are available on request from the corresponding author.

Conflicts of Interest: The authors declare no conflict of interest.

Appendix A

Figure A1 presents the correlation between LV/Ao angle and age. Figure A2 presents the correlation between sinus diameter and (a) total displacement and (b) distensibility.

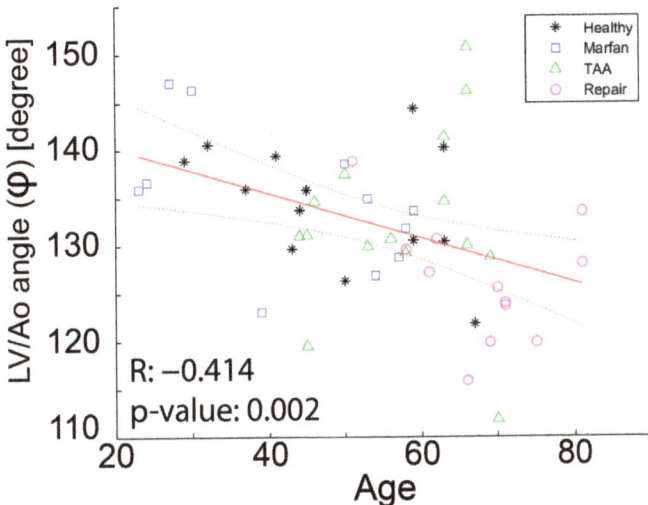

Figure A1. Scatter plot correlating LV/Ao angle and age. Solid and dotted red lines are fit and confidence bounds, respectively.

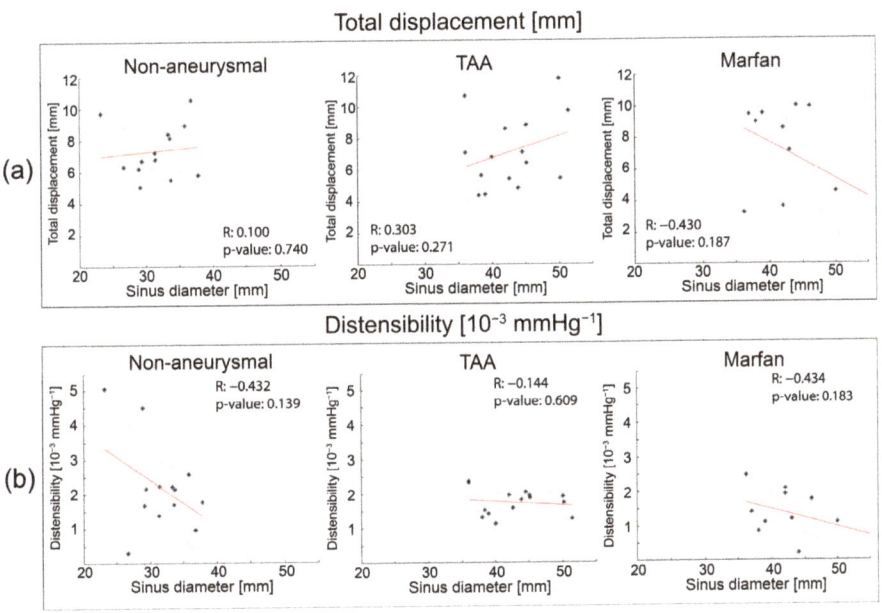

Figure A2. Scatter plot correlating (a) sinus diameter vs. total displacement and (b) sinus diameter vs. distensibility. Solid and dotted red lines are fit and confidence bounds, respectively.

References

1. Chau, K.H.; Elefteriades, J.A. Natural history of thoracic aortic aneurysms: Size matters, plus moving beyond size. *Prog. Cardiovasc. Dis.* **2013**, *56*, 74–80. [CrossRef]
2. Elefteriades, J.A.; Farkas, E.A. Thoracic aortic aneurysm: Clinically pertinent controversies and uncertainties. *J. Am. Coll. Cardiol.* **2010**, *55*, 841–857. [CrossRef] [PubMed]
3. Freeman, L.A.; Young, P.M.; Foley, T.A.; Williamson, E.E.; Bruce, C.J.; Greason, K.L. CT and MRI assessment of the aortic root and ascending aorta. *Am. J. Roentgenol.* **2013**, *200*, W581–W592. [CrossRef] [PubMed]
4. Desjardins, B.; Kazerooni, E.A. ECG-gated cardiac CT. *Am. J. Roentgenol.* **2004**, *182*, 993–1010. [CrossRef] [PubMed]
5. Beller, C.J.; Labrosse, M.R.; Thubrikar, M.J.; Robicsek, F. Role of aortic root motion in the pathogenesis of aortic dissection. *Circulation* **2004**, *109*, 763–769. [CrossRef] [PubMed]
6. Cutugno, S.; Agnese, V.; Gentile, G.; Raffa, G.M.; Wisneski, A.D.; Guccione, J.M.; Pilato, M.; Pasta, S. Patient-specific analysis of ascending thoracic aortic aneurysm with the living heart human model. *Bioengineering* **2021**, *8*, 175. [CrossRef]
7. Singh, S.; Xu, X.; Pepper, J.; Izgi, C.; Treasure, T.; Mohiaddin, R. Effects of aortic root motion on wall stress in the Marfan aorta before and after personalised aortic root support (PEARS) surgery. *J. Biomech.* **2016**, *49*, 2076–2084. [CrossRef]
8. Wei, W.; Evin, M.; Rapacchi, S.; Kober, F.; Bernard, M.; Jacquier, A.; Kahn, C.J.; Behr, M. Investigating heartbeat-related in-plane motion and stress levels induced at the aortic root. *BioMedical Eng. OnLine* **2019**, *18*, 1–15. [CrossRef]
9. Kozerke, S.; Scheidegger, M.B.; Pedersen, E.M.; Boesiger, P. Heart motion adapted cine phase-contrast flow measurements through the aortic valve. *Magn. Reson. Med. Off. J. Int. Soc. Magn. Reson. Med.* **1999**, *42*, 970–978. [CrossRef]
10. Burris, N.S.; Bian, Z.; Dominic, J.; Zhong, J.; Houben, I.B.; van Bakel, T.M.; Patel, H.J.; Ross, B.D.; Christensen, G.E.; Hatt, C.R. Vascular deformation mapping for CT surveillance of thoracic aortic aneurysm growth. *Radiology* **2022**, *302*, 218–225. [CrossRef]
11. Burris, N.S.; Hoff, B.A.; Kazerooni, E.A.; Ross, B.D. Vascular deformation mapping (VDM) of thoracic aortic enlargement in aneurysmal disease and dissection. *Tomography* **2017**, *3*, 163–173. [CrossRef] [PubMed]
12. Burris, N.S.; Hoff, B.A.; Patel, H.J.; Kazerooni, E.A.; Ross, B.D. Three-dimensional growth analysis of thoracic aortic aneurysm with vascular deformation mapping. *Circ. Cardiovasc. Imaging* **2018**, *11*, e008045. [CrossRef]
13. Rosset, A.; Spadola, L.; Ratib, O.J. OsiriX: An open-source software for navigating in multidimensional DICOM images. *J. Digit. Imaging* **2004**, *17*, 205–216. [CrossRef]
14. Zhong, J.; Bian, Z.; Hatt, C.R.; Burris, N.S. Segmentation of the thoracic aorta using an attention-gated u-net. In Proceedings of the Medical Imaging 2021: Computer-Aided Diagnosis, Online, 15–20 February 2021; pp. 147–153.
15. Groenink, M.; de Roos, A.; Mulder, B.J.; Spaan, J.A.; van der Wall, E.E. Changes in aortic distensibility and pulse wave velocity assessed with magnetic resonance imaging following beta-blocker therapy in the Marfan syndrome. *Am. J. Cardiol.* **1998**, *82*, 203–208. [CrossRef] [PubMed]
16. Kruskal, W.H.; Wallis, W.A. Use of ranks in one-criterion variance analysis. *J. Am. Stat. Assoc.* **1952**, *47*, 583–621. [CrossRef]
17. Izgi, C.; Nyktari, E.; Alpendurada, F.; Bruenger, A.S.; Pepper, J.; Treasure, T.; Mohiaddin, R. Effect of personalized external aortic root support on aortic root motion and distension in Marfan syndrome patients. *Int. J. Cardiol.* **2015**, *197*, 154–160. [CrossRef]
18. De Beaufort, H.W.; Conti, M.; Kamman, A.V.; Nauta, F.J.; Lanzarone, E.; Moll, F.L.; Van Herwaarden, J.A.; Auricchio, F.; Trimarchi, S. Stent-graft deployment increases aortic stiffness in an ex vivo porcine model. *Ann. Vasc. Surg.* **2017**, *43*, 302–308. [CrossRef]
19. Takeda, Y.; Sakata, Y.; Ohtani, T.; Tamaki, S.; Omori, Y.; Tsukamoto, Y.; Aizawa, Y.; Shimamura, K.; Shirakawa, Y.; Kuratani, T. Endovascular aortic repair increases vascular stiffness and alters cardiac structure and function. *Circ. J.* **2014**, *78*, 322–328. [CrossRef]
20. Ioannou, C.; Stergiopulos, N.; Katsamouris, A.; Startchik, I.; Kalangos, A.; Licker, M.; Westerhof, N.; Morel, D. Hemodynamics induced after acute reduction of proximal thoracic aorta compliance. *Eur. J. Vasc. Endovasc. Surg.* **2003**, *26*, 195–204. [CrossRef] [PubMed]
21. Tremblay, D.; Zigras, T.; Cartier, R.; Leduc, L.; Butany, J.; Mongrain, R.; Leask, R.L. A comparison of mechanical properties of materials used in aortic arch reconstruction. *Ann. Thorac. Surg.* **2009**, *88*, 1484–1491. [CrossRef]
22. Spadaccio, C.; Nappi, F.; Al-Attar, N.; Sutherland, F.W.; Acar, C.; Nenna, A.; Trombetta, M.; Chello, M.; Rainer, A.J. Old myths, new concerns: The long-term effects of ascending aorta replacement with dacron grafts. Not all that glitters is gold. *J. Cardiovasc. Transl. Res.* **2016**, *9*, 334–342. [CrossRef]
23. Baumgartner, C.; Matyas, G.; Steinmann, B.; Baumgartner, D. Marfan syndrome—A diagnostic challenge caused by phenotypic and genetic heterogeneity. *Methods Inf. Med.* **2005**, *44*, 487–497. [PubMed]
24. Seo, G.H.; Kim, Y.-M.; Kang, E.; Kim, G.-H.; Seo, E.-J.; Lee, B.H.; Choi, J.-H.; Yoo, H.-W. The phenotypic heterogeneity of patients with Marfan-related disorders and their variant spectrums. *Medicine* **2018**, *97*, e10767. [CrossRef]
25. de Wit, A.; Vis, K.; Jeremy, R.W. Aortic stiffness in heritable aortopathies: Relationship to aneurysm growth rate. *Heart Lung Circ.* **2013**, *22*, 3–11. [CrossRef] [PubMed]
26. van Andel, M.M.; de Waard, V.; Timmermans, J.; Scholte, A.J.; van den Berg, M.P.; Zwinderman, A.H.; Mulder, B.J.; Groenink, M. Aortic distensibility in Marfan syndrome: A potential predictor of aortic events? *Open Heart* **2021**, *8*, e001775. [CrossRef] [PubMed]
27. Kolipaka, A.; Illapani, V.S.P.; Kenyhercz, W.; Dowell, J.D.; Go, M.R.; Starr, J.E.; Vaccaro, P.S.; White, R.D. Quantification of abdominal aortic aneurysm stiffness using magnetic resonance elastography and its comparison to aneurysm diameter. *J. Vasc. Surg.* **2016**, *64*, 966–974. [CrossRef]

28. Perissiou, M.; Bailey, T.G.; Windsor, M.; Greaves, K.; Nam, M.C.; Russell, F.D.; O'Donnell, J.; Magee, R.; Jha, P.; Schulze, K.; et al. Aortic and systemic arterial stiffness responses to acute exercise in patients with small abdominal aortic aneurysms. *European J. Vasc. Endovasc. Surg.* **2019**, *58*, 708–718. [CrossRef]
29. van Disseldorp, E.M.; Petterson, N.J.; van de Vosse, F.N.; van Sambeek, M.R.; Lopata, R.G. Quantification of aortic stiffness and wall stress in healthy volunteers and abdominal aortic aneurysm patients using time-resolved 3D ultrasound: A comparison study. *Eur. Heart J. Cardiovasc. Imaging* **2019**, *20*, 185–191. [CrossRef]
30. Kwon, D.H.; Smedira, N.G.; Popovic, Z.B.; Lytle, B.W.; Setser, R.; Thamilarasan, M.; Schoenhagen, P.; Flamm, S.D.; Lever, H.M.; Desai, M.Y. Steep left ventricle to aortic root angle and hypertrophic obstructive cardiomyopathy: Study of a novel association using three-dimensional multimodality imaging. *Heart* **2009**, *95*, 1784–1791. [CrossRef]
31. Swinne, C.J.; Shapiro, E.P.; Jamart, J.; Fleg, J.L. Age-associated changes in left ventricular outflow tract geometry in normal subjects. *Am. J. Cardiol.* **1996**, *78*, 1070–1073. [CrossRef]
32. Cuomo, F.; Roccabianca, S.; Dillon-Murphy, D.; Xiao, N.; Humphrey, J.D.; Figueroa, C.A. Effects of age-associated regional changes in aortic stiffness on human hemodynamics revealed by computational modeling. *PLoS ONE* **2017**, *12*, e0173177. [CrossRef] [PubMed]
33. Hickson, S.S.; Butlin, M.; Graves, M.; Taviani, V.; Avolio, A.P.; McEniery, C.M.; Wilkinson, I.B. The relationship of age with regional aortic stiffness and diameter. *JACC Cardiovasc. Imaging* **2010**, *3*, 1247–1255. [CrossRef] [PubMed]
34. O'Rourke, M.F.; Nichols, W.W. Aortic diameter, aortic stiffness, and wave reflection increase with age and isolated systolic hypertension. *Hypertension* **2005**, *45*, 652–658. [CrossRef]
35. Cain, P.A.; Ahl, R.; Hedstrom, E.; Ugander, M.; Allansdotter-Johnsson, A.; Friberg, P.; Arheden, H. Age and gender specific normal values of left ventricular mass, volume and function for gradient echo magnetic resonance imaging: A cross sectional study. *BMC Med. Imaging* **2009**, *9*, 1–10. [CrossRef]
36. Port, S.; Cobb, F.R.; Coleman, R.E.; Jones, R.H. Effect of age on the response of the left ventricular ejection fraction to exercise. *N. Engl. J. Med.* **1980**, *303*, 1133–1137. [CrossRef] [PubMed]
37. Nollen, G.J.; Groenink, M.; Tijssen, J.G.; Van Der Wall, E.E.; Mulder, B.J. Aortic stiffness and diameter predict progressive aortic dilatation in patients with Marfan syndrome. *Eur. Heart J.* **2004**, *25*, 1146–1152. [CrossRef]
38. Vriz, O.; Driussi, C.; Bettio, M.; Ferrara, F.; D'Andrea, A.; Bossone, E. Aortic root dimensions and stiffness in healthy subjects. *Am. J. Cardiol.* **2013**, *112*, 1224–1229. [CrossRef]
39. Duprey, A.; Trabelsi, O.; Vola, M.; Favre, J.-P.; Avril, S. Biaxial rupture properties of ascending thoracic aortic aneurysms. *Acta Biomater.* **2016**, *42*, 273–285. [CrossRef]
40. Pichamuthu, J.E.; Phillippi, J.A.; Cleary, D.A.; Chew, D.W.; Hempel, J.; Vorp, D.A.; Gleason, T.G. Differential tensile strength and collagen composition in ascending aortic aneurysms by aortic valve phenotype. *Ann. Thorac. Surg.* **2013**, *96*, 2147–2154. [CrossRef]
41. Vianna, E.; Kramer, B.; Tarraf, S.; Gillespie, C.; Colbrunn, R.; Bellini, C.; Roselli, E.E.; Cikach, F.; Germano, E.; Emerton, K.; et al. Aortic diameter is a poor predictor of aortic tissue failure metrics in patients with ascending aneurysms. *J. Thorac. Cardiovasc. Surg.* **2022**, in press. [CrossRef]
42. Weber, T.F.; Ganten, M.-K.; Böckler, D.; Geisbüsch, P.; Kauczor, H.-U.; von Tengg-Kobligk, H. Heartbeat-related displacement of the thoracic aorta in patients with chronic aortic dissection type B: Quantification by dynamic CTA. *Eur. J. Radiol.* **2009**, *72*, 483–488. [CrossRef]
43. Rengier, F.; Weber, T.F.; Henninger, V.; Böckler, D.; Schumacher, H.; Kauczor, H.-U.; von Tengg-Kobligk, H. Heartbeat-related distension and displacement of the thoracic aorta in healthy volunteers. *Eur. J. Radiol.* **2012**, *81*, 158–164. [CrossRef]
44. Moireau, P.; Xiao, N.; Astorino, M.; Figueroa, C.A.; Chapelle, D.; Taylor, C.A.; Gerbeau, J.-F. External tissue support and fluid–structure simulation in blood flows. *Biomech. Model. Mechanobiol.* **2012**, *11*, 1–18. [CrossRef]
45. Maeda, E.; Ando, Y.; Takeshita, K.; Matsumoto, T. Through the cleared aorta: Three-dimensional characterization of mechanical behaviors of rat thoracic aorta under intraluminal pressurization using optical clearing method. *Sci. Rep.* **2022**, *12*, 8632. [CrossRef] [PubMed]
46. Meierhofer, C.; Schneider, E.P.; Lyko, C.; Hutter, A.; Martinoff, S.; Markl, M.; Hager, A.; Hess, J.; Stern, H.; Fratz, S. Wall shear stress and flow patterns in the ascending aorta in patients with bicuspid aortic valves differ significantly from tricuspid aortic valves: A prospective study. *Eur. Heart J. Cardiovasc. Imaging* **2013**, *14*, 797–804. [CrossRef] [PubMed]
47. Nathan, D.P.; Xu, C.; Plappert, T.; Desjardins, B.; Gorman, J.H., III; Bavaria, J.E.; Gorman, R.C.; Chandran, K.B.; Jackson, B.M. Increased ascending aortic wall stress in patients with bicuspid aortic valves. *Ann. Thorac. Surg.* **2011**, *92*, 1384–1389. [CrossRef]
48. Nathan, D.P.; Xu, C.; Gorman III, J.H.; Fairman, R.M.; Bavaria, J.E.; Gorman, R.C.; Chandran, K.B.; Jackson, B.M. Pathogenesis of acute aortic dissection: A finite element stress analysis. *Ann. Thorac. Surg.* **2011**, *91*, 458–463. [CrossRef]
49. Di Martino, E.S.; Guadagni, G.; Fumero, A.; Ballerini, G.; Spirito, R.; Biglioli, P.; Redaelli, A. Fluid–structure interaction within realistic three-dimensional models of the aneurysmatic aorta as a guidance to assess the risk of rupture of the aneurysm. *Med. Eng. Phys.* **2001**, *23*, 647–655. [CrossRef] [PubMed]
50. Venkatasubramaniam, A.; Fagan, M.; Mehta, T.; Mylankal, K.; Ray, B.; Kuhan, G.; Chetter, I.; McCollum, P. A comparative study of aortic wall stress using finite element analysis for ruptured and non-ruptured abdominal aortic aneurysms. *Eur. J. Vasc. Endovasc. Surg.* **2004**, *28*, 168–176.

51. Martin, C.; Sun, W.; Elefteriades, J. Patient-specific finite element analysis of ascending aorta aneurysms. *Am. J. Physiol. Heart Circ. Physiol.* **2015**, *308*, H1306–H1316. [CrossRef]
52. Schwarze, M.L.; Shen, Y.; Hemmerich, J.; Dale, W. Age-related trends in utilization and outcome of open and endovascular repair for abdominal aortic aneurysm in the United States, 2001–2006. *J. Vasc. Surg.* **2009**, *50*, 722–729.e2. [CrossRef] [PubMed]

Disclaimer/Publisher's Note: The statements, opinions and data contained in all publications are solely those of the individual author(s) and contributor(s) and not of MDPI and/or the editor(s). MDPI and/or the editor(s) disclaim responsibility for any injury to people or property resulting from any ideas, methods, instructions or products referred to in the content.

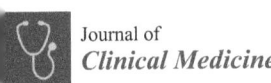

Article

Increased Aortic Exclusion in Endovascular Treatment of Complex Aortic Aneurysms [†]

Merel Verhagen [1], Daniel Eefting [1], Carla van Rijswijk [2], Rutger van der Meer [2], Jaap Hamming [1], Joost van der Vorst [1] and Jan van Schaik [1,*]

1 Department of Vascular Surgery, Leiden University Medical Center, 2333 ZA Leiden, The Netherlands; m.j.verhagen@lumc.nl (M.V.); d.eefting@lumc.nl (D.E.); j.f.hamming@lumc.nl (J.H.); j.r.van_der_vorst@lumc.nl (J.v.d.V.)
2 Department of Radiology, Leiden University Medical Center, 2333 ZA Leiden, The Netherlands; c.s.p.van_rijswijk@lumc.nl (C.v.R.); r.w.van_der_meer@lumc.nl (R.v.d.M.)
* Correspondence: j.van_schaik@lumc.nl
† Meeting presentation: This study was accepted for presentation at the European Society for Vascular Surgery (ESVS) Annual Meeting in Rome, Italy, 20–23 September 2022.

Abstract: Purpose: Perioperative risk assessments for complex aneurysms are based on the anatomical extent of the aneurysm and do not take the length of the aortic exclusion into account, as it was developed for open repair. Nevertheless, in the endovascular repair (ER) of complex aortic aneurysms, additional segments of healthy aorta are excluded compared with open repair (OR). The aim of this study was to assess differences in aortic exclusion between the ER and OR of complex aortic aneurysms, to subsequently assess the current classification for complex aneurysm repair. Methods: This retrospective observational study included patients that underwent complex endovascular aortic aneurysm repair by means of fenestrated endovascular aneurysm repair (FEVAR), fenestrated and branched EVAR (FBEVAR), or branched EVAR (BEVAR). The length of aortic exclusion and the number of patent segmental arteries were determined and compared per case in ER and hypothetical OR, using a Wilcoxon signed-rank test. Results: A total of 71 patients were included, who were treated with FEVAR (n = 44), FBEVAR (n = 8), or BEVAR (n = 19) for Crawford types I (n = 5), II (n = 7), III (n = 6), IV (n = 7), and V (n = 2) thoracoabdominal or juxtarenal (n = 44) aneurysms. There was a significant increase in the median exclusion of types I, II, III, IV, and juxtarenal aneurysms ($p < 0.05$) in ER, compared with hypothetical OR. The number of patent segmental arteries in the ER of type I–IV and juxtarenal aneurysms was significantly lower than in hypothetical OR ($p < 0.05$). Conclusion: There are significant differences in the length of aortic exclusion between ER and hypothetical OR, with the increased exclusion in ER resulting in a lower number of patent segmental arteries. The ER and OR of complex aortic aneurysms should be regarded as distinct modalities, and as each approach deserves a particular risk assessment, future efforts should focus on reporting on the extent of exclusion per treatment modality, to allow for appropriate comparison.

Keywords: complex aortic aneurysm; endovascular repair; open repair; aortic exclusion; Crawford classification

1. Introduction

The current classification for complex aortic aneurysms is based on the anatomical extent of the aneurysm. With the management of complex aortic aneurysms always having been associated with significant rates of adverse outcomes, the purpose of the original Crawford classification was to recognize differences in the intra- and postoperative risks of complications and mortality in the open repair of these aneurysms [1]. Based on the anatomical dimensions, aortic aneurysms were categorized in types I–IV, with Safi et al. later adding type V [2,3], which contributed greatly to standardized reporting in complex aortic surgery.

With the availability of endovascular repair for complex aortic aneurysms, management options have significantly increased as more frail patients can be considered for surgery [4,5]. The treatment modality offers therapeutic options for patients unfit for open surgery due to decreased cardio-pulmonary stress, blood loss, and surgical trauma [6,7]. However, endovascular treatment leads to an increase in aortic exclusion compared with open repair, as a result of additional segments of healthy aorta being sacrificed in order to ensure adequate proximal and distal seal [8–10]. As a consequence of the increased extent of aortic exclusion in endovascular repair, the Crawford classification, based on the anatomical extent of the aneurysm, might not provide for an accurate assessment of full aortic exclusion in endovascular repair. Imaginably, this could have significant consequences for reporting on complex aortic aneurysm repair, and the subsequent assessment of treatment options and prognostic risks. There is currently no widely adopted system to specify aortic exclusion in the endovascular repair of complex aortic aneurysms, resulting in a heterogeneity among methods used to report on the extent of treated aorta [11–14].

This study primarily aimed to evaluate differences in the length of aortic exclusion in the open and endovascular repair of complex aortic aneurysms, as well as differences in the loss of patent segmental arteries and treated visceral arteries, to subsequently reflect on the suitability of the current classification system in the endovascular era.

2. Materials and Methods

2.1. Study Design and Patient Cohort

A single center retrospective observational study was performed, which was presented to the Medical Ethics committee who waived the need for medical ethical approval under Dutch law. Patients that were primarily treated for a complex aortic aneurysm, by means of fenestrated endovascular aneurysm repair (FEVAR), combined fenestrated and branched EVAR (FBEVAR), or branched EVAR (BEVAR), at the department of Vascular Surgery between 2013 and 2020, were included in the study. Patients with connective tissue disease, as well as patients without a postoperative computed tomography angiography (CTA) follow up, were excluded. The primary outcomes of this study included the length of excluded aorta in hypothetical open and actual endovascular repair of complex aortic aneurysms, the number of patent segmental arteries, and the number of renal and visceral arteries that had to be treated in both treatment modalities.

2.2. Patient and Aneurysm Characteristics

Complex aortic aneurysms were categorized as juxtarenal aneurysms [15], or according to the Crawford classification in the case of thoracoabdominal aneurysms (TAAA), ranging from Crawford type I to type V [16]. Preoperative data on patient demographics, comorbidities, aneurysm characteristics, and postoperative data on early outcomes were collected. Retrospective analysis of 1 mm thin slice images of the preoperative, and the first postoperative, CTA was performed. Endovascular exclusion was determined by creating central luminal line reconstructions using 3-mensio vascular™ (Pie Medical Imaging, Maastricht, The Netherlands). The length of aortic exclusion in hypothetical open aortic repair was determined using the same central luminal line reconstructions, measuring the aorta between the hypothetical proximal clamping site and the aortic bifurcation. The hypothetical cross clamping location for an open approach was discussed and determined by two vascular surgeons (JS and JV). The length of the endovascular aortic exclusion was determined by measuring the aorta from the proximal covered seal of the stent graft up to the anatomical aortic bifurcation, as no segmental arteries originate from the common iliac artery. Patent segmental arteries were assessed by scoring the number of contrast-filled segmental arteries throughout the entire aorta, both pre- and postoperatively in 'open' and endovascular repair. Similarly, the number of treated visceral arteries was assessed by determining the number of visceral arteries that would need to be treated in 'open repair' (e.g., through clamping or reinsertion), and that were intraluminally manipulated in endovascular repair (e.g., through wire manipulation for visceral vessel stenting).

2.3. Perioperative Management

Patients were treated with custom-made or off-the-shelf endografts obtained from Cook Medical® (Bloomington, IN, USA), Medtronic© (Northridge, CA, USA), or Terumo Aortic© (Inchinnan, UK). The type of device was selected according to the patients' anatomy and urgency of the procedure. The endografts were designed according to the instructions for use (IFU) with intentional proximal and distal sealing zone lengths of at least 25 mm, taking into consideration the aortic diameter, mural thrombus, and eccentric wall dilatation. All elective procedures for TAAA were planned as staged procedures.

Patients were treated by a dedicated team of vascular surgeons and interventional radiologists, experienced in performing open and endovascular complex aortic repair. A standardized protocol was used to prevent the occurrence of spinal cord ischemia (SCI), consisting of spinal drainage and periprocedural neuromonitoring (e.g., motor-evoked potentials and somatosensory-evoked potentials). Carotid subclavian bypass was performed in all cases where proximal sealing necessitated coverage of the left subclavian artery. To provide for a durable distal seal, bi-iliac distal landing was performed in a substantial part of the patients. Postoperative management in TAAA repair consisted of spinal drainage during the first 24–72 h after the procedure. A mean arterial pressure (MAP) of 75 mmHg was maintained postoperatively, and hemoglobin was kept above 7 mmol/L. All patients included were followed up and underwent a CTA within 6 weeks after the (finalizing) procedure.

2.4. Statistical Analyses

Continuous data were reported as mean and standard deviation. Categorical data were presented as prevalence in the population by reporting absolute numbers and percentages. For aortic exclusion in open or endovascular approach, as well as for the number of patent segmental arteries, data were reported as median and interquartile ranges [IQR]. A Wilcoxon signed-rank test was used to compare the length of exclusion and patent segmental arteries in 'open' and endovascular repair. A p-value of < 0.05 was considered significant. Analyses were performed in collaboration with a medical statistician, using IBM SPSS software.

3. Results

Between May 2013 and September 2021, 74 patients underwent endovascular treatment of a complex aortic aneurysm, of which 71 patients were included in this study. Three patients were excluded due to the absence of a postoperative CTA, which was due to periprocedural mortality (n = 2) and following patients' explicit request for follow-up with duplex ultrasound (n = 1). The mean age of the study population was 73 years (±6.1), with 81.7% being male (Table 1). There were five patients with a Crawford type I, seven with a type II, six with a type III, seven with a type IV, and two with a type V TAAA, and forty-four patients had a juxtarenal aneurysm. The mean maximal aneurysm diameter was 64.6 mm (±10 mm). A total of forty-four patients were treated by means of FEVAR (62%), eight by means of FBEVAR (11.2%), and nineteen with BEVAR (26.8%). There were three emergency procedures.

Table 1. Characteristics of included patients treated by means of FEVAR, FBEVAR, or BEVAR for a complex aortic aneurysm.

Characteristics	Title 2
Patients (n)	71
Aneurysm extent (n)	
• Crawford type I	5
• Crawford type II	7
• Crawford type III	6
• Crawford type IV	7
• Crawford type V	2
• Juxtarenal	44
Maximal aortic aneurysm diameter (mm) (mean, SD)	64.6 (10.0)
Aneurysm etiology (%)	
• Post-dissection aneurysm	2.8
• Atherosclerosis	93
• Unknown	4.2
Procedures (n, %)	71
• FEVAR	44 (62)
1 or 2 fenestrations	35
3 or 4 fenestrations	9
• FBEVAR	8 (11.2)
• BEVAR	19 (26.8)
1 or 2 branches	0
3 branches	5
4 branches	14
Priority (n, % emergency)	3 (4.2)
Postoperative complications (%)	
• Renal complications	18.3
Temporary	15.5
Permanent	2.8
• Intestinal ischemia	4.2
• Spinal cord ischemia	8.5
30-day mortality (%)	4.2

3.1. Aortic Exclusion in Open Versus Endovascular Repair

The median length of the excluded aorta in type I TAAAs was 279 mm [186, 303 mm] in 'open' versus 388 mm [325, 432 mm] in endovascular treatment ($p < 0.05$) (Figure 1a and Supplementary Table S1). For type II aneurysms, the median length was 418 mm [356, 434 mm] compared with 485 mm [425–498 mm] in 'open' and endovascular repair, respectively ($p < 0.05$). For type III aneurysms, 'open' treatment excluded a median length of 311 mm [226, 423 mm] compared with 403 mm [354, 489 mm] in endovascular repair ($p < 0.05$). The estimated length of exclusion was 202 mm [144, 259 mm] in 'open' repair versus 291 mm [244, 353 mm] in the endovascular repair of type IV aneurysms ($p < 0.05$) and 174 mm (28 mm) in 'open' compared with 308 mm (81 mm) in the endovascular repair of type V aneurysms ($p > 0.05$). For juxtarenal aneurysms, the median length in 'open' treatment was 145 mm [121, 161 mm] versus 207 mm [182, 223 mm] in endovascular repair ($p < 0.05$).

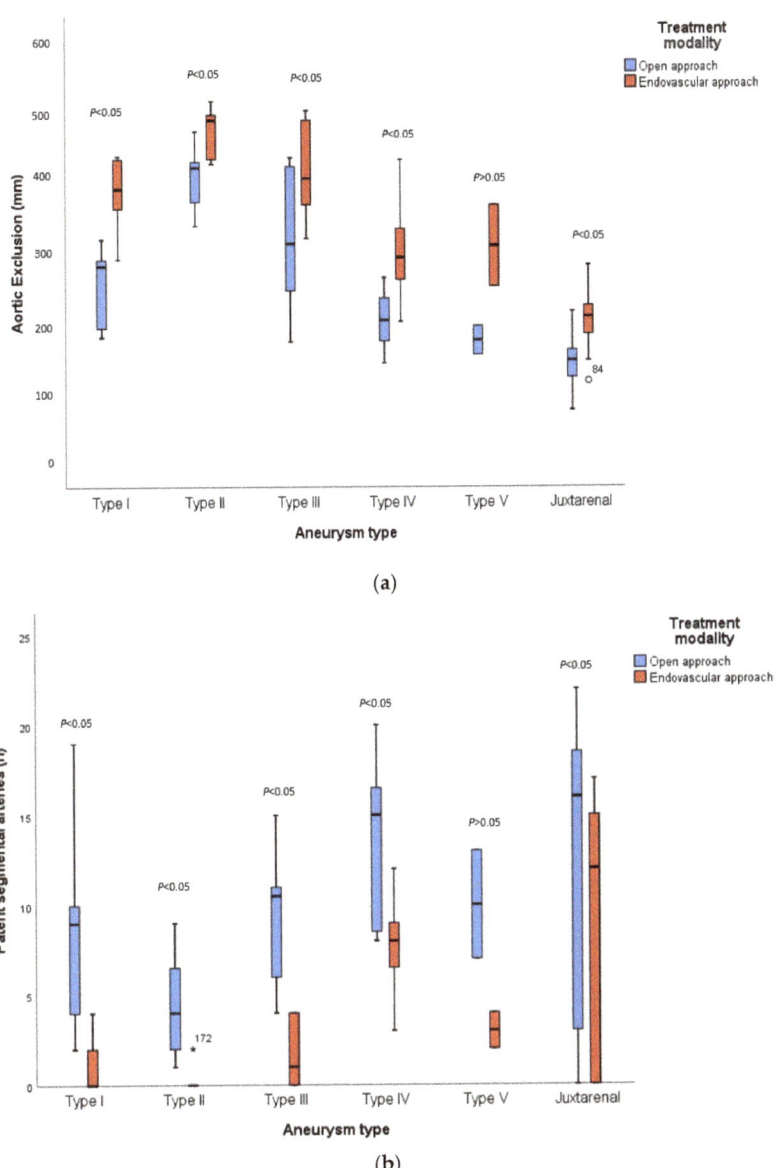

Figure 1. (a) differences in the median length of aortic exclusion in 'open' versus endovascular repair; (b) differences in patent segmental arteries in 'open' versus endovascular repair.

3.2. Patent Segmental Arteries in Open and Endovascular Repair

For Crawford type I aneurysms, in hypothetical open repair, a median of 9 [3, 14.5] patent segmental arteries would remain (Figure 1b and Supplementary Table S1), compared with 0 [0, 3] patent segmental arteries in endovascular treatment ($p < 0.05$). There were a median of 4 [2, 7] patent segmental arteries in 'open' versus 0 [0, 0] in endovascular repair of type II aneurysms ($p < 0.05$), and 10.5 [5.5, 12] versus 1 [0, 4] in type III aneurysms.

For the type IV TAAAs, there were 15 [8–17] patent segmental arteries in 'open' treatment, compared with 8 [5, 10] segmental arteries in endovascular repair ($p < 0.05$).

A mean of 10 (4.2) segmental arteries were patent in hypothetical open repair versus 3 (1.4) in endovascular repair ($p > 0.05$). Lastly, there were a median of 16 [2.5, 18.75] patent segmental arteries in the 'open' repair of juxtarenal aneurysms, compared with 12 [0, 15] in endovascular repair ($p < 0.05$).

3.3. Treated Visceral Arteries

In Crawford type I, II, III, IV, and V aortic aneurysms, there is no difference in the number of treated visceral arteries in 'open' or endovascular repair as all four are necessarily included in the repair (Supplementary Table S1). In the 'open' repair of juxtarenal aneurysms, four visceral arteries would have to be treated in one case (n = 1; 2.3% of all cases), two arteries in sixteen cases (n = 16; 36.3%), one artery in eight cases (n = 8, 18.2%), and zero arteries in the 'open' repair of nineteen cases (n = 19; 43.2%), averaging one visceral vessel per case. In the endovascular repair of these juxtarenal aneurysms, there were four treated arteries in ten cases (n = 10; 22.7%), three visceral arteries in twenty four cases (n = 24; 54.5%), two arteries in six cases (n = 6; 13.6%), and one artery in four cases (n = 4; 9.1%), averaging 2.9 visceral vessels per case.

4. Discussion

This study identified significant differences in the length of aortic exclusion between endovascular and hypothetical open treatment of TAA and juxtarenal aneurysms. Increased exclusion in endovascular repair inadvertently resulted in a lower number of patent intercostal and lumbar arteries. The endovascular treatment of juxtarenal aneurysms led to a higher number of treated visceral arteries, compared with open repair.

Based on our results, it can be concluded that the length of aortic tissue treated endovascularly is not comparable to the original anatomical extent of a complex aortic aneurysm, which has traditionally formed the basis for the Crawford classification. Examples of differences between the anatomical extent of an aneurysm, the extent of aortic repair in open, and the length of aortic exclusion in endovascular repair are illustrated in Figure 2. It could be argued that, when assessing the extent of aortic exclusion in endovascular repair for different types of complex aortic aneurysms more closely, the endovascular length of exclusion matches the anatomical extent of a different Crawford type. For instance, when performing endovascular repair of a juxtarenal aneurysm, the extent of this repair, which may often require four fenestrations, matches the anatomical extent of a Crawford type IV (Figure 3). Similarly, when using FEVAR to repair a Crawford type IV, the proximal seal might result in aortic exclusion matching the anatomical extent of a Crawford type III. Imaginably, this makes it questionable whether the clinical outcomes of open and endovascular repair of a Crawford type IV TAAA can be compared at all, as both treatment modalities consider widely varying lengths of aortic exclusion.

Our results are supported by recent work by Oderich et al. that underlines the importance of reporting on the extent of aortic exclusion in the endovascular repair of thoracoabdominal aneurysms, since the added seal for stent grafts differs from the would-be surgical anastomosis [8]. Oderich et al. recommend using a numerical system to indicate zones required for endovascular treatment and to calculate the estimated segments covered as a result of aortic exclusion to ultimately facilitate proper reporting on outcome and risk assessment, thereby facilitating comparison and benchmarking. Our study confirms this theoretical concept in an observational clinical setting: when comparing the zones required for the anastomosis in open repair or the sealing in endovascular repair for different types of complex aortic aneurysms according to the numerical system, similar correlations between the extent of open and endovascular exclusion are found. Another idea could be to revise the traditional Crawford classification, to make it applicable to both treatment modalities, by differentiating between conventional O-Crawford (for open repair) and E-Crawford (for endovascular repair). This way, as illustrated in Figure 3, an O-Crawford type IV would be considered an E-Crawford type III.

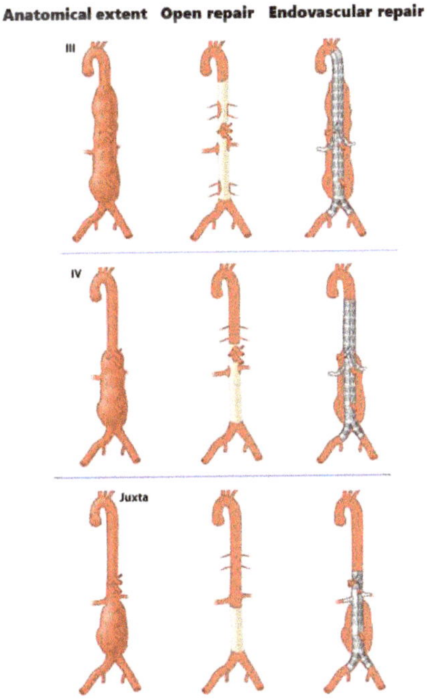

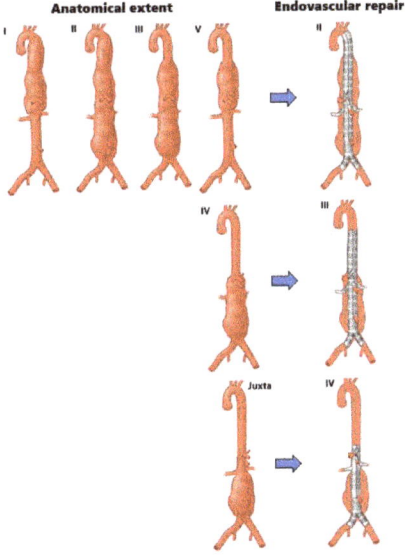

Figure 2. Examples of differences in anatomical extent and aortic exclusion in open and endovascular repair of three types of complex aortic aneurysms.

Figure 3. Illustration of how endovascular treatment of TAA and juxtarenal aneurysms may lead to a length of aortic exclusion that is comparable to the (anatomical) extent of Crawford types II, III, and IV.

Three other studies have focused on differences in aneurysm extent and aortic exclusion in complex endovascular aortic treatment. A study by Feezor et al. centered on thoracic endovascular repair, by identifying the length of a thoracic EVAR (TEVAR) graft as a significant risk factor for the incidence of SCI [17]. Gallitto et al. focused on custom-made FEVAR, portraying a mean additional aortic coverage of 48 mm proximally in juxta-, pararenal aneurysms and type IV TAAAs, with no significant effect on clinical outcomes [12]. Most segmental arteries were sacrificed in the repair of type IV aneurysms. These results align with our findings that, in accordance with a relatively small increase in aortic exclusion as a result of FEVAR instead of open repair, few segmental arteries were sacrificed. The difference in treated visceral arteries was not discussed. Lastly, Bertoglio et al. reported a greater sacrifice of healthy aortic tissue and intercostal arteries in TAAAs treated with an off-the-shelf branched device, compared with open repair [11]. As these devices nearly always require an additional proximal thoracic stent, these results cannot be compared to cases treated with custom-made branched devices. Further research should focus on a comparison of stent types and design strategies.

In the treatment of complex aortic aneurysms, a dilemma may arise between providing for a durable treatment and the increased risk of SCI, as a result of pursuing the IFUs or adjusting for anatomical aspects of the aneurysm. Imaginably, increased aortic exclusion entails an increased risk for SCI, yet the incidence of this complication depends on many other risk factors as well [18]. It is worthwhile appreciating the large disparities in the open and endovascular treatment of complex aneurysms. For instance, open repair includes the option of the reimplantation of segmental arteries, which is not possible in endovascular treatment. On the other hand, in open repair there is the postoperative risk of para-anastomotic aneurysm development, especially in the case of a proximal anastomosis close to the healthy aorta [19]. Also, open repair is more frequently associated with intra-, and postoperative systemic hypoperfusion due to blood loss or a more severe systemic inflammatory response, in turn increasing the risk of SCI [20,21]. Endovascular repair allows for staged treatment, possibly stimulating the collateral recruitment of spinal perfusion [18,22,23]. The current literature is not conclusive as of yet, with studies that report long proximal landing zones in fenestrated and branched EVAR resulting in low rates of SCI [24–26]. This is opposed to other studies that identified a relation between fenestrated grafts with a coverage of over 52 mm above the celiac artery and an increased risk of SCI [13]. As a result, the clinical consequence of preserving, for instance, 16 segmental arteries in the open, compared with 12 in the endovascular, repair of juxtarenal aneurysms, as was found in this study, is unknown.

Regarding the association between aortic exclusion and the risk of visceral complications in open or endovascular repair, various aspects are of influence, such as intra- or extraluminal manipulation of visceral or renal arteries. Endovascular treatment encompassing multiple fenestrations or branches can be demanding as it implies extensive intraluminal wire manipulation [27], whereas in open repair of TAAA, the selective perfusion of visceral and renal arteries is the golden standard. Imaginably, wall thrombus or irregular aortic diameters may lead to the application of three or four fenestrations in the case of juxtarenal aneurysm repair, as opposed to suprarenal clamping alone in open repair. A tendency to apply an increased number of fenestrations in the endovascular repair of aneurysms with similar anatomy over time has been described in experienced centers, illustrating how the complexity of the devices is evolving [13]. Despite extensive endovascular repair being safe, there have been concerns about more fenestrations increasing the risks for, amongst others, visceral complications, apart from the known prolonged operating and fluoroscopy time [9,27]. This is supported by a series of 610 patients undergoing endovascular repair for a juxtarenal or thoracoabdominal aneurysm, in which Mastracci et al. found that, with the increasing complexity of the devices, there was an accompanying increase in celiac occlusions and the need for reinterventions [13].

As for type V TAAAs and juxtarenal aneurysms, it should be noted that open repair is still a treatment to consider when looking at durability and long-term outcomes [21,28].

Work by Michel et al., for instance, has shown open repair to be cost-effective, compared with endovascular repair with F-/B-EVAR [29]. To conclude, taking into consideration how the risks of complications, such as SCI or visceral occlusions, are influenced by many different factors, as well as the aspects of durability and costs, open and endovascular treatments should be regarded as distinct modalities, each with their particular risk assessment.

Limitations

As this study was primarily intended to assess differences in aortic exclusion, in the number of patent segmental arteries and in the number of visceral arteries treated for both open and endovascular repair, a statistical assessment of the relation between aortic exclusion and clinical outcomes per Crawford type was beyond the scope of this study. To compare treatment modalities, a case-matched analysis of endovascular and open treatment of TAAAs was discussed but was deemed unreliable, due to the often unique anatomical features of complex aneurysms and heterogenous patient characteristics. This study served as the first exploration of an idea, and estimating hypothetical open repair was considered a suitable method for serving our research goal. Yet, the results of our study could be limited by the subjectivity of the assessment of the hypothetical open repair, as well as by the possibility of a difference in the intended clamp position and the eventual anastomosis (e.g., which changed as a result of anatomical factors perioperatively). Nevertheless, the extent of open repair was determined simultaneously by two vascular surgeons, experienced in the open and endovascular treatment of TAAAs, as this would normally be decided upon during a preoperative multidisciplinary team meeting. As the option to reimplant segmental arteries in the open repair of Crawford type I, II and III aneurysms is decided on perioperatively, this was not included in the assessment of patent segmental arteries in hypothetical open repair. Also, it should be noted that in the beginning of the complex aortic program at our hospital, 2-FEVAR procedures were performed, whereas today, according to advancing insights, these repairs are avoided. Nevertheless, data on 2-FEVARS were included in the data. Finally, the statistical power of the results is limited by the small groups of patients per Crawford type. This relates specifically to the type V TAAAs, of which a limited number of cases were included.

5. Conclusions

There are significant differences in lengths of aortic exclusion, patent segmental arteries, and the number of visceral arteries treated between the endovascular and hypothetical open repair of complex aortic aneurysms. The anatomical extent of these aneurysms does not match the length of aortic exclusion in endovascular repair, which might limit the suitability of a classification and subsequent risk assessment that was originally meant for an open repair of TAAA. Considering the differences in operation technique and the length of aortic exclusion, endovascular and open treatment of complex aneurysms should be considered as distinct treatment modalities. Future efforts should focus on uniformity in reporting on the extent of exclusion per treatment strategy, to further explore the consequences of these differences for clinical outcomes.

Supplementary Materials: The following supporting information can be downloaded at: https://www.mdpi.com/article/10.3390/jcm12154921/s1, Supplementary Table S1. Length of aortic exclusion, number of patent segmental arteries and the number of manipulated visceral arteries in hypothetical open repair and endovascular complex aortic aneurysm repair.

Author Contributions: Conceptualization and study design, J.v.S., J.v.d.V., and M.V.; software, J.v.S., J.v.d.V., and M.V.; data analysis and interpretation, M.V., D.E., C.v.R., R.v.d.M., J.H., J.v.d.V., and J.v.S.; data curation, M.V..; writing—original draft preparation, M.V.; writing—review and editing, M.V., D.E., C.v.R., R.v.d.M., J.H., J.v.d.V., and J.v.S. All authors equally contributed to revising the final manuscript. All authors have read and agreed to the published version of the manuscript.

Funding: The authors received no financial support for the research, authorship, and/or publication of this article.

Institutional Review Board Statement: This study was conducted in accordance with the Declaration of Helsinki, and approved by the Institutional Review Board and the Ethics Committee of Leiden University Medical Center (G20.148; 23rd of October 2020).

Informed Consent Statement: Informed consent was obtained from all subjects involved in this study.

Data Availability Statement: Not applicable.

Acknowledgments: The authors extend their special thanks to Manon Zuurmond, from the Leiden University Medical Center, for providing the illustrations.

Conflicts of Interest: The authors declare no conflict of interest.

References

1. Crawford, E.S.; Crawford, J.L.; Safi, H.J.; Coselli, J.S.; Hess, K.R.; Brooks, B.; Norton, H.J.; Glaeser, D.H. Thoracoabdominal aortic aneurysms: Preoperative and intraoperative factors determining immediate and long-term results of operations in 605 patients. *J. Vasc. Surg.* **1986**, *3*, 389–404. [CrossRef]
2. Safi, H.J.; Miller, C.C., 3rd. Spinal cord protection in descending thoracic and thoracoabdominal aortic repair. *Ann. Thorac. Surg.* **1999**, *67*, 1937–1939, discussion 1938–1953. [CrossRef] [PubMed]
3. Safi, H.J.; Winnerkvist, A.; Miller, C.C., 3rd; Iliopoulos, D.C.; Reardon, M.J.; Espada, R.; Baldwin, J.C. Effect of extended cross-clamp time during thoracoabdominal aortic aneurysm repair. *Ann. Thorac. Surg.* **1998**, *66*, 1204–1209. [CrossRef] [PubMed]
4. Starnes, B.W.; Caps, M.T.; Arthurs, Z.M.; Tatum, B.; Singh, N. Evaluation of the learning curve for fenestrated endovascular aneurysm repair. *J. Vasc. Surg.* **2016**, *64*, 1219–1227. [CrossRef]
5. Ziganshin, B.A.; Elefteriades, J.A. Surgical management of thoracoabdominal aneurysms. *Heart* **2014**, *100*, 1577–1582. [CrossRef]
6. Mastracci, T.M.; Greenberg, R.K.; Hernandez, A.V.; Morales, C. Defining high risk in endovascular aneurysm repair. *J. Vasc. Surg.* **2010**, *51*, 1088–1095.e1081. [CrossRef] [PubMed]
7. Greenberg, R.K.; Lu, Q.; Roselli, E.E.; Svensson, L.G.; Moon, M.C.; Hernandez, A.V.; Dowdall, J.; Cury, M.; Francis, C.; Pfaff, K.; et al. Contemporary analysis of descending thoracic and thoracoabdominal aneurysm repair: A comparison of endovascular and open techniques. *Circulation* **2008**, *118*, 808–817. [CrossRef] [PubMed]
8. Oderich, G.S.; Forbes, T.L.; Chaer, R.; Davies, M.G.; Lindsay, T.F.; Mastracci, T.; Singh, M.J.; Timaran, C.; Woo, E.Y.; Writing Committee, G. Reporting standards for endovascular aortic repair of aneurysms involving the renal-mesenteric arteries. *J. Vasc. Surg.* **2021**, *73*, 4S–52S. [CrossRef]
9. Oderich, G.S.; Ribeiro, M.; Hofer, J.; Wigham, J.; Cha, S.; Chini, J.; Macedo, T.A.; Gloviczki, P. Prospective, nonrandomized study to evaluate endovascular repair of pararenal and thoracoabdominal aortic aneurysms using fenestrated-branched endografts based on supraceliac sealing zones. *J. Vasc. Surg.* **2017**, *65*, 1249–1259.e1210. [CrossRef]
10. Konstantinou, N.; Antonopoulos, C.N.; Jerkku, T.; Banafsche, R.; Kolbel, T.; Fiorucci, B.; Tsilimparis, N. Systematic review and meta-analysis of published studies on endovascular repair of thoracoabdominal aortic aneurysms with the t-Branch off-the-shelf multibranched endograft. *J. Vasc. Surg.* **2020**, *72*, 716–725.e711. [CrossRef]
11. Bertoglio, L.; Cambiaghi, T.; Ferrer, C.; Baccellieri, D.; Verzini, F.; Melissano, G.; Chiesa, R.; Tshomba, Y. Comparison of sacrificed healthy aorta during thoracoabdominal aortic aneurysm repair using off-the-shelf endovascular branched devices and open surgery. *J. Vasc. Surg.* **2018**, *67*, 695–702. [CrossRef]
12. Gallitto, E.; Faggioli, G.; Pini, R.; Logiacco, A.; Mascoli, C.; Fenelli, C.; Abualhin, M.; Gargiulo, M. Proximal Aortic Coverage and Clinical Results of the Endovascular Repair of Juxta-/Para-renal and Type IV Thoracoabdominal Aneurysm with Custom-made Fenestrated Endografts. *Ann. Vasc. Surg.* **2021**, *73*, 397–406. [CrossRef] [PubMed]
13. Mastracci, T.M.; Eagleton, M.J.; Kuramochi, Y.; Bathurst, S.; Wolski, K. Twelve-year results of fenestrated endografts for juxtarenal and group IV thoracoabdominal aneurysms. *J. Vasc. Surg.* **2015**, *61*, 355–364. [CrossRef] [PubMed]
14. Diamond, K.R.; Simons, J.P.; Crawford, A.S.; Arous, E.J.; Judelson, D.R.; Aiello, F.; Jones, D.W.; Messina, L.; Schanzer, A. Effect of thoracoabdominal aortic aneurysm extent on outcomes in patients undergoing fenestrated/branched endovascular aneurysm repair. *J. Vasc. Surg.* **2021**, *74*, 833–842.e832. [CrossRef]
15. Wanhainen, A.; Verzini, F.; Van Herzeele, I.; Allaire, E.; Bown, M.; Cohnert, T.; Dick, F.; van Herwaarden, J.; Karkos, C.; Koelemay, M.; et al. Editor's Choice—European Society for Vascular Surgery (ESVS) 2019 Clinical Practice Guidelines on the Management of Abdominal Aorto-iliac Artery Aneurysms. *Eur. J. Vasc. Endovasc. Surg.* **2019**, *57*, 8–93. [CrossRef] [PubMed]
16. Riambau, V.; Bockler, D.; Brunkwall, J.; Cao, P.; Chiesa, R.; Coppi, G.; Czerny, M.; Fraedrich, G.; Haulon, S.; Jacobs, M.J.; et al. Editor's Choice—Management of Descending Thoracic Aorta Diseases: Clinical Practice Guidelines of the European Society for Vascular Surgery (ESVS). *Eur. J. Vasc. Endovasc. Surg.* **2017**, *53*, 4–52. [CrossRef]
17. Feezor, R.J.; Martin, T.D.; Hess, P.J., Jr.; Daniels, M.J.; Beaver, T.M.; Klodell, C.T.; Lee, W.A. Extent of aortic coverage and incidence of spinal cord ischemia after thoracic endovascular aneurysm repair. *Ann. Thorac. Surg.* **2008**, *86*, 1809–1814, discussion 1814. [CrossRef]

18. Dijkstra, M.L.; Vainas, T.; Zeebregts, C.J.; Hooft, L.; van der Laan, M.J. Editor's Choice—Spinal Cord Ischaemia in Endovascular Thoracic and Thoraco-abdominal Aortic Repair: Review of Preventive Strategies. *Eur. J. Vasc. Endovasc. Surg.* **2018**, *55*, 829–841. [CrossRef]
19. Serizawa, F.; Ohara, M.; Kotegawa, T.; Watanabe, S.; Shimizu, T.; Akamatsu, D. The Incidence of Para-Anastomotic Aneurysm After Open Repair Surgery for Abdominal Aortic Aneurysm Through Routine Annual Computed Tomography Imaging. *Eur. J. Vasc. Endovasc. Surg.* **2021**, *62*, 187–192. [CrossRef]
20. Maurel, B.; Delclaux, N.; Sobocinski, J.; Hertault, A.; Martin-Gonzalez, T.; Moussa, M.; Spear, R.; Le Roux, M.; Azzaoui, R.; Tyrrell, M.; et al. The impact of early pelvic and lower limb reperfusion and attentive peri-operative management on the incidence of spinal cord ischemia during thoracoabdominal aortic aneurysm endovascular repair. *Eur. J. Vasc. Endovasc. Surg.* **2015**, *49*, 248–254. [CrossRef]
21. Verhoeven, E.L.; Katsargyris, A.; Bekkema, F.; Oikonomou, K.; Zeebregts, C.J.; Ritter, W.; Tielliu, I.F. Editor's Choice—Ten-year Experience with Endovascular Repair of Thoracoabdominal Aortic Aneurysms: Results from 166 Consecutive Patients. *Eur. J. Vasc. Endovasc. Surg.* **2015**, *49*, 524–531. [CrossRef] [PubMed]
22. Etz, C.D.; Zoli, S.; Mueller, C.S.; Bodian, C.A.; Di Luozzo, G.; Lazala, R.; Plestis, K.A.; Griepp, R.B. Staged repair significantly reduces paraplegia rate after extensive thoracoabdominal aortic aneurysm repair. *J. Thorac. Cardiovasc. Surg.* **2010**, *139*, 1464–1472. [CrossRef]
23. Bischoff, M.S.; Brenner, R.M.; Scheumann, J.; Zoli, S.; Di Luozzo, G.; Etz, C.D.; Griepp, R.B. Staged approach for spinal cord protection in hybrid thoracoabdominal aortic aneurysm repair. *Ann. Cardiothorac. Surg.* **2012**, *1*, 325–328. [PubMed]
24. Haulon, S.; Tyrrell, M.R.; Fabre, D. Critical points from the reporting standards for endovascular aortic repair of aneurysms involving the renal-mesenteric arteries. *J. Vasc. Surg.* **2021**, *73*, 1S–3S. [CrossRef] [PubMed]
25. Schanzer, A.; Beck, A.W.; Eagleton, M.; Farber, M.A.; Oderich, G.; Schneider, D.; Sweet, M.P.; Crawford, A.; Timaran, C.; Consortium, U.S.M.F.B.A.R. Results of fenestrated and branched endovascular aortic aneurysm repair after failed infrarenal endovascular aortic aneurysm repair. *J. Vasc. Surg.* **2020**, *72*, 849–858. [CrossRef] [PubMed]
26. Van Calster, K.; Bianchini, A.; Elias, F.; Hertault, A.; Azzaoui, R.; Fabre, D.; Sobocinski, J.; Haulon, S. Risk factors for early and late mortality after fenestrated and branched endovascular repair of complex aneurysms. *J. Vasc. Surg.* **2019**, *69*, 1342–1355. [CrossRef]
27. Manning, B.J.; Agu, O.; Richards, T.; Ivancev, K.; Harris, P.L. Early outcome following endovascular repair of pararenal aortic aneurysms: Triple- versus double- or single-fenestrated stent-grafts. *J. Endovasc. Ther.* **2011**, *18*, 98–105. [CrossRef]
28. Rao, R.; Lane, T.R.; Franklin, I.J.; Davies, A.H. Open repair versus fenestrated endovascular aneurysm repair of juxtarenal aneurysms. *J. Vasc. Surg.* **2015**, *61*, 242–255. [CrossRef]
29. Michel, M.; Becquemin, J.P.; Marzelle, J.; Quelen, C.; Durand-Zaleski, I.; participants, W.T. Editor's Choice—A Study of the Cost-effectiveness of Fenestrated/branched EVAR Compared with Open Surgery for Patients with Complex Aortic Aneurysms at 2 Years. *Eur. J. Vasc. Endovasc. Surg.* **2018**, *56*, 15–21. [CrossRef]

Disclaimer/Publisher's Note: The statements, opinions and data contained in all publications are solely those of the individual author(s) and contributor(s) and not of MDPI and/or the editor(s). MDPI and/or the editor(s) disclaim responsibility for any injury to people or property resulting from any ideas, methods, instructions or products referred to in the content.

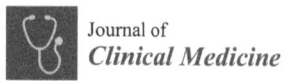

Article

Nonsurgical Repair of the Ascending Aorta: Why Less Is More

Xun Yuan [1,2], Xiaoxin Kan [3,4], Zhihui Dong [3], Xiao Yun Xu [4] and Christoph A. Nienaber [1,2,*]

1. Cardiology and Aortic Centre, Royal Brompton & Harefield Hospitals, Guy's and St Thomas' NHS Foundation Trust, London SW3 6NP, UK; x.yuan@rbht.nhs.uk
2. National Heart and Lung Institute, School of Medicine, Imperial College London, London SW3 6LY, UK
3. Center for Vascular Surgery and Wound Care, Jinshan Hospital, Fudan University, Shanghai 201508, China; x.kan17@imperial.ac.uk (X.K.); dong.zhihui@zs-hospital.sh.cn (Z.D.)
4. Department of Chemical Engineering, Imperial College London, London SW7 2BX, UK; yun.xu@imperial.ac.uk
* Correspondence: c.nienaber@rbht.nhs.uk

Abstract: *Objective:* Advanced endovascular options for acute and chronic pathology of the ascending aorta are emerging; however, several problems with stent grafts placed in the ascending aorta have been identified in patients unsuitable for surgical repair, such as migration and erosion at aorta interface. *Method:* Among the six cases analysed in this report, three were treated with a stent graft in the ascending aorta to manage chronic dissection in the proximal aorta; dimensions of those stent grafts varied between 34 and 45 mm in diameter, and from 77 to 100 mm in length. Three patients, matched by age, sex and their nature of pathology, were subjected to the focal closure of a single communicating entry by the use of an occluding device (Amplatzer ASD and PFO occluders between 14 and 18 mm disc diameter) with similar Charlson comorbidity score. *Results:* Both conceptually different nonsurgical management strategies were technically feasible; however, with stent grafts, an early or delayed erosion to full re-dissection was documented with stent grafts, in contrast to complete seal, with an induced remodelling and a long-term survival after the successful placing of coils and occluder devices. Moreover, aortic root motion was not impaired by the focal occlusion of a communication with an occluder, while free motion was impeded after stent graft placement. *Conclusions:* The intriguing observation in our small series was that stent grafts placed in the ascending aorta portends the risk of an either early (post-procedural) or delayed migration and erosion of aortic tissues at the landing site or biological interface between 12 and 16 months after the procedure, a phenomenon not seen with the use of focal occluding devices up to 5 years of follow-up. Obviously, the focal approach avoids the erosion of the aortic wall as the result of minimal interaction with the biological interface, such as a diseased aortic wall. Potential explanations may be related to a reduced motion of the aortic root after the placement of stent graft in the ascending aorta, whereas the free motion of aortic root was preserved with an occluder. The causality of erosion may however not be fully understood, as besides the stiffness and radial force of the stent graft, other factors such as the induced inflammatory reactions of aortic tissue and local adhesions within the chest may also play a role. With stent grafts failing to portend long-term success, they may still have a role as a temporizing solution for elective surgical conversion. Larger datasets from registries are needed to further explore this evolving field of interventions to the ascending aorta.

Keywords: ascending aorta; endovascular repair; stent graft; vascular occluder; false lumen; aortic remodelling; FLIRT

Citation: Yuan, X.; Kan, X.; Dong, Z.; Xu, X.Y.; Nienaber, C.A. Nonsurgical Repair of the Ascending Aorta: Why Less Is More. *J. Clin. Med.* **2023**, *12*, 4771. https://doi.org/10.3390/jcm12144771

Academic Editors: Martin Teraa, Constantijn E.V.B. Hazenberg and Carlo Setacci

Received: 12 June 2023
Revised: 4 July 2023
Accepted: 17 July 2023
Published: 19 July 2023

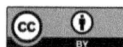

Copyright: © 2023 by the authors. Licensee MDPI, Basel, Switzerland. This article is an open access article distributed under the terms and conditions of the Creative Commons Attribution (CC BY) license (https://creativecommons.org/licenses/by/4.0/).

1. Introduction

Advanced endovascular options for the acute and chronic pathology of the ascending aorta are emerging and have reached the clinical arena [1,2]. Observations in small case series and registries have identified several problems with stent grafts placed in the ascending aorta in patients who are not candidates for surgical repair, such as migration and erosion at the stent graft and aorta interface [3–7]. One of the reasons for those serious complications is related to the three-dimensional movement of the ascending aorta in the thoracic cage and the subsequent friction between the ends of a placed stent graft and the ascending aorta [4,8,9]. Although early success has been described in selected patients with focal aneurysmatic transformation or chronic localised dissection by virtue of sealing the entry to either false lumen or aneurysmatic space [10], longer-term observations have at best shown a temporizing effect when using stent graft in this area [11]. In the acute/subacute setting, case reports and the ARISE trial have failed to show a lasting positive effect [3,4].

While stent grafts placed into the ascending aorta have been associated with migration and erosion, various reports on the focal patching of entry tears using septal occluders or occluder-like instruments [5,6] have shown promise with no midterm erosion or migration [6]. In this paper, we test the hypothesis whether sealing an entry tear or communication between true and false lumen by an occluder device would lead to similar or better results than stent grafts placed in the ascending aorta in patients with focal aneurysmatic disease or chronic aortic dissection. For this pilot study, three consecutive patients who underwent endovascular stenting in the ascending aorta were compared to three patients subjected to focal entry closure by an occluding device, and followed over 5 years.

2. Methods

2.1. Study Design

Our analysis is based on a retrospective matched cohort (head-to-head) comparison of two methods to isolate the false lumen in inoperative patients with a proximal type of aortic dissection. All patients had a DeBakey type II pathology with a focal dissection in the ascending aorta.

2.2. Demographics

Patients who underwent nonsurgical repair for chronic pathology in the ascending aorta had been considered unsuitable for surgical repair, with the idea to seal the entry tear of communication to a false lumen in chronic type A dissection by an interventional procedure under general anaesthesia; none of the 6 patients were treated in the acute phase of dissection. Among all six cases analysed in this report, 3 patients were treated with a stent graft in the ascending aorta (with 2 males and 1 female patient) at an average age of 77.7 ± 1.53 years; dimensions of those stent grafts varied between 34 and 45 mm, while varying in length from 77 to 100 mm. Three patients matched by age, sex and nature of pathology were subjected to the focal closure of communicating entry by use of an occluding device (Amplatzer ASD and PFO occluders between 14 and 18 mm disc diameter); there were also 2 males and 1 female patient aged 79.3 ± 5.13 years (Table 1). The Charlson comorbidity score was high in both groups, ranging between 3 and 9 in the stent graft group versus 4 and 5 in the comparator.

Table 1. Demographics and procedure details.

	Group I—Stent Graft Patient 1	Patient 2	Patient 3		Group II—Occluding Device Patient 4	Patient 5	Patient 6	
Demographics								
Age at procedure (years)	76	78	79	77.7 ± 1.53	75	85	78	79.3 ± 5.13
Gender	Female	Female	Male		Female	Female	Male	
Hypertension	Yes	No	Yes		Yes	No	Yes	
Diabetes	No	No	No		No	No	No	
Charlson comorbidity index	9	3	4		5	4	4	
EuroScore II	20.4	5.84	4.88		31.41	11.47	23.94	
Procedure details								
Total diameter of Asc. Ao. (mm)	55	50	66		66	62	42	
Max diameter of false lumen (mm)	29	25	55		46	53	10	
Number of entry tear(s)	1	1	1		1	1	1	
Devices	Zenith® TX2®	Gore Tag®	Gore CTag active control		Coils + Amplatzer PFO occluder	Coils + Occlutech ASD occluder	Coils + Amplazter ASD occluder	
Device dimension (mm)	34 × 77	37 × 100	45 × 100		18	14	14	
General anaesthesia	Yes	Yes	Yes		Yes	Yes	Yes	
Procedure time (mins)	64	319	174	185 ± 127	180	157	120	152 ± 30
Total contrast (mL)	70	140	190	133 ± 60	60	140	170	123 ± 56
Total radiation dose (uGym^2)	523.92	6289.09	17,901.52	8238 ± 8851	14,708.06	11,697.69	21,561.91	15,989 ± 5055
Procedure outcome	Successful	Successful	Unsuccessful		Successful	Successful	Successful	
Hospital stays (days)	9	6	19	11 ± 6	4	6	3	4 ± 1

2.3. Procedural Details

Technical and procedural details are individually listed in Table 1. Both with the placement of stent graft and with occluder deployment, a wide range of procedural time and radiation burden was documented; however, there was a trend towards a shorter hospital stay and use of resources with occluder devices than with stent grafts due to the fully percutaneous approach. Conversely, for TEVAR procedures in collaboration with vascular surgeons, access was established by surgical cutdown to the femoral artery. For the respective interventions, either commercially available stent grafts were used (Zenith® TX2® COOK® Medical, GoreTag® or CTag) or commercially available ASD and PFO occluders (Occlutech® or Amplatzer™). Initial intraprocedural success was seen in all patients with early failure in 1 case after stent graft and late failure in 2 cases after stent graft, essentially using technology and techniques as previously published elsewhere [5,12].

CT images prior to TEVAR were reviewed by experienced radiologists and the size of the stent graft was chosen based on the measurement of pre-TEVAR CT images. The proximal sealing zone was determined at a level at least 2 cm apart from the entry in the dissection lamella. Stent graft dimensions were determined by the estimated true lumen diameter at proximal sealing segment. All TEVAR procedures were performed under general anaesthesia, allowing for vascular cutdown in the groin to expose the femoral artery for access. A pigtail catheter was inserted over a guide wire via a 6 French introducer, then exchanged to a stiff wire over pigtail catheter in the true lumen of the ascending aorta. Digital subtraction angiography (DSA) imaging via the pigtail catheter was used to check the dissection and confirm the location and proximal sealing zone. After exchange for DrySeal introducer, the delivery system for a proximal stent graft was inserted over a Lunderquist wire (Boston Scientific, Marlborough, MA, USA) and positioned carefully under fluoroscopy. To ensure the designated satisfactory landing position, the stent graft was deployed under rapid right ventricular pacing to reduce systolic blood pressure to 60 bpm during launch. DSA was repeated after launch of stent graft to document stent graft placement and sealing of the communication between true and false lumen. After the angiographic image acquisition, all instruments and introducers were removed, followed by a surgical repair of the femoral artery access.

Prior to the use of a focal ASD or PFO occluding device, similar with TEVAR, pre-procedural CT images were reviewed by experienced radiologists, and details of focal dissection, width and depth of false lumen, and the diameter of the dissected aorta were measured from appropriate CT angiographic images. The size of any given occluder was chosen based on both the diameter of the communication (or entry) and the depth of false lumen to accommodate the distal disc of an occluder device in the false lumen, thus determining the required dimension to seal the communication between true and false lumen. The waist of ADS/PFO occluder device was smaller than the diameter of the diameter of focal entry tear. Via percutaneous approach from a femoral artery, a coronary multi-purpose catheter was utilised to identify and navigate the focal dissection lesion and advance the tip into false lumen under fluoroscopy. As a first step, some coils were advanced via the multi-purpose catheter into the false lumen (to promote later thrombus formation); secondly, a normal exchange length of 0.035 inches of wire was advanced in the false lumen over the multi-purpose catheter, which was then removed in exchange for a delivery sheath for the occluder. Deployment of the distal umbrella in the false lumen followed by the deployment of the proximal umbrella in the true lumen was subsequently monitored by fluoroscopy and documented on a final DSA run to prove the exact placement and sealing of the communication.

2.4. Medication

All patients were treated simultaneously for underlying chronic arterial hypertension by a combination of at least three different drugs, assuring a low normal blood pressure; there were no obvious differences between groups (Table 2).

Table 2. Follow-up details.

	Group I—Stent Graft			Group II—Occluding Device		
	Patient 1	Patient 2	Patient 3	Patient 4	Patient 5	Patient 6
Medication						
Beta-blocker	Bisoprolol	Bisoprolol	Bisoprolol	None	Bisoprolol	None
ACEi/ARB	None	None	None	None	Ramipril	Ramipril
CCB	Amlodipine	None	Amlodipine	Amlodipine	Amlodipine	None
Anticoagulant	None	None	Apixaban	None	Rivaroxaban	None
Antiplatelet	None	Aspirin	None	Aspirin	None	Aspirin
Adverse event						
Device-related complication	SINE	SINE	Migration	No	No	No
Re-intervention	No	No	Yes	No	No	No
Survival						
At 1 year	Yes	Yes	Yes	Yes	Yes	Yes
At 5 years	No	Yes	Yes	Yes	Yes	Yes
Follow-up duration (months)	18	86	47	79	76	72

2.5. Follow-Up and Survival

A 5-year follow-up was documented for all six patients. Clinical surveillance was conducted in all patients over 5 years with annual clinical appointments, including echocardiographic assessment and contrast-enhanced CT imaging (Table 2).

2.6. Motion Analysis

For each patient, pre- and post-procedural DSA images were adopted to perform quantitative analysis of device-induced aortic motion alteration. The two-dimensional DSA images were acquired at a frame rate of 4 frames per second during an average scan time of 5.5 s (minimum 3 s). Hence, for an individual scan, a minimum of 12 frames were obtained and analysed. The open-sourced medical image analysis package 3D Slicer was adopted for marking the spatial position of anatomical landmarks on DSA images.

DSA images were analysed frame by frame by following the methodology described in a previous study [13]. The base of 2 aortic sinuses shown on DSA images were marked as reference points, while the mid-point of the two reference points was used to represent the location of the aortic root in the current frame (Figure 1). After marking mid-points in all frames during the total scanning time, the maximum distance of all mid-points were calculated as the maximum motion range of aortic root by using MATLAD (MathWorks, Natick, MA, USA). The extent of aortic root motion before and after each intervention is listed in Table 3 and illustrated in Figure 1.

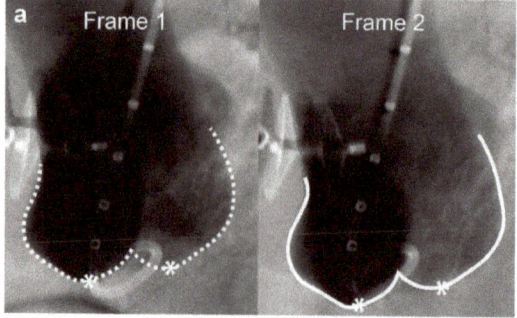 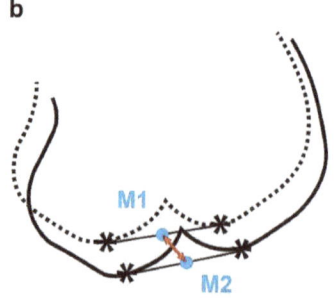

Figure 1. Illustration of the measurement of aortic root motion from DSA images. (a) For each angiographic frame, reference points at the base of aortic sinuses were marked. (b) The mid-points of the reference points were calculated and adopted to represent the position of aortic root in each frame. Maximum distance between the mid-points was measured as the maximum aortic root motion within the total scanning time.

Table 3. Maximum aortic root motion under aortogram and motion changed before and after procedure.

Displacement (mm)	Group I—Stent Graft			Group II—Occluding Device		
	Patient 1	Patient 2	Patient 3	Patient 4	Patient 5	Patient 6
Pre-procedure	6.84	8.51	6.78	5.59	3.23	13.3
Post-procedure	3.16	7.53	4.01	5.23	3.66	15.6
Motion changed	−53.8%	−11.5%	−40.9%	−6.41%	+13.2%	+17.4%

3. Results

Both conceptually different nonsurgical management strategies are illustrated in typical case examples; Figure 2 shows a case of a stent graft placed in an ascending aorta while Figure 3 illustrates the focal sealing of an entry tear by the use of an Amplatzer™ occluder device in a similar setting of proximal communication in type A aortic dissection. Note the early erosion to full re-dissection in contrast to complete seal and induced remodelling after the placement of an occluder device.

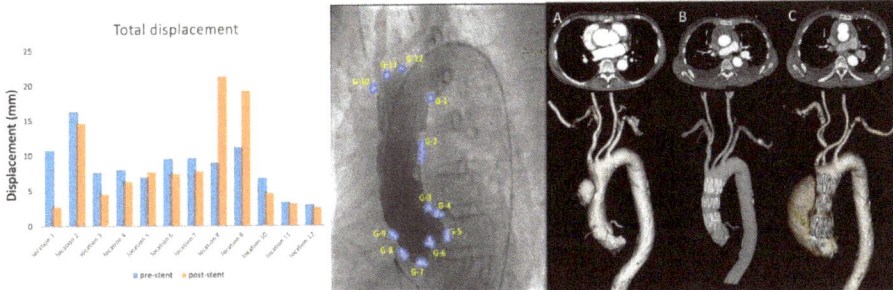

Figure 2. Aortic root motion for a patient treated with a stent graft in the ascending aorta. The composite illustration shows numeric values of displacement at each reference point before and after the placement of a stent graft on the left. The centre piece shows one given angiographic frame with attached reference points; and on the right, the reconstructed CT angiographic images are depicted before the endovascular intervention (**A**), with the stent graft in place (**B**); and finally, 16 months after the intervention (**C**), the creation of a re-dissection from a stent graft-induced erosion is revealed.

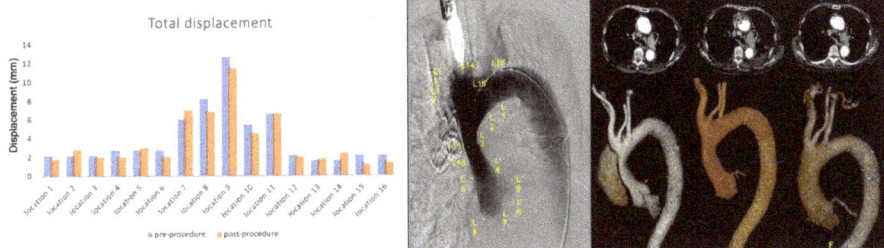

Figure 3. Aortic root motion in a patient treated with an ASD occlude and additional coils to seal localised ascending aortic dissection. The composite illustration shows the numeric values of displacement at each reference point before and after placement of an ASD occluder on the left. The centre piece shows one patient given an angiographic frame after coils were placed in the false lumen, and the complete occlusion of the entry tear by the use of double umbrella occluder; on the right, note the reconstructed CT angiographic images demonstrating the complete occlusion of any communication to the false lumen, successful remodelling over 3 months from before the endovascular intervention with no evidence of any remaining false lumen.

Demographic and procedural details are summarised in Table 1. Group 1 (stent graft) was similar to group 2 (focal use of occluding device) with regard to age, gender distribution and nature of pathology. Patients in both groups were unsuitable for open surgical repair, considering their high comorbidity profile by the Charlton score and EuroScore II. The Charlson comorbidity index ranged from 3 to 9 in group 1, and 4 to 5 in group 2; and EuroScore II ranged from 4.88 to 20.4 in group I, compared with 11.47 to 31.41 in group 2. The total diameter of ascending aorta was similar in both groups. Every patient has one proximal entry tear in the aorta and could therefore be considered for DeBakey II aortic dissection.

Procedural details were similar between groups in view of the use of general anaesthesia time, procedural duration and the amount of contrast dye used; there was a trend towards a higher radiation burden in cases undergoing interventional occluder placement (as a less standardised method). However, the patients receiving an occluder device enjoyed a shorter hospital stay due to the total percutaneous procedure with an approximal 4 ± 1 days compared to the stent graft group with 11 ± 6 days (Table 1). An immediate procedural success was seen in two of the three patients undergoing stent graft placement compared to the three cases undergoing interventional occluder placement. The hospital stay in group 1 was longer compared with group 2 (occluder devices), owing to surgical cutdown to the femoral artery for large bore access.

The post-intervention medication used in each patient and the follow-up outcomes are summarised in Table 2. The medication and combination of drugs were essentially similar between groups. While reinterventions were necessary after stent graft placement, such as conversion to open surgery, no reintervention was required in patients after the placement of an occluder device (group 2) over the entire follow-up period of 5 years with completed false lumen thrombosis and remodelling (Figure 3). In contrast, two cases developed stent-induced new entry tear (SINE), and one case was unsuccessful due to peri-procedural stent graft migration in group 1. The outcomes in terms of survival pattern reveal one death and one conversion to open surgery after stent grafting (group 1), while the mortality and reintervention rates in group 2 were zero over at least 5 years. Despite of the need for conversion to open surgery, group 1 patients survived at least 1 year with one death soon after 1 year. Figures 2 and 3 display a typical example from each group, also highlighting the similarity of the pathologies treated.

The extent of aortic root motion before and after either stent graft placement of occluder deployment is listed individually in Table 3 and summarised in Figure 4; the graphical display illustrates that aortic root motion was not impaired by the focal occlusion of a communication with an occluder and was similar before and after the intervention in all three cases on the line of identity. Conversely, with a stent graft, the free motion of the aortic root was found to be impeded with markedly less motion after stent graft placement than before in all three cases (Figure 4).

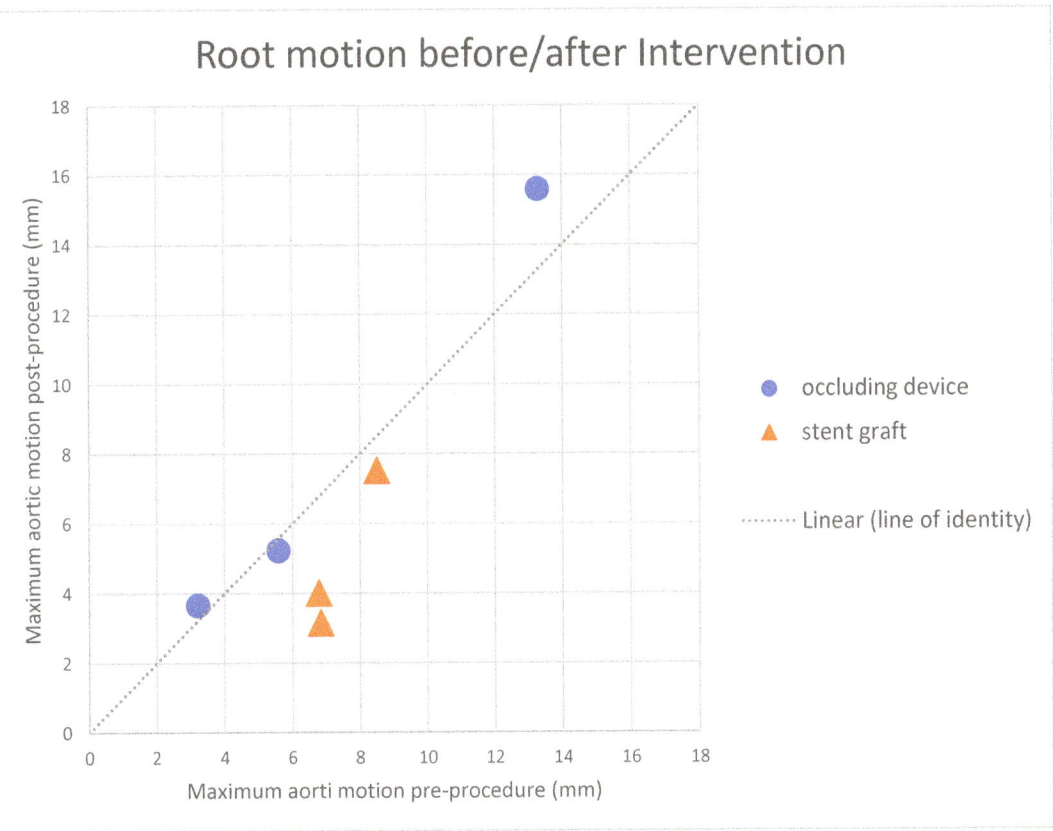

Figure 4. This graph illustrates the motion of the aortic root before and after the placement of either a stent graft or an occluder device; the ratio of motion (before and after each intervention) reveals that no patients fitted with an occluder revealed any significant impairment of motion as they are located on the line of identity (marked in blue). Conversely, with a stent graft placed in the ascending aorta, post-interventional aortic motion was impaired to varying extents in those three patients (in orange).

4. Discussion

Our comparison between two nonsurgical strategies to address the ascending aorta in selected patients unsuitable for open repair has shown that the focal closure and sealing of entry sites is technically feasible in the chronic dissection of the ascending aorta. Both the focal use of occluders and the short stent graft aim for the same goal: to depressurise the false lumen by closing entry tears, thereby initiating thrombosis and the remodelling of the false lumen in the setting of chronic ascending aortic dissection. While the concept of sealing entry tears by the use of stent grafts has been successfully shown in the descending aorta (e.g., in type B dissection) its application to pathologies in the ascending aorta is at best controversial [14,15]; the concept of the focal occlusion of entry tears by the use of occluders and coils as a primary strategy is new and limited in case reports [5,6]; there seems to be a consensus that only patients with a prohibitively high risk for open surgery may be candidates for any interventional approach in this setting, as in our observational series of six cases.

The intriguing observation in our small series was that stent grafts placed in the ascending aorta portend the risk of either an early (post-procedural) or a delayed migration and erosion of aortic tissues at the landing site or biological interface between 12 and 16 months, a phenomenon not seen with the use of focal occluding devices up to 5 years of follow-up. While all three patients after stent graft treatment required either immediate or late surgical conversion (with one death), patients selected for occluder devices (including coils) to seal entry points demonstrated remodelling and survived >5 years with no need for further intervention. Obviously, the focal approach avoids the migration and erosion of the aortic wall as the result of minimal interaction with the biological interface, e.g., the diseased aortic wall. Moreover, a complete seal and an induced thrombosis of the false lumen with subsequent remodelling were demonstrated in all three cases of ascending aortic pathology (Figure 3). While those observations in a small set of patients are quite interesting, explanations are not entirely clear yet and rather speculative, but conceptual differences in the approaches may provide at least some answers. Radial force may play a role in stent grafts and may impact the interface between stent grafts and native aortic walls which are likely to cause erosion, particularly with relatively rigid devices such as Zenith® TX2®.

Our analysis of aortic root motion in the chest before and after each intervention had clearly revealed some degree of a reduced motion of the aortic root after the placement of a stent graft in the ascending aorta, whereas the free motion of the root was preserved after sealing an entry with an occluder (Figure 4); this signal was consistent and clearly separated the two groups with regard to post-procedural aortic motion, and may play a predisposing role for aortic wall erosion observed after stent graft placement. The causality of erosion may however not be fully understood yet, as besides the stiffness of the stent graft, other factors such as the stent-induced inflammatory reactions of aortic tissue and local adhesions within the chest may also play a role.

Conversely, with the use of a focal closure of an entry tear, the synchronic swinging motion of the aortic root remains uninhibited and may avoid the untoward consequences of stent grafts in the ascending aorta. In fact, the extent of aortic root motion was identical before and after the placement of coils and occluders (Table 3), thereby minimizing or completely avoiding any friction at the interface between occluder and biological tissue, and promoting instead the integration of coils and occluder into the healing process of the aortic tissue. The fundamental problem associated with the placement of a stent graft into the ascending aorta in dissection had been recognised previously [7,9,16] as any device would always be placed in diseased or even dissected tissue even if initial seal could be achieved; even with technological advances and a dedicated stent graft designed for the ascending aorta, its use in acute dissection was not approved (ARISE study and others). While stent grafts failed to portend a long-term success, they could at best be characterised as a temporizing solution for elective surgical conversion. Whether the concept of an endo-Bentall with an integrated aortic valve as an anker point (instead of landing a stent graft in diseased tissue) would solve the problem of stent-induced erosion in a mobile ascending aorta remains to be determined; today, this concept appears unlikely to be widely adopted as it comes with the sacrifice of the native aortic valve [14,17,18].

Although the early experience with the focal occlusion of entries in (essentially chronic) cases unfit for open surgery is promising, this "focal concept" targeting a mayor entry tear needs to be scrutinised in larger series or registries. So far, the experience is limited to a few patients, although with no failure yet, thus constituting a highly selective group of patients (or selection bias). Moreover, procedures were performed in a highly specialised centre by super-specialised operators, and yet, were also associated with a rather extensive radiation burden and duration; in addition, in the early stage of the learning curve, all procedures were performed under general anaesthesia, and thus needed streamlining. Nevertheless, new interventional approaches to address difficult scenarios in the setting of proximal dissection are feasible and should be documented and meticulously followed in international registries (as randomised trials are unlikely to materialise for various reasons).

With better diagnostics and initial management, the aortovascular community is likely to be seeing more cases of proximal aortic dissection that are not candidates of classic surgical aortic repair; demographic changes will also increase the number of patients for whom open surgery is no option. At the very least, experienced aortic centres with a multidisciplinary team approach should be open to new solutions for old problems; those places should feel the some responsibility to advance clinical research and create strategies in unchartered territories at best with a background of a profound understanding of disease and healing processes.

5. Limitations

This is a small retrospective cohort study that compares two different concepts, which of course need to be subjected to the scrutiny of a larger registry or even a randomised comparison (with a further improvement of the technologies used). Moreover, aortic root motion was analysed based on 2D DSA images rather than 4D MRI [19,20] or ECG-gated retrospective CT, which could be more accurate in a temporal–spatial tracking manner.

Author Contributions: Conceptualization, C.A.N. and X.Y.X.; methodology, X.Y. and X.K.; software, X.K.; formal analysis, X.K.; investigation, X.Y.; resources, Z.D.; data curation, C.A.N., X.Y. and X.K.; writing—original draft preparation, X.Y. and C.A.N.; writing—review and editing, C.A.N. and X.Y.X.; supervision, C.A.N., X.Y.X. and Z.D. All authors have read and agreed to the published version of the manuscript.

Funding: This research received no external funding.

Institutional Review Board Statement: Ethical review and approval were waived for this study due to retrospective study on existing anonymised data, no patient involved or impact on their management.

Informed Consent Statement: Patient consent was waived due to reusing anonymised data, no patient identifiable data presented.

Data Availability Statement: The data presented in this study are available on request from the corresponding author.

Acknowledgments: The authors acknowledge the Lee Family Scholarship for the support of Xun Yuan.

Conflicts of Interest: The authors declare no conflict of interest.

References

1. Isselbacher, E.M.; Preventza, O.; Hamilton Black, J., 3rd; Augoustides, J.G.; Beck, A.W.; Bolen, M.A.; Braverman, A.C.; Bray, B.E.; Brown-Zimmerman, M.M.; Chen, E.P.; et al. 2022 ACC/AHA Guideline for the Diagnosis and Management of Aortic Disease: A Report of the American Heart Association/American College of Cardiology Joint Committee on Clinical Practice Guidelines. *Circulation* **2022**, *146*, e334–e482. [CrossRef] [PubMed]
2. Atkins, A.D.; Reardon, M.J.; Atkins, M.D. Endovascular Management of the Ascending Aorta: State of the Art. *Methodist DeBakey Cardiovasc. J.* **2023**, *19*, 29–37. [CrossRef] [PubMed]
3. Roselli, E.E.; Atkins, M.D.; Brinkman, W.; Coselli, J.; Desai, N.; Estrera, A.; Johnston, D.R.; Patel, H.; Preventza, O.; Vargo, P.R.; et al. ARISE: First-In-Human Evaluation of a Novel Stent Graft to Treat Ascending Aortic Dissection. *J. Endovasc. Ther.* **2022**, *30*, 15266028221095018. [CrossRef] [PubMed]
4. Yuan, X.; Kan, X.; Xu, X.Y.; Nienaber, C.A. Finite element modeling to predict procedural success of thoracic endovascular aortic repair in type A aortic dissection. *JTCVS Tech.* **2020**, *4*, 40–47. [CrossRef] [PubMed]
5. Yuan, X.; Mitsis, A.; Semple, T.; Castro Verdes, M.; Cambronero-Cortinas, E.; Tang, Y.; Nienaber, C.A. False lumen intervention to promote remodelling and thrombosis-The FLIRT concept in aortic dissection. *Catheter. Cardiovasc. Interv.* **2018**, *92*, 732–740. [CrossRef] [PubMed]
6. Yuan, X.; Mitsis, A.; Mozalbat, D.; Nienaber, C.A. Novel Endovascular Management of Proximal Type A (DeBakey II) Aortic Dissection With a Patent Foramen Ovale Occluder. *J. Endovasc. Ther.* **2017**, *24*, 809–813. [CrossRef] [PubMed]
7. Sengupta, S.; Yuan, X.; Maga, L.; Pirola, S.; Nienaber, C.; Xiao, X. Aortic haemodynamics and wall stress analysis following arch aneurysm repair using a single-branched endograft. *Front. Cardiovasc. Med.* **2023**, *10*, 1125110. [CrossRef] [PubMed]
8. Yuan, X.; Kan, X.; Xu, X.Y.; Nienaber, C. Identifying and quantifying the 4D motion of aortic root. *J. Am. Coll. Cardiol.* **2021**, *77*, 1832. [CrossRef]
9. Kan, X.; Yuan, X.; Salmasi, M.Y.; Moore, J.; Sasidharan, S.; Athanasiou, A.; Xu, X.Y.; Nienaber, C.A. Comprehensive Mechanical Modelling of Thoracic Endovascular Aortic Repair in Type A Aortic Dissection. *Circulation* **2021**, *144*, A10478. [CrossRef]
10. Castro Verdes, M.; Yuan, X.; Li, W.; Senior, R.; Nienaber, C.A. Aortic intervention guided by contrast-enhanced transoesophageal ultrasound whist waiting for cardiac transplantation: A case report. *Eur. Heart J. Case Rep.* **2021**, *5*, ytaa485. [CrossRef] [PubMed]

11. Banathy, A.K.; Khaja, M.S.; Williams, D.M. Update on Trials & Devices for Endovascular Management of the Ascending Aorta and Arch. *Tech. Vasc. Interv. Radiol.* **2021**, *24*, 100756. [CrossRef] [PubMed]
12. Nienaber, C.A.; Sakalihasan, N.; Clough, R.E.; Aboukoura, M.; Mancuso, E.; Yeh, J.S.; Defraigne, J.O.; Cheshire, N.; Rosendahl, U.P.; Quarto, C.; et al. Thoracic endovascular aortic repair (TEVAR) in proximal (type A) aortic dissection: Ready for a broader application? *J. Thorac. Cardiovasc. Surg.* **2017**, *153*, S3–S11. [CrossRef] [PubMed]
13. Beller, C.J.; Labrosse, M.R.; Thubrikar, M.J.; Robicsek, F. Role of aortic root motion in the pathogenesis of aortic dissection. *Circulation* **2004**, *109*, 763–769. [CrossRef] [PubMed]
14. Gouveia, E.M.R.; Stana, J.; Prendes, C.F.; Kolbel, T.; Peterss, S.; Stavroulakis, K.; Rantner, B.; Pichlmaier, M.; Tsilimparis, N. Current state and future directions of endovascular ascending and arch repairs: The motion towards an endovascular Bentall procedure. *Semin. Vasc. Surg.* **2022**, *35*, 350–363. [CrossRef] [PubMed]
15. Czerny, M.; Schmidli, J.; Adler, S.; van den Berg, J.C.; Bertoglio, L.; Carrel, T.; Chiesa, R.; Clough, R.E.; Eberle, B.; Etz, C.; et al. Editor's Choice—Current Options and Recommendations for the Treatment of Thoracic Aortic Pathologies Involving the Aortic Arch: An Expert Consensus Document of the European Association for Cardio-Thoracic Surgery (EACTS) & the European Society for Vascular Surgery (ESVS). *Eur. J. Vasc. Endovasc. Surg.* **2019**, *57*, 165–198. [CrossRef] [PubMed]
16. Suh, G.K.; Bondesson, J.; Zhu, Y.D.; Nilson, M.C.; Roselli, E.E.; Cheng, C.P. Ascending Aortic Endograft and Thoracic Aortic Deformation After Ascending Thoracic Endovascular Aortic Repair. *J. Endovasc. Ther.* **2023**. online ahead of print. [CrossRef] [PubMed]
17. Felipe Gaia, D.; Bernal, O.; Castilho, E.; Baeta Neves Duarte Ferreira, C.; Dvir, D.; Simonato, M.; Honorio Palma, J. First-in-Human Endo-Bentall Procedure for Simultaneous Treatment of the Ascending Aorta and Aortic Valve. *JACC Case Rep.* **2020**, *2*, 480–485. [CrossRef] [PubMed]
18. Kern, M.; Hauck, S.R.; Dachs, T.M.; Haider, L.; Stelzmuller, M.E.; Ehrlich, M.; Loewe, C.; Funovics, M.A. Endovascular repair in type A aortic dissection: Anatomical candidacy for currently manufactured stent grafts and conceptual valve-carrying devices for an Endo-Bentall procedure. *Eur. J. Cardio-Thorac. Surg.* **2023**, *63*, ezad085. [CrossRef] [PubMed]
19. Oberhuber, A.; Schabhasian, D.; Kohlschmitt, R.; Rottbauer, W.; Orend, K.H.; Rasche, V. The bird beak configuration has no adverse effect in a magnetic resonance functional analysis of thoracic stent grafts after traumatic aortic transection. *J. Vasc. Surg.* **2015**, *61*, 365–373. [CrossRef] [PubMed]
20. Rasche, V.; Oberhuber, A.; Trumpp, S.; Bornstedt, A.; Orend, K.H.; Merkle, N.; Rottbauer, W.; Hoffmann, M. MRI assessment of thoracic stent grafts after emergency implantation in multi trauma patients: A feasibility study. *Eur. Radiol.* **2011**, *21*, 1397–1405. [CrossRef] [PubMed]

Disclaimer/Publisher's Note: The statements, opinions and data contained in all publications are solely those of the individual author(s) and contributor(s) and not of MDPI and/or the editor(s). MDPI and/or the editor(s) disclaim responsibility for any injury to people or property resulting from any ideas, methods, instructions or products referred to in the content.

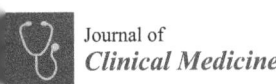

Article

The Correlation of Aortic Neck Angle and Length in Abdominal Aortic Aneurysm with Severe Neck Angulation for Prediction of Intraoperative Neck Complications and Postoperative Outcomes after Endovascular Aneurysm Repair

Khamin Chinsakchai [1,*], Thana Sirivech [1], Frans L. Moll [2], Sasima Tongsai [3] and Kiattisak Hongku [1]

1 Division of Vascular Surgery, Department of Surgery, Faculty of Medicine Siriraj Hospital, Mahidol University, Bangkok 10700, Thailand; dent1234thanatoy@gmail.com (T.S.); kiattisak.hongku@gmail.com (K.H.)
2 Vascular Surgery Department, University Medical Center Utrecht, 3584 Utrecht, The Netherlands; fransmoll50@gmail.com
3 Research Department, Faculty of Medicine Siriraj Hospital, Mahidol University, Bangkok 10700, Thailand; sasima.ton@mahidol.edu
* Correspondence: khamin.chi@mahidol.edu; Tel.: +66-2-419-8021; Fax: +66-2-412-9160

Abstract: Objectives: Endovascular aneurysm repair (EVAR) in a hostile neck has been associated with adverse outcomes. We aimed to determine the association of infrarenal aortic neck angle and length and establish an optimal cutoff value to predict intraoperative neck complications and postoperative outcomes. Methods: This was a retrospective review of patients with an intact infrarenal abdominal aortic aneurysm (AAA) with severe neck angulation (>60 degrees) who underwent EVAR from October 2010 to October 2018. Demographic data, aneurysm morphology, and operative details were collected. The ratio of neck angle and length was calculated as the optimal cutoff value of the aortic neck angle-length index. The patients were categorized into two distinct groups using latent profile analysis, a statistical technique employed to identify concealed subgroups within a larger population by examining a predetermined set of variables. Intraoperative neck complications, adjunct neck procedures, and early and late outcomes were compared. Results: 115 patients were included. Group 1 (G1) had 95 patients with an aortic neck angle-length index ≤ 4.8, and Group 2 (G2) had 20 patients with an aortic neck angle-length index > 4.8. Demographic data and aneurysm morphology were not significantly different between groups except for neck length ($p < 0.001$). G2 had more intraoperative neck complications than G1 (21.1% vs. 55%, $p = 0.005$). Adjunctive neck procedures were more common in G2 (18.9% vs. 60%, $p < 0.001$). The thirty-day mortality rate was not statistically different. G1 patients had a 5-year proximal neck re-intervention-free rate comparable to G2 patients (93.7% G1 vs. 87.5% G2, $p = 0.785$). The 5-year overall survival rate was not statistically different (59.9% G1 vs. 69.2% G2, $p = 0.891$). Conclusions: Patients with an aortic neck angle-length index > 4.8 are at greater risk of intraoperative neck complications and adjunctive neck procedures than patients with an aortic neck angle-length index ≤ 4.8. The 5-year proximal neck re-intervention-free rate and the 5-year survival rate were not statistically different. Based on our findings, this study suggests that the aortic neck angle-length index is a reliable predictor of intraoperative neck complications during EVAR in AAA with severe neck angulation.

Keywords: abdominal aortic aneurysm; severe neck angulation; neck length; index; outcomes

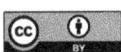

1. Introduction

Endovascular aneurysm repair (EVAR) is now performed in up to 44% of abdominal aortic aneurysm (AAA) surgeries outside the instructions for use, mostly due to hostile aortic neck anatomies [1]. Two of the most important predictors of EVAR failure in AAA are infrarenal aortic neck angulation [2,3] and short aortic neck [4,5], conditions that are associated with a significantly higher rate of early and late-type 1A endoleak.

As per the expert panel's assessment of EVAR's hostile neck definition, a severe neck angulation is deemed to be present when the infrarenal neck angulation exceeds 60 degrees, while a neck length of less than 10 mm is classified as a short neck [1].

While some studies have reported good early and mid-term outcomes in AAA with severely infrarenal neck angulation [6,7], this condition has a tendency to develop type 1A endoleaks during long-term follow-up [8]. The correlation between the severely infrarenal neck angulation and neck length for AAA treated with EVAR has not been studied.

Therefore, we investigated whether the index of infrarenal aortic neck angulation and length has any effect on intraoperative complications and outcomes after EVAR. We aimed to determine the association of infrarenal aortic neck angle in severely angulated aortic neck and length to find the optimal cutoff value for prediction of intraoperative neck complications after EVAR and to compare early and late outcomes between groups classified by the aortic neck angle-length index.

2. Materials and Methods

2.1. Patient Selection

All intact infrarenal AAA patients with severe neck angulation (infrarenal neck angle greater than 60°) who underwent standard EVAR at our institute between October 2010 and October 2018 were enrolled in this study. Patients who lacked preoperative computed tomographic angiography (CTA) data were excluded. The study protocol was approved by the Siriraj Institutional Review Board (SIRB) (COA no. Si 499/2018). Data were collected from a prospectively maintained AAA database through a retrospective review of medical records. Demographic data and clinical-specific profiles were recorded including age, sex, and medical co-morbidities. In addition, the American Society of Anesthesiologists (ASA) physical status classification estimated by an anesthesiologist was also documented.

2.2. Preoperative CT Scan Measurement

Preoperative assessment of aneurysm morphology was performed using a multidetector CTA with thin-slice (1 mm) imaging. Accurate measurements were determined using post-processing 3D imaging software, such as Osirix MD 13.0.0 (Pixemo, Geneva, Switzerland). The aortic neck angle and length measurements were determined by two observers (KC and TS). The two investigators performed the angle and length measurements independently and in a random order. Infrarenal aortic neck angulation was defined as the maximal angle from all views between the proximal aortic neck and the longitudinal axis of the aneurysm [9]. Infrarenal aortic neck length was defined as the first diameter showing growth of 10% over the diameter at the most caudal renal artery [10]. A conical neck was defined as a gradual neck dilatation of ≥ 2 mm within the first 10 mm after the most caudal renal artery [11]. Other AAA morphologies were recorded including maximal diameter, suprarenal neck angulation, $\geq 50\%$ circumferential proximal neck thrombus (≥ 2 mm thick), $\geq 50\%$ calcified proximal neck, and AAA length (the length from the lowest renal artery to aortic bifurcation). For determination of intraobserver reliability, the co-author (TS) measured both the infrarenal aortic neck angle and neck length twice with an interval of 1 to 2 weeks. The aortic neck angle and neck length were measured by two observers (KC and TS) to evaluate the interobserver reliability. Details of these measurements were reviewed separately without the knowledge of the clinical outcomes of the patients to avoid measurement bias.

2.3. Definitions and Outcomes Measurement

The aortic neck angle-length index was calculated using the average of the infrarenal neck angle (degree) divided by the average of the infrarenal aortic neck length (millimeter) (Figure 1). Intraoperative neck complications were detected by completion angiography after the endografts were deployed completely. We focused on four types of intraoperative neck complications. A type 1A endoleak was defined as the extravasation of contrast between the prosthesis and aneurysm wall from the proximal neck [12]. Endograft migration was determined by the displacement of the stent graft caudally, measuring the distance from the lowest renal artery and the most cephalad portion of the stent graft > 10 mm [12]. Renal artery occlusion was defined as partial or complete occlusion of one or bilateral renal arteries. Aortic dissection was determined as retrograde aortic dissection.

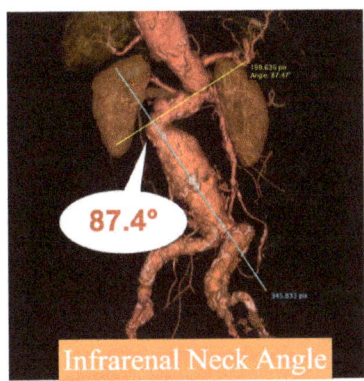 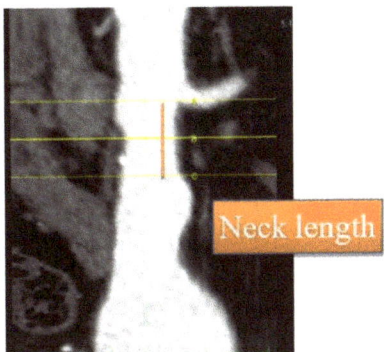

$$= \frac{\text{Infrarenal Neck Angle (degrees)}}{\text{Infrarenal Neck Length (millimeters)}}$$

Figure 1. How to calculate an optimal cutoff value of the aortic neck angle-length index.

Intraoperative adjunctive neck procedure was defined as any other procedure designed to augment the effects of the principal procedure, especially for management of intraoperative neck complications or otherwise unsatisfactory outcomes such as proximal extension cuff and Palmaz stent placement (Cordis Corp., Miami Lakes, FL, USA). Operative details were composed of the brand of aortic stent graft product, procedure time (minutes), fluoroscopic time (minutes), volume of contrast usage (milliliters), and intraoperative blood loss (milliliters).

In-hospital death or any death or complications occurring during the first 30-day postoperative period were analyzed. Complications were defined according to a previous report by Chaikof et al. [12].

All patients undergoing EVAR were followed according to a predetermined protocol that included a CTA at 1, 6, and 12 months, and then every 12 months thereafter. In patients with stage IV or V chronic kidney disease (eGFR < 30 mL/min per 1.73 m^2), the aortic stent graft was evaluated via standard duplex ultrasound performed by a radiologist. All radiologic exams conducted after endovascular repair were reviewed for migration, endoleaks, graft limb occlusions, aneurysm sac size, and re-interventions.

2.4. Statistical Analysis

The required sample size for point biserial correlation was conducted in G*Power 3.1.9.2 using a significance level of 0.05, a power of 0.90, a medium effect size ($\rho = 0.3$), and a two-tailed test. Given the absence of a definitive rule for determining sample size in latent profile analysis, Wurpts et al. [13] have recommended a minimum of 100 subjects as a reasonable sample size. Consequently, all subjects meeting the inclusion criteria were recruited. Building upon this assumption, the desired sample size for our study was determined to be 109.

Data were recorded and analyzed using PASW Statistics 18.0 (SPSS Inc., Chicago, IL, USA). Descriptive statistics were used to describe demographic and clinical characteristics. For normal distribution data, quantitative variables were described using mean and standard deviation (SD), while non-normal distribution data were described using median and range. Qualitative data were expressed by number and percentage. An intraclass correlation coefficient (ICC) was used to evaluate intraobserver reliability using a two-way mixed effects model and interobserver reliability using a two-way random effects model. A latent profile analysis (LPA) was used to classify groups of patients based on aortic neck angle-length index using the R package mclust [14]. LPA is a method that aims to identify latent subpopulations within a larger population by analyzing a specific set of variables. LPA assumes that individuals can be classified into different categories with varying probabilities, each characterized by unique combinations of personal and/or environmental attributes [15]. Four indices were used to select the correct number of latent classes, i.e., log-likelihood, Bayesian information criterion (BIC), integrated complete-data likelihood, and bootstrap likelihood ratio test (BLRT). Lower BIC and integrated complete-data likelihood values coupled with higher log-likelihood values show and indicate a better-fitting model. The BLRT was used to compare successive models, where a significant change in −2 log-likelihood indicated that the model with the greater number of classes provided a better fit to the data. Point biserial correlation coefficient (r_{pb}) was used to examine the relationship between the aortic neck angle-length index score and two classes of aortic neck angle-length groups classified by LPA. In comparison between two groups, the Pearson chi-square test, Yates' continuity correction, or Fisher's exact test was performed for qualitative variables, and the independent sample t-test or Mann-Whitney U test was used for quantitative variables with means or medians, as appropriate. The Kaplan-Meier method was performed to estimate overall survival time and re-intervention free time. The log-rank test or Breslow test was used to compare overall survival and re-intervention free time between aortic neck angle-length index groups. All tests were considered statistically significant with a p-value less than 0.05.

3. Results

From October 2010 to October 2018, 759 patients were diagnosed with intact AAA at our institution. Open surgical repair, fenestrated or chimney EVAR procedure, and AAA without severely angulated infrarenal neck were excluded. One hundred and fifty-five of these patients presented with a severely angulated neck of AAA treated with EVAR. Forty patients were not included in this study due to lack of preoperative CTA ($n = 30$), using other brands of aortic stent graft (Nelix, AFX, Ovation, and Gore Excluder, $n = 7$), using funnel technique ($n = 2$), and previous open surgical repair ($n = 1$). In total, 115 patients were enrolled in our study.

3.1. Intraobserver and Interobserver Reliability

Intraobserver reliability of the author on aortic neck length had an ICC of 0.988 (95% CI; 0.982–0.992) and infrarenal angle showed excellent reliability with an ICC of 0.986 (95% CI; 0.981–0.991). Interobserver reliability of two observers on neck length showed excellent and moderate reliability with an ICC of 0.969 (95% CI; 0.954–0.979) and aortic neck angle with an ICC of 0.739 (95% CI; 0.632–0.816).

3.2. Aortic Neck Angle-Length Index

The aortic neck angle-length index was calculated from the average of the infrarenal neck angle (degree) divided by the average neck length (millimeter) for each patient (Figure 1). The median of the aortic neck angle-length index was 3.2 (range 1.1–14.3). LPA classified the aortic neck angle-length index into two groups, i.e., aortic neck angle-length index ≤ 4.8 [Group 1, (G1)] and aortic neck angle-length index > 4.8 [Group 2, (G2)], which represented 95 (82.6%) and 20 (17.4%) patients, respectively. The relationship between the aortic neck angle-length index score and two classes of aortic neck angle-length groups was high with r_{pb} of 0.780 (95% CI: 0.704–0.857). There were no statistically significant differences in demographic variables (Table 1). Most of the patients were male (70.5% G1 and 80% G2), and the mean patient age was 77.1 ± 6.4 (G1) and 75.7 ± 7.2 (G2) years, respectively. Hypertension was the most common comorbidity, presented in almost three-quarters (80% G1 and 75% G2), followed by dyslipidemia (45.3% G1 and 40% G2).

Table 1. Demographic data and clinical characteristics.

Baseline Characteristics	Group 1 ANAL Index ≤ 4.8 (n = 95)	Group 2 ANAL Index > 4.8 (n = 20)	p Value
Age, mean ± SD years	77.1 ± 6.4	75.7 ± 7.2	0.360
Male gender, no. (%)	67 (70.5%)	16 (80%)	0.559
Cardiac disease, no. (%)	31 (32.6%)	4 (20%)	0.396
COPD, no. (%)	14 (14.7%)	1 (5%)	0.463
Hypertension, no. (%)	76 (80%)	15 (75%)	0.762
Dyslipidemia, no. (%)	43 (45.3%)	8 (40%)	0.885
Chronic kidney disease, no. (%)	23 (24.2%)	2 (10%)	0.235
Diabetes mellitus, no. (%)	14 (14.7%)	1 (5%)	0.463
Cerebrovascular disease, no. (%)	13 (13.7%)	1 (5%)	0.458
ASA class II, no. (%)	22 (23.2%)	6 (30%)	0.674
ASA class III, no. (%)	71 (74.7%)	14 (70%)	0.674

Abbreviation: ANAL, aortic neck angle-length index; no., number; SD, standard deviation; COPD, chronic obstructive pulmonary disease, ASA, American Society of Anesthesiologists.

3.3. AAA Morphology

All patients had a fusiform-type aneurysm. There were no statistically significant differences in the median of the suprarenal neck angle (43.6° G1 vs. 40.5° G2, $p = 0.912$) or the mean of the infrarenal neck angle (82.9° G1 vs. 89.7° G2, $p = 0.108$). The aortic neck length was significantly shorter in Group 2 (34.1 mm vs. 14.0 mm, $p < 0.001$). The other aneurysm morphologies were not statistically significantly different (Table 2).

Table 2. Morphology of abdominal aortic aneurysm by aortic neck angle-length indexes.

Aneurysm Morphology	Group 1 ANAL Index ≤ 4.8 (n = 95)	Group 2 ANAL Index > 4.8 (n = 20)	p Value
AAA morphology, fusiform (%)	95 (100%)	20 (100%)	1.000
AAA length (mm), mean ± SD	127.7 ± 24.8	134.2 ± 24.6	0.285
AAA max. diameter (mm), mean ± SD	64.5 ± 14.6	66.6 ± 12.0	0.550
Suprarenal neck angle (°), median (min, max)	43.6 (0, 133.7)	40.5 (13.5, 91.3)	0.912
Infrarenal neck angle (°), mean ± SD	82.9 ± 17.1	89.7 ± 15.9	0.108
Neck length (mm), mean ± SD	34.1 ± 13.8	14.0 ± 3.7	<0.001
Neck calcification, no. (%)	4 (4.2%)	0 (0%)	1.000
Neck thrombus, no. (%)	6 (6.3%)	2 (10%)	0.626
Neck morphology, no. (%)			0.751
Cylindrical	74 (77.9%)	14 (70%)	
Conical	14 (14.7%)	4 (20%)	
Reverse conical	7 (7.4%)	2 (10%)	

Abbreviation: AAA, abdominal aortic aneurysm; ANAL, aortic neck angle-length index; mm, millimeter; no., number; SD, standard deviation.

3.4. Intraoperative Outcomes

For intraoperative outcomes (Table 3), Group 2 had significantly higher intraoperative neck complication rates than Group 1 (21.1% G1 vs. 55% G2, $p = 0.005$), especially type IA endoleaks (10.5% G1 vs. 40% G2, $p < 0.003$). There was no significant difference in endograft migration and renal artery coverage between the two ANAL index groups.

Table 3. Intraoperative details and outcomes between 2 groups of aortic neck angle-length indexes.

Variable	Group 1 ANAL Index ≤ 4.8 (n = 95)	Group 2 ANAL Index > 4.8 (n = 20)	p Value
Stent graft product, no. (%)			
Endurant	52 (54.7%)	11 (55%)	0.986
Zenith	39 (41.1%)	8 (40%)	0.986
Treovance	4 (4.2%)	1 (5%)	0.986
Intraoperative neck complications no. (%)	20 (21.1%)	11 (55%)	0.005
Type IA endoleak	10 (10.5%)	8 (40%)	0.003
Endograft migration	4 (4.2%)	1 (5%)	1.000
Type IA endoleak and endograft migration	4 (4.2%)	2 (10%)	0.279
Renal artery coverage	2 (2.1%)	0 (0%)	1.000
Adjunctive neck procedures, no. (%)	18 (18.9%)	12 (60%)	<0.001
Aortic cuff	7 (7.4%)	5 (25%)	0.034
Palmaz stent	9 (9.5%)	4 (20%)	0.237
Aortic cuff and Palmaz stent	2 (2.1%)	3 (15%)	0.036
Operative details			
Procedure time, mean ± SD (min.)	178.1 ± 63.5	206.0 ± 75.2	0.087
Fluoroscopic time (min.), median (min, max)	34.6 (15, 110)	40.1 (19, 97)	0.248
Volume of contrast usage (mL), median (min, max)	122 (28, 300)	142.5 (54, 470)	0.162
Blood loss (mL), median (min, max)	250 (50, 1500)	352.5 (75, 2000)	0.082

Abbreviation: ANAL, aortic neck angle-length index; mL, milliliter; no., number; SD, standard deviation.

In Group 2, the adjunctive neck procedures were performed significantly more frequently (18.9% G1 vs. 60% G2, $p < 0.001$). The proximal extension cuff placements were more common in Group 2 (7.4% G1 vs. 25% G2, $p = 0.034$), and Palmaz stent placements were more common in Group 2, but the difference was not statistically significant (9.5% G1 vs. 20% G2, $p = 0.237$).

3.5. Operative Details

The Endurant, Zenith, and Treovance devices were used to perform EVAR, and there were no statistically significant differences between the two groups. The mean of procedure time (minutes), fluoroscopic time, volume of contrast usage, and intraoperative blood loss were all higher in the aortic neck angle-length index > 4.8 (G2), but these did not reach statistical significance. Operative details are summarized in Table 3.

3.6. Early Postoperative Outcomes

There was no statistically significant difference in 30-day complications (30.5% G1 vs. 40% G2, $p = 0.575$) or in deployment-related complications (6.3% G1 vs. 10% G2, $p = 0.626$). In eight patients with deployment-related complications, two aortic dissections occurred within 30 days. One patient required open repair. Four patients had access site hematoma, and one required surgical evacuation. One patient had distal embolization, treated with transfemoral thromboembolectomy and another patient had a dissection of the right external iliac artery with conservative treatment.

There was one procedure-related death in Group 1 from a retrograde aortic dissection on postoperative day 8, and one patient in Group 2 died from severe colonic ischemia on postoperative day 2. There was no statistically significant difference in the 30-day mortality rate between the two groups (1.1% G1 vs. 5% G2, $p = 0.319$). Two patients in Group 1 died after 30 days, one from pulmonary infection with severe sepsis and another from multiple organ failure. One patient in Group 2 died from pulmonary infection with severe sepsis on postoperative day 85 (3.1% G1 vs. 10% G2, $p = 0.439$). The median length of stay was not statistically significantly different between the two groups (7 days, G1 vs. 8 days, G2, $p = 0.401$). Post-operative outcomes are shown in Table 4.

Table 4. Early postoperative outcomes between aortic neck angle-length indexes groups.

Post-Operative Outcomes	Group 1 ANAL Index ≤ 4.8 (n = 95)	Group 2 ANAL Index > 4.8 (n = 20)	p Value
30-day complication, no. (%)	29 (30.5%)	8 (40%)	0.575
Myocardial infarction	0 (0%)	1 (5%)	0.174
Congestive heart failure	3 (3.2%)	1 (5%)	0.540
Respiratory failure	2 (2.1%)	2 (10%)	0.139
Renal failure	5 (5.3%)	1 (5%)	1.000
Deployment-related complications, no. (%)	6 (6.3%)	2 (10%)	0.626
30-day mortality, no. (%)	1 (1.1%)	1 (5%)	0.319
In-hospital mortality *, no. (%)	3 (3.1%)	2 (10%)	0.439
Length of stay, (days) Median (min, max)	7 (2, 124)	8 (2, 85)	0.401

* In-hospital mortality was defined as death occurring during the hospital stay including 30-day mortality.

3.7. Late Outcomes

The median follow-up duration was 36.6 months (range: 1–110 months). During the 6-month follow-up, one case experienced graft limb occlusion which was subsequently managed through a femorofemoral polytetrafluoroethylene (PTFE) bypass graft procedure. In the 5-year proximal neck re-intervention-free rate, there was no statistically significant difference between the aortic neck angle-length index ≤ 4.8 group and the aortic neck angle-length index > 4.8 group (93.7% G1 vs. 87.5% G2, $p = 0.785$), (Figure 2). Four (4.2%) patients in Group 1 required proximal neck re-intervention due to a type 1A endoleak ($n = 3$) and a type 3B endoleak ($n = 1$). One patient had a type 3B endoleak at 15 months postoperatively at the main body of the stent graft due to the pressure effect of the Palmaz stent and was treated successfully with a proximal extension cuff. Three patients developed a type 1A endoleak during follow-up. One patient required an aortic extension cuff at four months and two patients needed a Palmaz stent at two and 24 months, respectively. In Group 2, one (5%) patient underwent a proximal extension cuff placement due to a ruptured AAA from a type 1A endoleak at 33 months postoperatively. There was no statistically significant difference in the 5-year overall survival rate between the two groups (59.9% G1 vs. 69.2% G2, $p = 0.337$), (Figure 3).

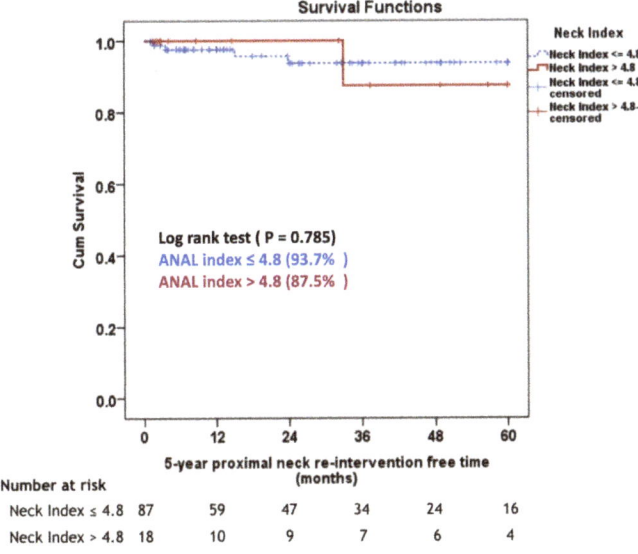

Figure 2. Five-year proximal neck re-intervention-free rate between 2 groups of aortic neck angle-length indexes. Abbreviation: ANAL, aortic neck angle-length index.

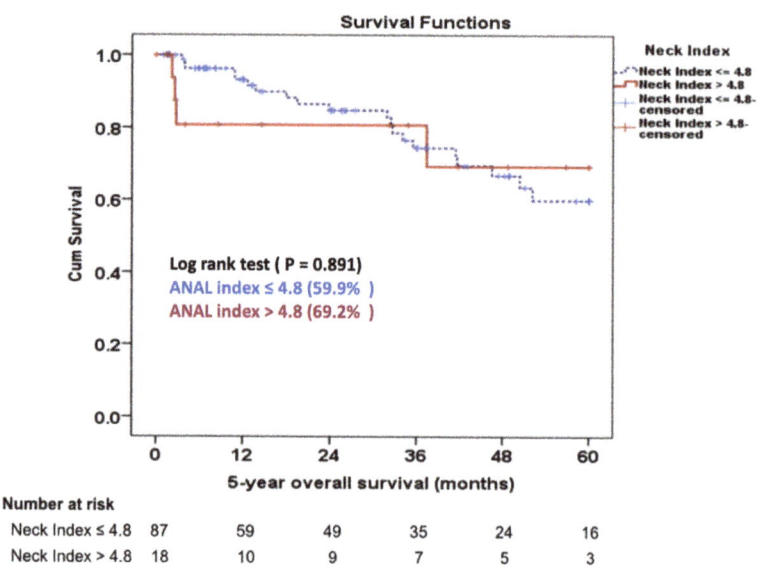

Figure 3. Five-year overall survival rate between aortic neck angle-length indexes groups. Abbreviation: ANAL, aortic neck angle-length index.

4. Discussion

The suitability of EVAR is usually based on the manufacturer's instructions for use. Strict adherence to the standard requirements generally leads to good outcomes. EVAR within a hostile neck anatomy, particularly in short and severe neck angulation, is associated with poor early and late outcomes [3,5]. One study of AAA with severely angulated necks revealed significant changes in velocity, flow streamline, pressure, and wall shear stress inside the aneurysm sac [16]. These findings provide valuable insights that can help predict the occurrence of ruptured AAA. We measured a correlation between aortic infrarenal neck angulation and aortic neck length, showing a higher rate of intraoperative neck complications and immediate adjunctive neck procedures in patients with an aortic neck angle-length index > 4.8. Nevertheless, there was no statistically significant difference in the rate of re-intervention or survival between the two groups at late follow-up.

The success of EVAR is largely dependent on the ability of the device to achieve proper fixation and seal [17]. However, inadequate fixation and seal, particularly at the proximal neck, can pose a significant risk of type 1A endoleaks and subsequent rupture of the AAA following EVAR. Researchers have conducted studies to explore predictive factors for AAA rupture. One study found that specific imaging markers obtained from CTA and characteristics of intraluminal thrombus morphology can be used to assess the risk of AAA rupture [18]. Another study focused on geometric parameters, such as the proximal neck angle, which is associated with aortic wall stress, as potential predictors of AAA rupture risk [19]. Additionally, research has shown that a neck length of <15 mm is associated with higher rates of early and late proximal type 1A endoleaks [5], while severe infrarenal neck angulation increases the likelihood of early type 1A endoleaks and graft migration [3]. Similarly, EVAR performed in the presence of a hostile neck morphology, characterized by a neck length of <10 mm and infrarenal neck angulation >60 degrees, has been found to be associated with a higher rate of intraoperative type 1A endoleaks and immediate adjunct neck procedures compared to cases with favorable aortic neck anatomy [11].

Our study provided additional insight into the effect of the aortic neck length and angulation on EVAR outcomes. Consistent with a recent meta-analysis, we found that patients with an aortic neck angle-length index > 4.8 (G2) have higher rates of immediate adjunct neck procedures in short aortic neck length < 15 mm, and/or neck angulation > 60 degrees [20]. No study has reported this association or proposed an optimal cutoff value of the aortic neck angle-length index for the prediction of intraoperative neck complications and immediate adjunct neck procedures after EVAR in AAA with severe neck angulation.

We found that patients with a short neck and an aortic neck angle-length index > 4.8 had significantly higher intraoperative neck complication rates (21% G1 vs. 55% G2, $p = 0.005$) and immediate adjunct neck procedures (18.9% G1 vs. 60% G2, $p < 0.001$). All patients in both groups with intraoperative type 1A endoleaks were successfully treated with a proximal extension cuff and/or Palmaz stent placement to achieve a proximal seal. This finding is consistent with the meta-analysis by Antoniou et al. [20] where adjunctive neck procedures were needed in 22% of AAA with hostile neck anatomy. In addition, short aortic neck length may be a crucial factor in determining neck complications and the requirement for adjunct neck procedures during EVAR in AAA with a severely angulated neck [5,21]. The findings of intraoperative neck complications in our study also support the repair of type 1A endoleaks with a large balloon-expandable Palmaz stent that Cox et al. [22] reported to be beneficial for use in hostile aortic neck, including proximal aortic neck angle > 60 degrees. Despite the danger of type 1A endoleaks, some studies [23,24] have suggested conservative management only in patients with anatomy considered suitable for EVAR, and if an adequately oversized stent graft had been optimally deployed. All type 1A endoleaks in our study developed in patients with severely angulated necks; therefore, we usually performed adjunct neck procedures for immediate type 1A endoleak repair.

Procedure time, fluoroscopic time, volume of contrast usage, and intraoperative blood loss were all higher in the aortic neck angle-length index > 4.8 group (G2), but without reaching statistical significance, perhaps due to an insufficient number of patients. Patients with aortic neck angle-length index > 4.8 (G2) had higher rates of intraoperative neck complications and needed more adjunctive neck procedures. Therefore, the procedure time, fluoroscopic time, contrast usage, and blood loss were higher than in the aortic neck angle-length index ≤ 4.8 (G1). A recently published study has also reported increases in these operative details in the presence of hostile neck anatomy [21].

No statistically significant difference in perioperative mortality was found between the two groups (1.1% G1 vs. 5% G2, $p = 0.319$), which agrees with earlier reports on hostile neck anatomy leading to 30-day mortality between 1.8% and 3% [11,25]. Within our study, there was an occurrence of graft limb occlusion in a single patient, which necessitated the implementation of a femorofemoral PTFE bypass graft procedure. In a separate investigation conducted by Catanese et al. [26], the incidence of limb graft occlusion following EVAR was reported to be 2.5% at a median postoperative day of 27. We observed that freedom from five-year re-intervention was in 93.7% of patients in the aortic neck angle-length index ≤ 4.8 (G1), and in 87.5% of the aortic neck angle-length index > 4.8 (G2), ($p = 0.785$). This is consistent with a study by Oliveira et al. [7] who reported a 95% freedom from four-year re-intervention in severely angulated neck and with Aburahma et al. [11] who reported an 85% freedom from four-year re-intervention in hostile aortic neck anatomy. The estimated overall survival rate at five years was 59.9% in patients with the aortic neck angle-length index ≤ 4.8 (G1), and 69.2% in the aortic neck angle-length index > 4.8 (G2), respectively ($p = 0.337$). Surprisingly, few studies have addressed long-term survival in AAA with severely angulated neck. Oliveira et al. [8] described 7-year survival rates of 44.3% for AAA with severely angulated neck.

Our study has certain limitations that should be acknowledged. Firstly, the small sample size, retrospective design, and observational nature of the study introduce inherent limitations, such as potential selection bias and reliance on existing data. This may affect the generalizability of our findings. Moreover, the inability to control for confounding variables may impact the validity of the observed associations. Additionally, it is important to note that not all patients included in the study had preoperative CT scans available, leading to potential information gaps. Furthermore, the utilization of different endograft devices for EVAR introduces a potential source of variability in our results. Lastly, it is worth mentioning that the study assessed outcomes only up to a 5-year follow-up period. As a result, the long-term effects and complications associated with EVAR in patients with severe neck angulation may not have been fully captured. A more comprehensive understanding of post-operative outcomes could be obtained by extending the follow-up duration.

5. Conclusions

Patients with an aortic neck angle-length index > 4.8 had a higher risk of intraoperative neck complications and adjunctive neck procedures compared with patients with an aortic neck angle-length index ≤ 4.8. The 5-year proximal neck re-intervention-free rate and the 5-year overall survival were not statistically different between groups. The aortic neck angle-length index is a reliable predictor of intraoperative neck complications and to prepare backup devices for immediate adjunct neck procedures during EVAR in AAA with a severely angulated neck.

Author Contributions: Conceptualization, K.C. and F.L.M.; Methodology, T.S., F.L.M., S.T. and K.H.; Software, S.T.; Validation, S.T.; Formal analysis, K.C., T.S., S.T. and K.H.; Investigation, T.S., F.L.M. and K.H.; Writing—original draft, T.S.; Writing—review & editing, K.C., F.L.M. and K.H.; Project administration, K.C. All authors have read and agreed to the published version of the manuscript.

Funding: This research did not receive any specific grant from funding agencies in the public, commercial, or not-for-profit sectors.

Institutional Review Board Statement: The study was conducted in accordance with the Declaration of Helsinki, and approved by the Institutional Review Board of the Siriraj Institutional Review Board (SIRB) (COA no. Si 499/2018 and Approval date: 15 August 2018) for studies involving humans.

Informed Consent Statement: Patient consent was waived due to the retrospective study.

Data Availability Statement: Data is unavailable due to privacy or ethical restrictions.

Acknowledgments: The authors would like to thank Surut Chalermjitt, Aphanan Phiromyaphorn, and Wannaporn Paemueang for their assistance with data collection. We also thank James Mark Simmerman, for his technical editing.

Conflicts of Interest: The authors declare no conflict of interest.

References

1. Marone, E.M.; Freyrie, A.; Ruotolo, C.; Michelagnoli, S.; Antonello, M.; Speziale, F.; Veroux, P.; Gargiulo, M.; Gaggiano, A. Expert Opinion on Hostile Neck Definition in Endovascular Treatment of Abdominal Aortic Aneurysms (a Delphi Consensus). *Ann. Vasc. Surg.* **2020**, *62*, 173–182. [CrossRef] [PubMed]
2. Rockley, M.; Hadziomerovic, A.; van Walraven, C.; Bose, P.; Scallan, O.; Jetty, P. A new "angle" on aortic neck angulation measurement. *J. Vasc. Surg.* **2019**, *70*, 756–761.e1. [CrossRef] [PubMed]
3. Hobo, R.; Kievit, J.; Leurs, L.J.; Buth, J. Influence of severe infrarenal aortic neck angulation on complications at the proximal neck following endovascular AAA repair: A EUROSTAR study. *J. Endovasc. Ther.* **2007**, *14*, 1–11. [CrossRef] [PubMed]
4. AbuRahma, A.F.; Campbell, J.; Stone, P.A.; Nanjundappa, A.; Jain, A.; Dean, L.S.; Habib, J.; Keiffer, T.; Emmett, M. The correlation of aortic neck length to early and late outcomes in endovascular aneurysm repair patients. *J. Vasc. Surg.* **2009**, *50*, 738–748. [CrossRef]
5. Leurs, L.J.; Kievit, J.; Dagnelie, P.C.; Nelemans, P.J.; Buth, J. Influence of infrarenal neck length on outcome of endovascular abdominal aortic aneurysm repair. *J. Endovasc. Ther.* **2006**, *13*, 640–648. [CrossRef]
6. Bastos Goncalves, F.; de Vries, J.P.; van Keulen, J.W.; Dekker, H.; Moll, F.L.; Van Herwaarden, J.A.; Verhagen, H.J.M. Severe proximal aneurysm neck angulation: Early results using the Endurant stentgraft system. *Eur. J. Vasc. Endovasc. Surg.* **2011**, *41*, 193–200. [CrossRef]
7. Oliveira, N.F.; Bastos Goncalves, F.M.; de Vries, J.P.; Ultee, K.H.J.; Werson, D.A.B.; Hoeks, S.E.; Moll, F.; Van Herwaarden, J.A.; Verhagen, H.J.M. Mid-Term Results of EVAR in Severe Proximal Aneurysm Neck Angulation. *Eur. J. Vasc. Endovasc. Surg.* **2015**, *49*, 19–27. [CrossRef]
8. Oliveira, N.F.; Gonçalves, F.B.; Hoeks, S.E.; van Rijn, M.J.; Ultee, K.; Pinto, J.P.; Raa, S.T.; van Herwaarden, J.A.; de Vries, J.-P.P.; Verhagen, H.J. Long-term outcomes of standard endovascular aneurysm repair in patients with severe neck angulation. *J. Vasc. Surg.* **2018**, *68*, 1725–1735. [CrossRef]
9. van Keulen, J.W.; Moll, F.L.; Tolenaar, J.L.; Verhagen, H.J.; van Herwaarden, J.A. Validation of a new standardized method to measure proximal aneurysm neck angulation. *J. Vasc. Surg.* **2010**, *51*, 821–828. [CrossRef]

10. Sweet, M.P.; Fillinger, M.F.; Morrison, T.M.; Abel, D. The influence of gender and aortic aneurysm size on eligibility for endovascular abdominal aortic aneurysm repair. *J. Vasc. Surg.* **2011**, *54*, 931–937. [CrossRef]
11. Aburahma, A.F.; Campbell, J.E.; Mousa, A.Y.; Hass, S.M.; Stone, P.A.; Jain, A.; Nanjundappa, A.; Dean, L.S.; Keiffer, T.; Habib, J. Clinical outcomes for hostile versus favorable aortic neck anatomy in endovascular aortic aneurysm repair using modular devices. *J. Vasc. Surg.* **2011**, *54*, 13–21. [CrossRef] [PubMed]
12. Chaikof, E.L.; Blankensteijn, J.D.; Harris, P.L.; White, G.H.; Zarins, C.K.; Bernhard, V.M.; Matsumura, J.S.; May, J.; Veith, F.J.; Fillinger, M.F.; et al. Reporting standards for endovascular aortic aneurysm repair. *J. Vasc. Surg.* **2002**, *35*, 1048–1060. [CrossRef] [PubMed]
13. Wurpts, I.C.; Geiser, C. Is adding more indicators to a latent class analysis beneficial or detrimental? Results of a Monte-Carlo study. *Front. Psychol.* **2014**, *5*, 920. [CrossRef] [PubMed]
14. Scrucca, L.; Fop, M.; Murphy, T.B.; Raftery, A.E. mclust 5: Clustering, Classification and Density Estimation Using Gaussian Finite Mixture Models. *R J.* **2016**, *8*, 289–317. [CrossRef] [PubMed]
15. Daniel Spurk, A.H.; Wang, M.; Valero, D.; Kauffeld, S. Latent profile analysis: A review and "how to" guide of its application within vocational behavior research. *J. Vocat. Behav.* **2020**, *120*, 130445.
16. Kaewchoothong, Y.A.N.; Assawalertsakul, T.; Nuntadusit, C.; Chatpun, S. Computational Study of Abdominal Aortic Aneurysms with Severely Angulated Neck Based on Transient Hemodynamics Using an Idealized Model. *Appl. Sci.* **2022**, *12*, 2113. [CrossRef]
17. De Bock, S.; Iannaccone, F.; De Beule, M.; Vermassen, F.; Segers, P.; Verhegghe, B. What if you stretch the IFU? A mechanical insight into stent graft Instructions For Use in angulated proximal aneurysm necks. *Med. Eng. Phys.* **2014**, *36*, 1567–1576. [CrossRef]
18. Arbănași, E.M.; Mureșan, A.V.; Coșarcă, C.M.; Arbănași, E.M.; Niculescu, R.; Voidăzan, S.T.; Ivănescu, A.D.; Hălmaciu, I.; Filep, R.C.; Mărginean, L.; et al. Computed Tomography Angiography Markers and Intraluminal Thrombus Morphology as Predictors of Abdominal Aortic Aneurysm Rupture. *Int. J. Environ. Res. Public. Health* **2022**, *19*, 15961. [CrossRef]
19. You, J.H.; Lee, C.W.; Huh, U.; Lee, C.S.; Ryu, D. Comparative Study of Aortic Wall Stress According to Geometric Parameters in Abdominal Aortic Aneurysms. *Appl. Sci.* **2021**, *11*, 3195. [CrossRef]
20. Antoniou, G.A.; Georgiadis, G.S.; Antoniou, S.A.; Kuhan, G.; Murray, D. A meta-analysis of outcomes of endovascular abdominal aortic aneurysm repair in patients with hostile and friendly neck anatomy. *J. Vasc. Surg.* **2013**, *57*, 527–538. [CrossRef]
21. Broos, P.P.; Stokmans, R.A.; van Sterkenburg, S.M.; Torsello, G.; Vermassen, F.; Cuypers, P.W.; van Sambeek, M.R.; Teijink, J.A. Performance of the Endurant stent graft in challenging anatomy. *J. Vasc. Surg.* **2015**, *62*, 312–318. [CrossRef] [PubMed]
22. Cox, D.E.; Jacobs, D.L.; Motaganahalli, R.L.; Wittgen, C.M.; Peterson, G.J. Outcomes of endovascular AAA repair in patients with hostile neck anatomy using adjunctive balloon-expandable stents. *Vasc. Endovasc. Surg.* **2006**, *40*, 35–40. [CrossRef] [PubMed]
23. Millen, A.M.; Osman, K.; Antoniou, G.A.; McWilliams, R.G.; Brennan, J.A.; Fisher, R.K. Outcomes of persistent intraoperative type Ia endoleak after standard endovascular aneurysm repair. *J. Vasc. Surg.* **2015**, *61*, 1185–1191. [CrossRef]
24. Bastos Gonçalves, F.; Verhagen, H.J.; Vasanthananthan, K.; Zandvoort, H.J.; Moll, F.L.; van Herwaarden, J.A. Spontaneous delayed sealing in selected patients with a primary type-Ia endoleak after endovascular aneurysm repair. *Eur. J. Vasc. Endovasc. Surg.* **2014**, *48*, 53–59. [CrossRef] [PubMed]
25. Torsello, G.; Troisi, N.; Donas, K.P.; Austermann, M. Evaluation of the Endurant stent graft under instructions for use vs off-label conditions for endovascular aortic aneurysm repair. *J. Vasc. Surg.* **2011**, *54*, 300–306. [CrossRef] [PubMed]
26. Catanese, V.; Sangiorgi, G.; Sotgiu, G.; Saderi, L.; Settembrini, A.; Donelli, C.; Martelli, E. Clinical and anatomical variables associated in the literature to limb graft occlusion after endovascular aneurysm repair compared to the experience of a tertiary referral center. *Minerva Chir.* **2020**, *75*, 51–59. (In English) [CrossRef] [PubMed]

Disclaimer/Publisher's Note: The statements, opinions and data contained in all publications are solely those of the individual author(s) and contributor(s) and not of MDPI and/or the editor(s). MDPI and/or the editor(s) disclaim responsibility for any injury to people or property resulting from any ideas, methods, instructions or products referred to in the content.

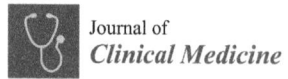
Journal of
Clinical Medicine

Review

Systematic Review and Meta-Analysis of the Incidence of Rupture, Repair, and Death of Small and Large Abdominal Aortic Aneurysms under Surveillance

Nicola Leone [1,2,*,†], Magdalena Anna Broda [1,3,†], Jonas Peter Eiberg [1,3,4] and Timothy Andrew Resch [1,3]

1. Department of Vascular Surgery, Rigshospitalet, 2200 Copenhagen, Denmark; magdalena.anna.broda.01@regionh.dk (M.A.B.); jonas.peter.eiberg@regionh.dk (J.P.E.); timothy.andrew.resch@regionh.dk (T.A.R.)
2. Department of Vascular Surgery, Ospedale Civile di Baggiovara, Azienda Ospedaliero-Universitaria di Modena, University of Modena and Reggio Emilia, 41126 Modena, Italy
3. Department of Clinical Medicine, Faculty of Health and Medical Sciences, University of Copenhagen, 1172 København, Denmark
4. Copenhagen Academy of Medical Education and Simulation (CAMES), 2100 København, Denmark
* Correspondence: nicola.leone.md@gmail.com
† These authors contributed equally to this work.

Abstract: Background: The ultimate goal of treating patients with abdominal aortic aneurysms (AAAs) is to repair them when the risk of rupture exceeds the risk of repair. Small AAAs demonstrate a low rupture risk, and recently, large AAAs just above the threshold (5.5–6.0 cm) seem to be at low risk of rupture as well. The present review aims to investigate the outcomes of AAAs under surveillance through a comprehensive systematic review and meta-analysis. Methods: PubMed, Embase, and the Cochrane Central Register were searched (22 March 2022; PROSPERO; #CRD42022316094). The Cochrane and PRISMA statements were respected. Blinded systematic screening of the literature, data extraction, and quality assessment were performed by two authors. Conflicts were resolved by a third author. The meta-analysis of prevalence provided estimated proportions, 95% confidence intervals, and measures of heterogeneity (I^2). Based on I^2, the heterogeneity might be negligible (0–40%), moderate (30–60%), substantial (50–90%), and considerable (75–100%). The primary outcome was the incidence of AAA rupture. Secondary outcomes included the rate of small AAAs reaching the threshold for repair, aortic-related mortality, and all-cause mortality. Results: Fourteen publications (25,040 patients) were included in the analysis. The outcome rates of the small AAA group (<55 mm) were 0.3% (95% CI 0.0–1.0; I^2 = 76.4%) of rupture, 0.6% (95% CI 0.0–1.9; I^2 = 87.2%) of aortic-related mortality, and 9.6% (95% CI 2.2–21.1; I^2 = 99.0%) of all-cause mortality. During surveillance, 21.4% (95% CI 9.0–37.2; I^2 = 99.0%) of the initially small AAAs reached the threshold for repair. The outcome rates of the large AAA group (>55 mm) were 25.7% (95% CI 18.0–34.3; I^2 = 72.0%) of rupture, 22.1% (95% CI 16.5–28.3; I^2 = 25.0%) of aortic-related mortality, and 61.8% (95% CI 47.0–75.6; I^2 = 89.1%) of all-cause mortality. The sensitivity analysis demonstrated a higher rupture rate in studies including <662 subjects, patients with a mean age > 72 years, >17% of female patients, and >44% of current smokers. Conclusion: The rarity of rupture and aortic-related mortality in small AAAs supports the current conservative management of small AAAs. Surveillance seems indicated, as one-fifth reached the threshold for repair. Large aneurysms had a high incidence of rupture and aortic-related mortality. However, these data seem biased by the sparse and heterogeneous literature overrepresented by patients unfit for surgery. Specific rupture risk stratified by age, gender, and fit-for-surgery patients with large AAAs needs to be further investigated.

Keywords: aortic pathology; aortic disease; aortic aneurysm; aneurysm; ruptured aneurysm; mortality

Citation: Leone, N.; Broda, M.A.; Eiberg, J.P.; Resch, T.A. Systematic Review and Meta-Analysis of the Incidence of Rupture, Repair, and Death of Small and Large Abdominal Aortic Aneurysms under Surveillance. *J. Clin. Med.* **2023**, *12*, 6837. https://doi.org/10.3390/jcm12216837

Academic Editors: Martin Teraa and Constantijn E.V.B. Hazenberg

Received: 5 September 2023
Revised: 24 October 2023
Accepted: 25 October 2023
Published: 29 October 2023

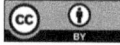

Copyright: © 2023 by the authors. Licensee MDPI, Basel, Switzerland. This article is an open access article distributed under the terms and conditions of the Creative Commons Attribution (CC BY) license (https://creativecommons.org/licenses/by/4.0/).

1. Introduction

Ruptured abdominal aortic aneurysms (AAAs) have a mortality rate of approximately 80% [1]. Although prophylactic endovascular aortic repair (EVAR) and open aortic repair (OAR) are valid treatment options, repair is not without risks of mortality and complications [2,3]. The ultimate goal of treating patients with abdominal aortic aneurysms (AAAs) is to repair them when the risk of rupture exceeds the risk of repair.

The association between diameter and rupture risk is well established, and randomized control trials (RCTs) have confirmed that the repair of AAAs smaller than 5.5 cm in maximum diameter should be avoided [4–6]. Based on these findings, the current guidelines suggest elective repair when the maximum anteroposterior aortic diameter is $\geq 5.0/5.5$ cm on ultrasound in women and men, or in cases of rapid growth (≥ 1 cm/year) [7]. However, these recommendations rely on outdated RCTs powered by historical, perhaps overestimated, AAA rupture data [8–10]. Furthermore, the RCTs were flawed by underestimating the surgical operative risk (UK SAT) and by using different methodologies for measuring AAA diameter (UK SAT and ADAM) [11,12]. This information is currently transposed into the National Institute for Health and Care Excellence (NICE) guidelines, confirming the absence of robust evidence to support the 5.5 cm threshold for men [13].

There has been a lack of population-based studies in the last two decades. Between 2009 and 2017, the National Health Service AAA Screening Programme (NAAASP) screened more than 18 65-year-old males with small AAAs (30–55 mm) [14]. The three-year cumulative incidence of rupture was approximately 0.6% [14]. According to a retrospective analysis of a large prospectively maintained database, the three-year cumulative incidence of rupture in patients with AAAs measuring 5.5–6.0 cm and 6.1–7.0 cm was 2.2% and 6.0%, respectively [15]. Thus, small AAAs demonstrate a low rupture risk, and much more surprisingly, large AAAs just above the threshold (5.5–6.0 cm) seem to be at low risk of rupture as well.

The risk of rupture has implications for patient counselling, surveillance protocols, and surgical decision-making. However, updated systematic reviews and meta-analyses summarising the modern outcomes of AAA surveillance are lacking. Therefore, this work aimed to perform a comprehensive systematic review of the evidence on AAA rupture risk and the rate of small AAAs reaching the threshold for repair, aortic-related mortality, and all-cause mortality after the year 2000.

2. Materials and Methods

The objectives and methodology of this project were prespecified in the International Prospective Register of Systematic Reviews (PROSPERO) under ID #CRD42022316094. This systematic review and meta-analysis was performed according to the Cochrane Collaboration and PRISMA statements [16]. The search was completed on 22 March 2022 in Medline, Embase, and CENTRAL (Cochrane Central Register of Controlled Trials), combining thesaurus and free text terms (untreated, nonoperative, risk, rupture, diameter, threshold, growth, size, fate, natural history, surveillance, screening, follow-up, AAA, and abdominal aortic aneurysm) with standard Boolean operators.

2.1. Study Selection and Inclusion Criteria

This systematic review evaluated all the available studies with the following inclusion criteria: (i) both men and women, or a single gender, older than 18 years and being part of all ethnic groups; (ii) with an abdominal aortic aneurysm (AAA) of any size (>30 mm; see the Section 2.3 for details); (iii) under surveillance/screening; (iv) with duplex ultrasound scans (DUS), computed tomography angiography (CTA), or magnetic resonance (MR) imaging; (v) reporting a rupture rate and/or rate of small aneurysms reaching the threshold for repair; (vi) with a follow-up initiated after the year 2000. Interventional or observational and prospective or retrospective study designs were considered eligible.

Meta-analysis and reviews were excluded using the 'Publication type' option. Exclusion criteria included: (i) studies not reporting the rate of rupture or the baseline size of the small aneurysm reaching the threshold for repair; (ii) studies reporting on aortic ectasia or on aortic segments other than abdominal; (iii) studies focusing on operative management; and (iv) follow-ups initiated before the year 2000. Authors responsible for either included or excluded papers were not contacted. No language or other constraints were applied.

2.2. Data Collection Process and Quality

The literature search result was uploaded and managed through Covidence systematic review Software, Veritas Health Innovation, Melbourne, Australia (available at www.covidence.org), allowing two authors (N.L. and M.A.B.) to perform a blinded systematic screening of the literature search result. A senior author (T.A.R.) resolved disagreements. Each title and abstract were evaluated for inclusion/exclusion criteria. Studies assessed as having an eligible abstract underwent a blinded full-text screening. Finally, the screening authors extracted data from included publications using a data collection form that was established a priori following an internal discussion. A study quality assessment (the Quality Appraisal Checklist from the Institute of Health Economics) [17] was performed simultaneously. For the primary outcome, publication and reporting biases were assessed by evaluating funnel plot asymmetry. Egger's test was used to evaluate small study effect biases.

2.3. Outcomes and Definitions

The primary outcome was the incidence of AAA ruptures during surveillance. Secondary outcomes were (i) the rate of small AAAs reaching the threshold for repair, (ii) aortic-related mortality, and (iii) all-cause mortality.

As suggested by the current guidelines, an AAA was defined as a dilation of ≥ 30 mm [7]. Aneurysms were classified as small if the diameter ranged between 30 and 55 mm, considering that in this case prophylactic repair is not recommended [7]. Correspondingly, a large AAA was defined as a diameter exceeding 55 mm. The rate of small AAAs reaching the threshold for repair was extracted by the current authors as presented in the literature. Aortic-related mortality accounts for death caused by the aneurysm directly (rupture) or indirectly (e.g., infection). All-cause mortality includes all etiologies leading to death. The thought behind presenting overlapping diameter groups was to evaluate eventual differences between diameter subgroups; e.g., the small AAA group outcomes might be overshadowed by the inclusion of very small aneurysms (<40 mm) in contrast with the 40–55 mm subgroup. The outcomes were aggregated, analysed, and presented according to baseline size ranges when a minimum of three publications were available.

There were no attempts to contact primary authors to better clarify the threshold for repair details (e.g., which guidelines were applied, how many patients were women, treatment of different aneurysm morphology at different thresholds, etc.) nor the causes of aortic-related mortality and all-cause mortality. All variables included in the data collection form have been specified in Table A1.

2.4. Data Synthesis and Analysis

The outcomes were gathered as proportions for the quantitative analysis. For instance, the small AAA estimate proportion of rupture was calculated by dividing the number of ruptured AAAs ranging from 30 to 55 mm by the total number of patients in the subgroup. This provided the data for pooling proportions in a meta-analysis of multiple studies. Data presented as median and interquartile range were converted into means and standard deviation, according to Hozo and colleagues [18]. The primary outcome was displayed as a forest plot for the size ranges of interest. The 95% confidence interval (95% CI) was based on the Wilson score. The Freeman-Tukey transformation (double arcsine transformation) was applied to avoid negative proportions in the CI (CI range 0–100%) [19]. The heterogeneity of the included studies was managed using the random-effects model [20]. The heterogeneity coming from different studies was examined by either inspecting the scatter in the data points and the CIs overlap as well as by performing I^2 statistics [21]. Sensitivity analysis was performed for the primary outcome of the most frequently reported size group (30–55 mm) regarding female gender, smokers, study sample size, and mean age of included patients. The cut-offs for meta-regressions were based on median values. Statistical analysis was performed with STATA 15.1 (StataCorp College Station, TX, USA).

3. Results

The literature search resulted in 11,315 references after the removal of duplicates (Figure 1).

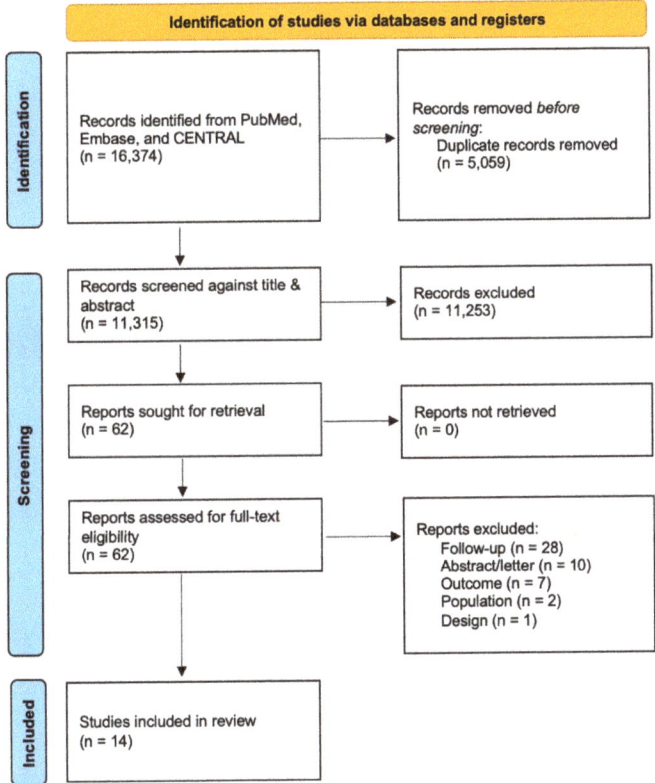

Figure 1. PRISMA flow diagram.

Of the 62 full texts considered for inclusion, 28 were excluded because the follow-up initiated before the year 2000; ten were congress abstracts or correspondences; seven did not match the present outcomes of interest; two reported on populations not suitable for inclusion; and one was excluded based on study design (Table A2). Overall, 31,432 participants were reported in the 14 included studies [6,14,15,22–32]. However, the number of patients eligible for analysis in the present meta-analysis was 25,040 due to loss of follow-up (n = 1933), sub-populations not matching the inclusion criteria, and other causes of withdrawal. Nine (64%) publications were European [14,26,28,30,31]; one was a multicenter study including European and western Asian hospitals [6]; and the remaining four publications were from New Zealand (n = 1, 7.2%), Australia (n = 1, 7.2%), the United States of America (n = 1, 7.2%), and Qatar (n = 1, 7.2%) [15,23,25,27]. The baseline and specific details for each included study have been displayed in Tables 1 and 2.

Table 1. General information from the fourteen studies included in the meta-analysis.

Author and Publication Year	Country	Journal	Study Period—y	Aim	AAA [a]	Male/Female [a]	Age—y [b]	Follow-Up—y [b]
Cao 2011 [6]	Europe and Western Asia	EJVES	2004–2008	Surveillance vs. EVAR for small AAAs	178	172/6	68.8	2.6
Buckenham 2007 [23]	New Zealand	NZMJ	2000–2005	Surveillance programme based on the UK SAT	198	148/50	72	1.6
Söderberg 2017 [26]	Sweden	EJVES	2007–2014	5-year natural history of sub-AAAs and AAAs in 70-year-old women	19	0/19	70.0	5.0
Scott 2016 [28]	UK	EJVES	2006–2013	Survival from AAAs not undergoing immediate repair	138	115/23	77.0	2.3
Oliver-Williams 2019 [14]	UK	Circulation	2009–2017	Safety of men under surveillance in NAAASP	18,652	18,652/0	66.8	2.7
Noronen 2013 [31]	Finland	EJVES	2000–2012	Fate of an AAA meeting treatment criteria but not the operative requirements	154	106/48	79.6	1.6
Lim 2015 [30]	UK	EJVES	2001–2013	Examine men from the GASP	59	59/0	71.0	-
Lancaster 2022 [15]	USA	JVS	2003–2020	Impact of large AAA sizes on the incidence of rupture and mortality	3248	2312/936	83.6	3.6
Hultgren 2020 [29]	Sweden	Angiology	2010–2017	Long-term follow-up of men in a population-based regional screening programme	662	662/0	65.0	4.7
Golledge 2019 [25]	Australia	EJVES	2002–2017	Determine whether AAA-related clinical events were lower in patients under metformin	1080	881/199	73.4	2.6
Ghulam 2017 [32]	Denmark	EJVES	2013–2015	Surveillance of small AAAs with a new, non-invasive 3D-US	179	146/33	74.1	1
Elmallah 2018 [22]	Ireland	Vascular	2006–2017	Outcome of conservative management of large AAAs unfit for surgery	76	54/22	80.0	2.1
Al-Thani 2014 [27]	Qatar	Angiology	2004–2008	Outcomes of AAAs incidentally discovered	55	50/11	67.0	3.0
MA3RS Investigators 2017 [24]	UK	Circulation	2012–2014	Determine whether USPIO-enhanced MRI could predict the rate of AAA expansion, rupture, or surgical repair	342	292/50	73.1	2.7

[a] Data are presented as counts; [b] Data are presented as means. AAA, abdominal aortic aneurysm; NZMJ, New Zealand Medical Journal; UK SAT, United Kingdom Small Aneurysm Trial; EJVES, European Journal for Vascular and Endovascular Surgery; NAAASP, National Health Service AAA Screening Programme; JVS, Journal for Vascular Surgery; 3D-US, three-dimensional ultrasound; USPIO, ultrasmall superparamagnetic iron oxide; MRI, magnetic resonance imaging.

Table 2. Outcomes data extracted from the 14 studies included in the meta-analysis.

Author and Publication Year	Size Range—mm	AAA [a]	Rupture [b]	Threshold for Repair [b]	Aortic Mortality [b]	All-Cause Mortality [b]
Cao 2011 [6]	41–54	178	2 (1.2)	75 (42.1)	1 (0.6)	8 (4.5)
Buckenham 2007 [23]	30–55	198	3 (1.5)	52 (26.3)	5 (2.5)	23 (11.6)
Söderberg 2017 [26]	30–55	19	1 (5.2)	6 (31.6)	1 (5.2)	2 (10.5)
Scott 2016 [28]	>55	138	37 (26.8)	-	37 (26.8)	71 (51.4)
Oliver-Williams 2019 [14]	(i) 30–55 (ii) 30–44 (iii) 45–54 (iv) 50–54	(i) 18,652 (ii) 16,430 (iii) 2222 (iv) 769	(i) 31 (0.2) (ii) 20 (0.1) (iii) 11 (0.5) (iv) 3 (0.4)	(i) 1314 (7.0) (ii) - (iii) - (iv) -	(i) 29 (0.2) (ii) 19 (0.1) (iii) 10 (0.5) (iv) -	(i) 980 (5.3) (ii) 912 (5.6) (iii) 68 (3.1) (iv) 15 (2.0)
Noronen 2013 [31]	(i) >55 (ii) 55–60 (iii) 61–70 (iv) >70	(i) 154 (ii) 74 (iii) 57 (iv) 23	(i) 56 (36.4) (ii) - (iii) - (iv) -	-	(i) - (ii) 31 (41.9) (iii) 25 (43.8) (iv) 10 (43.5)	(i) 120 (77.9) (ii) - (iii) - (iv) -
Lim 2015 [30]	>55	59	10 (16.9)	-	10 (16.9)	30 (50.8)
Lancaster 2022 [15]	>50	3 248	216 (6.7)	-	-	756 (23.3)
Hultgren 2020 [29]	(i) 30–55 (ii) 30–39 (iii) 40–49 (iv) 45–50 (v) >50	(i) 579 (ii) 472 (iii) 107 (iv) 35 (v) 76	(i) 0 (0) (ii) 0 (0) (iii) 0 (0) (iv) 0 (0) (v) 2 (2.6)	(i) 42 (7.3) (ii) 9 (1.9) (iii) 33 (30.8) (iv) 0 (0) (v) -	(i) - (ii) - (iii) - (iv) - (v) 1 (1.3)	(i) - (ii) - (iii) - (iv) - (v) -
Golledge 2019 [25]	30–55	952	-	442 (46.4)	12 (1.3)	321 (33.7)
Ghulam 2017 [32]	30–55	179	0	13 (7.3)	0	3 (1.7)
Elmallah 2018 [22]	>55	76	16 (21.1)	-	15 (19.7)	49 (64.5)
Al-Thani 2014 [27]	>70	14	8 (57.1)	-	-	6 (42.9)
MA3RS Investigators 2017 [24]	(i) 40–49 (ii) >50	(i) 187 (ii) 155	(i) 4 (2.1) (ii) 98 (63.2)	(i) 38 (20.3) (ii) -	(i) 4 (2.1) (ii) 13 (8.4)	(i) 20 (10.7) (ii) 28 (18.1)

[a] Data are presented as counts; [b] Data are presented as counts and percentages calculated on the included number of AAAs per specific size range. AAA, abdominal aortic aneurysm.

The quality appraisal is summarised in Table A3. The project has evolved since its initial inception due to the absence of a homogeneous statistical measure of the rupture risk and the heterogeneity of size thresholds reported in the literature. Specifically, a direct comparison of subgroups just below and above the threshold for repair was not possible due to the absence of data.

The pooled estimate of subjects' mean age was 74.0 years (95% CI 68.7–79.3; I^2 = 91.7%) [6,14,15,22–32]. The female proportion was 17.4% (95% CI 6.0–32.8; I^2 = 99.7%) [6,14,15,22–32]. The patients had a mean follow-up of 2.2 years (95% CI 1.4–3.1; I^2 = 81.6%) [6,15,22–29,31,32]. One study did not report the mean or median follow-up duration [30]. The proportions of current-, previous-, and never-smokers were 44.8% (95% CI 34.0–55.7; I^2 = 99.2%), 26.2% (95% CI 13.7–41.1; I^2 = 99.7%), and 11.6% (95% CI 8.7–14.9; I^2 = 96.1%), respectively [6,14,15,22,24–29,32]. However, the sum of the three smoking statuses does not reach

100% because the statuses were heterogeneously reported and different publications were used to estimate the single variable.

3.1. Patients with Small AAAs

The overall outcomes of the small aneurysm group (30–55 mm) as well as the mid-sized AAAs (40–55 mm) are shown in Table 3. Seven publications reported on the primary outcome of patients with small aneurysms [6,14,23,24,26,29,32]. One additional study also published the secondary outcomes of small aneurysms [25].

Table 3. Outcomes of pooled estimates for the major size ranges.

	Rupture [a]	Repair Threshold [a]	Aortic Mortality [a]	All-Cause Mortality [a]
30–55 mm	N = 19,992 e = 41 0.3 | 0.0–1.0 | 76.4 [6,14,23,24,26,29,32]	N = 20,944 e = 1982 21.4 | 9.0–37.2 | 99.3 [6,14,23–26,29,32]	N = 20,365 e = 52 0.6 | 0.0–1.9 | 87.2 [6,14,23–26,32]	N = 20,365 e = 1357 9.6 | 2.2–21.1 | 99.0 [6,14,23–26,32]
40–55 mm	N = 3498 e = 20 0.6 | 0.1–1.6 | 57.7 [6,14,24,29]	N = 507 e = 170 33.7 | 20.1–48.9 | 91.9 [6,24,29]	N = 3356 e = 15 0.7 | 0.0–2.1 | 71.1 [6,14,24]	N = 3356 e = 111 5.4 | 1.7–10.9 | 90.6 [6,14,24]
>55 mm	N = 427 e = 119 25.7 | 18.0–34.3 | 72.0 [22,28,30,31]	-	N = 273 e = 62 22.1 | 16.5–28.3 | 25.0 [22,28,30]	N = 427 e = 270 61.8 | 47.0–75.6 | 89.1 [22,28,30,31]

N, population available for the specific outcome; e, number of events; ES%, estimate proportion; 95% CI, 95% confidence interval. [a] Data are presented as ES% | 95% CI | I^2.

A total of 19,992 small AAAs were analyzed. The incidence of AAA rupture in patients with small AAAs was 0.3% (n = 41 ruptures), with a slight increase in mid-sized AAAs to 0.6% (n = 20 ruptures; subgroup total number of 3498 patients), over a mean follow-up of 2.3 years (95% CI 1.1–3.5; I^2 = 88.3%). The small AAA group rupture incidence has been graphically illustrated as a forest plot (Figure 2). The corresponding funnel plot demonstrated a fair distribution on average, and Egger's test p-value was higher than 0.05, suggesting the absence of publication biases (Figure 3). The aortic and all-cause deaths were 52 and 1357 vs. 15 and 111 for the 30–55 mm and the 40–55 mm groups, respectively. These data led to 0.6% and 9.6% vs. 0.7% and 5.4% estimated proportions of aortic and all-cause mortality for the 30–55 mm and the 40–55 mm groups, respectively; see Table 3 for details.

The rupture proportion of 30–39 mm AAAs was 0.0% (95% CI 0.0–0.8), and the rate of those reaching the threshold for repair was 1.9% (95% CI 0.9–3.6) during a mean follow-up time of 4.7 years (95% CI 2.6–6.8), according to the single study reporting the subgroup's outcomes [29]. The rupture proportion in the 30–44 mm subgroup was similar to the one reported for the 30–39 mm subgroup, 0.1% (95% CI 0.1–0.2) [14] within the mean 2.7-year follow-up. The same single publication reported the 30–44 mm subgroup having an aortic-related and all-cause mortality of 0.1% (95% CI 0.1–0.2) and 5.6% (95% CI 5.2–5.9), respectively [14].

All studies reporting the outcomes of 40–49 mm, 45–50 mm, 45–54 mm, and 50–54 mm AAAs were merged under the 40–55 mm size range. Specific outcomes for these groups have been detailed in Table A4.

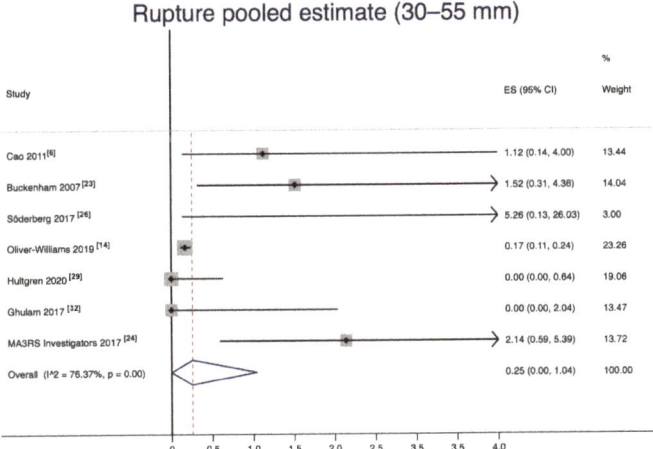

Figure 2. Small abdominal aortic aneurysm pooled estimate of rupture incidence. The vertical dotted line represents the mean proportion of all studies. The black horizontal lines represents the confidence interval of each single study [6,14,23,24,26,29,32].

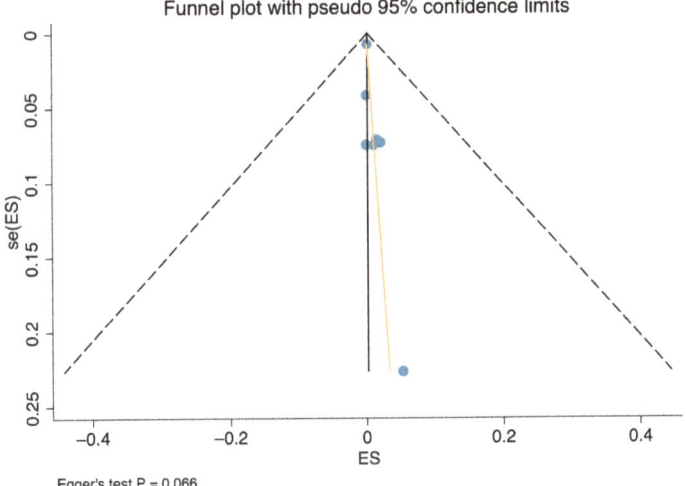

Figure 3. Funnel plot and Egger's test of small abdominal aortic aneurysm pooled estimate of rupture incidence.

3.2. Patients with Large AAAs

The outcomes of patients with large AAAs (>55 mm) are displayed in Table 3. Four publications reported on rupture, aortic-related mortality, and all-cause mortality of large AAAs [22,28,30,31]. Three studies used a different threshold for large aneurysms > 50 mm, demonstrating a pooled estimate of rupture of 19.0% (95% CI 0.0–60.4; I^2 = 99.2%) [15,24,29] over a mean follow-up of 2.2 years (95% CI 1.6–2.8; I^2 = 0.0%). Both primary and secondary outcomes of large AAA subgroups were scarcely reported, leading us to analyse the outcomes of the following sub-groups: 55–60 mm, 61–70 mm, and >70 mm (Table A4). One publication reported the rupture rate for AAAs > 70 mm (57.1%; 95% CI 28.9–82.3) [27] over a mean follow-up of three years. The aortic mortality rate was 41.9% (95% CI 30.5–53.9),

43.9% (95% CI 30.7–57.6), and 43.5% (95% CI 23.2–65.5) for 55–60, 61–70, and >70 mm AAAs, respectively, according to the only publication reporting on this outcome [31]. Primary and secondary outcome data were not available for the remaining size ranges.

3.3. Sensitivity Analysis

The results of the sensitivity analysis have been graphically depicted in Figure 4.

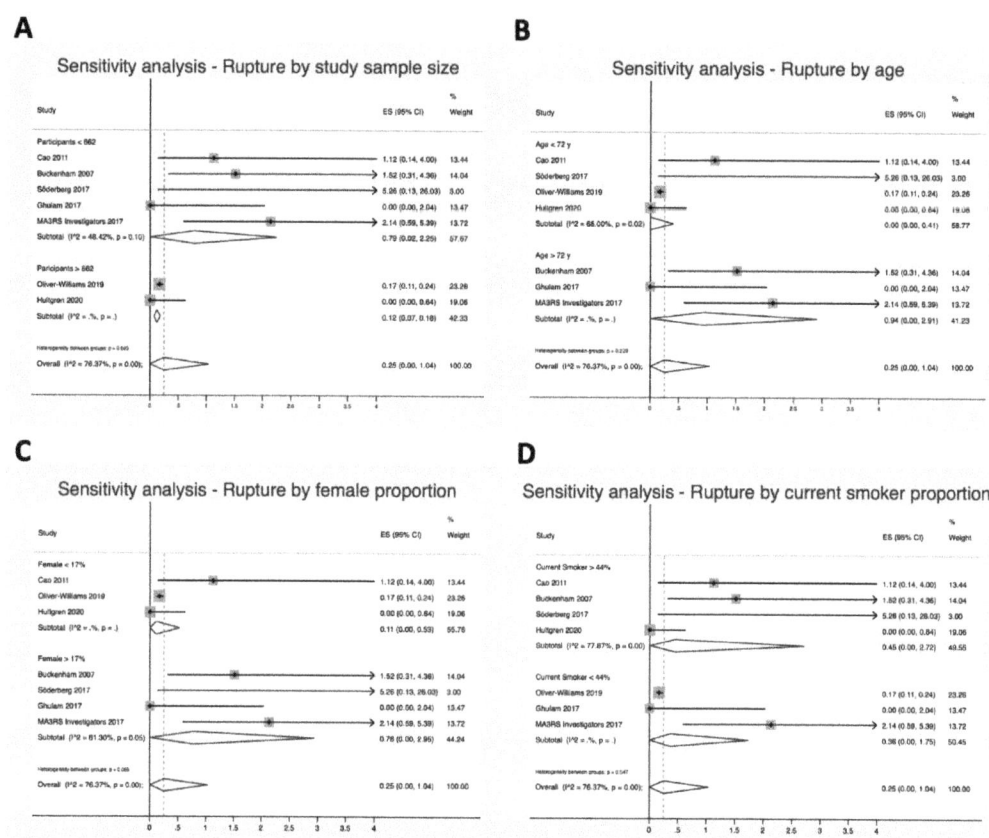

Figure 4. Sensitivity analysis of small abdominal aortic aneurysm pooled estimate rupture (**A**) by sample size (< vs. >662 patients), (**B**) by mean age (< vs. >72 years old), (**C**) by female proportion (< vs. >17%), and (**D**) by current smoker proportion (< vs. >44%). The vertical dotted line represents the mean proportion of all studies. The black horizontal lines represents the confidence interval of each single study [6,14,23,24,26,29,32].

Overall, the study sample size, mean age, proportion of females, and proportion of current smokers were used for the sensitivity analysis of the seven publications reporting on small aneurysms [6,14,23,24,26,29,32]. The rupture proportion was higher in studies including <662 subjects (0.8% vs. 0.1%; heterogeneity between groups, $p = 0.003$). Furthermore, the rupture proportion was higher within studies including patients with a mean age > 72 years (0.9% vs. 0.0%; heterogeneity between groups, $p = 0.22$). A proportion of female patients exceeding 17% and of current smokers > 44% demonstrated higher estimates of rupture: 0.8% vs. 0.1% (heterogeneity between groups, $p = 0.059$) and 0.5% vs. 0.4% (heterogeneity between groups, $p = 0.55$), respectively.

4. Discussion

This meta-analysis confirmed a low incidence of rupture amongst patients with small AAAs (30–55 mm, 0.3%) with a slight increase for patients with mid-sized small AAAs (40–55 mm, 0.6%) over a mean follow-up of 2.3 years. One-fifth (21%) of patients with small AAAs reached the threshold for repair during the same time period. Aortic-related mortality in patients with small AAAs was rare (0.6%), in contrast to all-cause mortality (10%). These results align with the previously published pooled outcomes of small aneurysms, mainly including subjects enrolled before the year 2000 [33]. The rarity of rupture and aortic mortality, as opposed to the non-negligible all-cause mortality, supports non-operative management of small AAAs. The rupture incidence among large aneurysm (>55 mm) patients was 26% over a mean follow-up period of 2.2 years. Of patients with large AAAs, 22% died following an aortic-related complication. The all-cause mortality estimate for this subgroup of patients was 62%. The large AAA rupture rate was higher than the 19% found by Parkinson and colleagues that pooled results of large AAAs turned down from elective repair [34]. We do not have a clear explanation for this; however, several biases and confounders should be considered. First, it is challenging to define the cause of death in patients dying outside healthcare facilities, especially in retrospective studies. Second, the risk of rupture might be exponential, but the pivot point needs further investigation.

Lancaster and colleagues estimated three-year cumulative rupture risks of 2.2%, 6.0%, and 18.4% for AAAs measuring 55–60 mm, 61–70 mm, and >70 mm, respectively [15]. Large population-based screening studies presented a significantly lower rupture rate compared with smaller, observational studies [14,29]. The rupture rates estimated in the present meta-analysis were higher in studies presenting a mean patient age > 72 years (Figure 4B) and with a female proportion > 17% (Figure 4B). The higher risk of rupture associated with ageing seems easily understandable. On the other hand, the higher risk of rupture in those studies, including a relevant number of women, deserves careful discussion. It should be noticed that females with 50–55 mm AAAs seem to be at higher risk of rupture compared with males with 55–60 mm AAAs, 3.4% vs. 2.2%, respectively [15]. However, the 50 mm cut-off for women is debated, and conflicting findings have been found recently [35,36]. Some colleagues strongly support the above-mentioned cut-off as opposed to others proposing a 52 mm threshold [35,36]. To conclude, most published studies support a lower threshold for elective AAA repair in females, eventually meaning that different screening protocols might be required. These results stand in contrast with conducting population screening on 65-year-old men only [14,29].

Thirteen years have passed since Powell et al. [33] published a systematic review on rupture rates of small aneurysms. Still, after all this time, the most relevant finding we can confirm is the scarcity of high-quality evidence investigating the modern fate of AAAs. Nine years have passed since the last systematic review reporting on large aneurysms deemed unfit for elective repair [34]. Our literature search showed more than eleven thousand potential studies, yet the eligibility assessment resulted in a very low number of included studies (n = 14). In addition, the absence of specific reporting standards yields a huge heterogeneity among the papers. We have found twelve different size thresholds, making the pooling process very challenging. Even the definition of a large aneurysm was not uniform, with some studies using a 50 mm cut-off instead of the 55 mm suggested by the guidelines.

The reasoning behind the year 2000 cut-off was the substantial improvement in cardiovascular medical management during the last two decades. A recent meta-analysis confirmed the mortality reduction in AAA patients receiving statins [37]. Metformin treatment showed similar benefits in a prospective study from Australia investigating predictors of AAA outcomes [25]. Stronger evidence is expected to come from an ongoing randomised trial (MAAAGI) [38]. Unfortunately, the extracted publications commonly waived a detailed report of the medications given to the patients, and we were unable to further study this topic.

4.1. Limitations

The most relevant limitation in analysing the AAA natural history literature was the lack of homogeneous, high-level, well-powered studies. Assessment of rupture and cause of death is a critical issue, considering that most of the included studies waived the methods employed to ascertain the event's cause. Hultgren and colleagues pointed out this issue, concluding that the low autopsy rate leads to a 'difficult and imprecise' evaluation of the causes of death in such studies [29]. Screening studies focusing on small aneurysms have been performed on relatively young male patients, overshadowing the AAA natural history in the female gender, which has still not been adequately investigated. The rate of repair before reaching the counselled threshold and the number of AAAs not receiving surgery after reaching the threshold were not available. In addition, female-specific size definitions, repair thresholds, and ruptures were commonly not reported, hindering the present authors from providing gender-detailed data. Studies on large aneurysms included patients deemed unfit for surgery, likely biasing the data for fit, less comorbid, and younger patients with large AAAs. Also, there is a lack of data divided by large aneurysm subgroups. An additional limitation is the common avoidance of reporting methods to ascertain the causes of mortality. Similarly, the repair threshold has not been clearly reported, biasing its interpretation. Yet, the pooling process was challenging, with a low number of items per size range likely leading to huge heterogeneity. Also, analysis became more difficult when meta-regressions were performed due to the non-systematic reporting of comorbidities and medical therapies. For this reason, we did not pursue some of the secondary analyses originally planned. As less than ten studies were included in the final analysis, the results should be interpreted with caution. The mean estimated follow-up was short (2.2 years) and stands in contrast to the disease's natural history. The diagnostic technique varied significantly, and the measuring methodologies (e.g., leading edge to leading edge, inner or outer diameter, etc.) were commonly waived. To conclude, most AAA publications focused on EVAR during the last few decades.

4.2. Gaps in Knowledge and Future Perspectives

- Reporting standards defining either the outcomes or the size thresholds are needed.
- Age-stratified rupture risk should be investigated.
- Women deserve gender-focused studies.
- The outcomes of large, fit-for-surgery AAA patients are unknown.
- Repair indications in specific subgroups, such as females and rapid growth, should be further pioneered.
- A new trial using artificial intelligence might improve measuring standardisation, either in the case of computed tomography or duplex ultrasound.

5. Conclusions

The rarity of rupture and aortic mortality supports the ongoing guidelines to avoid prophylactic repair of small AAAs (<55 mm). Surveillance of small AAAs seems indicated, considering that one-fifth of patients reach the threshold for repair. The pooled estimate of ruptures and aortic mortality in patients with large aneurysms ($\geq$55 mm) was high, though such crude stratification of size seems unnuanced. There is recent evidence showing that AAAs measuring 55–60 mm in males and 50–55 mm in females might have a reasonably low rupture risk. The modern fate of AAAs is not studied adequately in prospective, controlled trials, and further scientific efforts must be undertaken.

Author Contributions: Conceptualization, N.L. and T.A.R.; methodology, N.L.; software, N.L. and M.A.B.; validation, J.P.E. and T.A.R.; formal analysis, N.L.; investigation, N.L. and M.A.B.; data curation, N.L. and M.A.B.; writing—original draft preparation, N.L. and M.A.B.; writing—review and editing, N.L., M.A.B., J.P.E. and T.A.R.; visualisation, N.L. and M.A.B.; supervision, J.P.E. and T.A.R.; project administration, N.L. All authors have read and agreed to the published version of the manuscript.

Funding: This research received no external funding.

Institutional Review Board Statement: Not applicable.

Informed Consent Statement: Not applicable.

Data Availability Statement: Data are available on a reasonable request to the corresponding author.

Acknowledgments: The authors thank the Medical Research Library of the Rigshospitalet for the scientific support provided during the literature search.

Conflicts of Interest: The authors declare no conflict of interest.

Appendix A

Table A1. Variables extracted from included studies.

	Variables	Type
General	First author name and year of publication	String
	Title	String
	Journal	String
	Study aim	String
	Country	String
	European	Binary
	Study period	String
Methods	Population description (small aneurysms under surveillance, large aneurysms deemed unfit for surgery, aneurysms under surveillance)	Categorical
	Design (RCT, observational, other)	Categorical
	Prospective	Binary
	Multicenter	Binary
	Inclusion criteria	String
	Exclusion criteria	String
	Type of imaging	Categorical
Quality appraisal	Consecutive recruitment	Categorical
	Completeness of baseline characteristics description	Categorical
	Completeness of inclusion/exclusion statement	Categorical
	Entering the study at a similar point in the disease	Binary
	Clarity of intervention/outcome description	Categorical
	Clarity of co-intervention/secondary outcome description	Categorical
	Outcome measures established a priori	Categorical
	Outcome assessors blinded to intervention	Categorical
	Outcomes measured using appropriate objective/subjective methods	Categorical
	Measures made before and after the intervention—Multiple measures over time	Categorical
	Appropriateness/completeness of the statistical analysis	Categorical
	Appropriateness of the follow-up length	Categorical
	Report of losses to follow-up	Binary
	Use of random variability estimates	Categorical
	Conclusions supported by results	Categorical
	Declaration of competing interests and sources of support	Binary
Outcomes	Number of participants	Continuous
	Number of losses to follow-up	Continuous
	Male/Female	Continuous
	Mean (standard deviation) or median (IQR range) of:	
	• Length of follow-up	Continuous
	• Age	
	Smokers, non-smokers, and previous smokers proportion	Continuous
	Specific outcomes collected for each size threshold (numbers):	
	• Patients	
	• Rupture	Continuous
	• Reaching the threshold for repair	
	• Aortic-related death	
	• All-cause death	

Table A2. Excluded studies after full-text screening.

	Follow-Up Being Initiated Before the Year 2000
1	Vega de Céniga et al. Analysis of expansion patterns in 4–4.9 cm abdominal aortic aneurysms. Ann Vasc Surg. 2008;22(1):37–44.
2	Vallabhaneni SR. Final follow-up of the Multicentre Aneurysm Screening Study (MASS) randomized trial of abdominal aortic aneurysm screening (Br J Surg 2012; 99: 1649–1656). Br J Surg. 2012;99(12):1656.
3	Lederle et al. Multicentre study of abdominal aortic aneurysm measurement and enlargement. Br J Surg. 2015;102(12):1480–7.
4	Brown PM, Sobolev B, Zelt DT. Selective management of abdominal aortic aneurysms smaller than 5.0 cm in a prospective sizing program with gender-specific analysis. J Vasc Surg. 2003;38(4):762–5.
5	Lederle et al. Rupture rate of large abdominal aortic aneurysms in patients refusing or unfit for elective repair. Journal of the American Medical Association. 2002;287(22):2968–72.
6	Brown LC, Powell JT. Risk factors for aneurysm rupture in patients kept under ultrasound surveillance. UK Small Aneurysm Trial Participants. Annals of surgery. 1999;230(3):289-96; discussion 296-7.
7	Aziz et al. Four-year follow up of patients with untreated abdominal aortic aneurysms. ANZ J Surg. 2004;74(11):935–40.
8	Valentine et al. Watchful waiting in cases of small abdominal aortic aneurysms—Appropriate for all patients? Journal of Vascular Surgery. 2000;32(3):441–50.
9	Tambyraja et al. Non-operative management of high-risk patients with abdominal aortic aneurysm. Eur J Vasc Endovasc Surg. 2003;26(4):401–4.
10	Devaraj et al. Ultrasound surveillance of ectatic abdominal aortas. Ann R Coll Surg Engl. 2008;90(6):477–82.
11	Schlösser et al. Growth predictors and prognosis of small abdominal aortic aneurysms. Journal of Vascular Surgery. 2008;47(6):1127–33.
12	Scott et al. Randomized clinical trial of screening for abdominal aortic aneurysm in women. British Journal of Surgery. 2002;89(3):283–5.
13	Brady et al. Abdominal aortic aneurysm expansion: Risk factors and time intervals for surveillance. Circulation. 2004;110(1):16–21.
14	Vega de Céniga et al. Growth rate and associated factors in small abdominal aortic aneurysms. Eur J Vasc Endovasc Surg. 2006;31(3):231–6.
15	Powell et al. Rupture rates of small abdominal aortic aneurysms: A systematic review of the literature. Journal of Vascular Surgery. 2011;53(1):249.
16	Thompson et al. Growth rates of small abdominal aortic aneurysms correlate with clinical events. Br J Surg. 2010;97(1):37–44.
17	Propranolol for small abdominal aortic aneurysms: results of a randomized trial. J Vasc Surg. 2002;35(1):72–9.
18	Heikkinen et al. The fate of AAA patients referred electively to vascular surgical unit. Scandinavian Journal of Surgery. 2002;91(4):345–52.
19	Veith et al. Conservative observational management with selective delayed repair for large abdominal aortic aneurysms in high risk patients. J Cardiovasc Surg (Torino). 2003;44(3):459–64.
20	Powell et al. The natural history of abdominal aortic aneurysms and their risk of rupture. Acta chirurgica Belgica. 2001;101(1):11-16.
21	Filardo et al. Immediate open repair vs. surveillance in patients with small abdominal aortic aneurysms: survival differences by aneurysm size. Mayo Clinic proceedings. 2013;88(9):910-919.
22	Mosorin et al. The use of statins and fate of small abdominal aortic aneurysms. Interact Cardiovasc Thorac Surg. 2008;7(4):578–81.
23	Brown et al. The risk of rupture in untreated aneurysms: the impact of size, gender, and expansion rate. J Vasc Surg. 2003;37(2):280–4.
24	Kurvers et al. Discontinuous, staccato growth of abdominal aortic aneurysms. J Am Coll Surg. 2004;199(5):709–15.
25	Powell et al. Final 12-year follow-up of surgery versus surveillance in the UK Small Aneurysm Trial. British Journal of Surgery. 2007;94(6):702–8.
26	Powell et al. Long-term outcomes of immediate repair compared with surveillance of small abdominal aortic aneurysms. New England journal of medicine. 2002;346(19):1445-1452.
27	Solberg et al. Increased growth rate of abdominal aortic aneurysms in women. The Tromsø study. Eur J Vasc Endovasc Surg. 2005;29(2):145–9.
28	Ahmad et al. How Quickly Do Asymptomatic Infrarenal Abdominal Aortic Aneurysms Grow and What Factors Affect Aneurysm Growth Rates? Analysis of a Single Centre Surveillance Cohort Database. Eur J Vasc Endovasc Surg. 2017;54(5):597–603.

Table A2. Cont.

	Congress abstracts or correspondences
1	Chang et al. Natural History of Abdominal Aortic Aneurysm Expansion: Fifteen-Year Analysis of Nearly 15,000 Patients Under Surveillance in a Large, Integrated Health System. Journal of Vascular Surgery. 2020;72(1):e74–5.
2	Duncan et al. The Subaneursymal Aorta — A Ten Year Perspective from a Single Centre. European journal of vascular and endovascular surgery. 2019;58(6):e21-e22.
3	Bogdanovic et al. Semi-automatic measurement of external and luminal diameter predicts the four-year prognosis of small abdominal aortic aneurysms. Arteriosclerosis, Thrombosis, and Vascular Biology. 2018;38.
4	Lee et al. Growth Rates of Small Abdominal Aortic Aneurysms Identified in a Contemporary Practice. Journal of Vascular Surgery. 2020;72(3):321–2.
5	Haveman et al. Multicentre Aneurysm Screening S. Multicentre Aneurysm Screening Study (MASS). In: Lancet. England; 2003. p. 1058.
6	Vega de Ceniga et al. Outcomes in a Prospective Cohort of Octogenarian and Nonagenarian Patients Diagnosed With a Small (<55 Mm) Abdominal Aortic Aneurysm: Rupture, Growth to a Large (>=55 Mm) Size and Mortality Rates. European Journal of Vascular and Endovascular Surgery. 2019;58(6):e603.
7	Clarke et al. Turndown for Abdominal Aortic Aneurysm Intervention: A Five Year Follow Up Study. European Journal of Vascular and Endovascular Surgery. 2020;60(2):e57.
8	Lancaster et al. The Natural History of Large Abdominal Aortic Aneurysms in Patients Without Timely Repair: Implications for Rupture and Mortality. Journal of Vascular Surgery. 2020;72(3):e315.
9	Berntsen et al. Familial Abdominal Aortic Aneurysms Don't Occur Earlier in Life, Neither do they Progress More Rapidly—Observations from Two Population Based Screening Trials. European Journal of Vascular and Endovascular Surgery. 2019;58(6):e555.
10	Brunner-Ziegler et al. Longterm evaluation on the impact of thrombus formation on the course of abdominal aortic diameter expansion. Vasa—Journal of Vascular Diseases. 2013;42:14–5.
	Not reporting outcomes of interest
1	Kristensen et al. Glycated Hemoglobin Is Associated With the Growth Rate of Abdominal Aortic Aneurysms: a Substudy From the VIVA (Viborg Vascular) Randomized Screening Trial. Arteriosclerosis, thrombosis, and vascular biology. 2017;37(4):730-736.
2	da Silva et al. The similarities and differences among patients with abdominal aortic aneurysms referred to a tertiary hospital and found at necropsy. Vascular. 2015;23(4):411–8.
3	Badger et al. Surveillance strategies according to the rate of growth of small abdominal aortic aneurysms. Vasc Med. 2011;16(6):415–21.
4	Itoga et al. Metformin prescription status and abdominal aortic aneurysm disease progression in the U.S. veteran patient population. Journal of Vascular Surgery. 2018;67(6):e52.
5	Yau et al. Surveillance of small aortic aneurysms does not alter anatomic suitability for endovascular repair. J Vasc Surg. 2007;45(1):96–100.
6	Lindholt et al. Survival, prevalence, progression and repair of abdominal aortic aneurysms: Results from three randomised controlled screening trials over three decades. Clinical Epidemiology. 2020;12:95–103.
7	Golledge et al. Association between metformin prescription and growth rates of abdominal aortic aneurysms. Br J Surg. 2017;104(11):1486–93.
	Populations not suitable for inclusion
1	Hansen et al. Natural history of thoraco-abdominal aneurysm in high-risk patients. Eur J Vasc Endovasc Surg. 2010;39(3):266–70.
2	Chun et al. Risk of developing an abdominal aortic aneurysm after ectatic aorta detection from initial screening. J Vasc Surg. 2020;71(6):1913–9.
	Study design
1	Skibba et al. Reconsidering gender relative to risk of rupture in the contemporary management of abdominal aortic aneurysms. J Vasc Surg. 2015;62(6):1429–36.

Table A3. Study quality analysis according to the Quality Appraisal Checklist from the Institute of Health Economics.

Study Objective		
1.	Was the hypothesis/aim/objective of the study clearly stated?	Yes [6,14,15,22–32] Partial No
Study design		
2.	Was the study conducted prospectively?	Yes [6,14,15,22–26,29,30,32] Unclear No [27,28,31]
3.	Were the cases collected in more than one centre?	Yes [6,14,15,24–26,29] Unclear No [22,23,27,28,30–32]
4.	Were patients recruited consecutively?	Yes [24,27,29–32] Unclear [6,14,15,22,23,25,26,28] No
Study population		
5.	Were the characteristics of the patients included in the study described?	Yes [6,15,22–30,32] Partial [14,31] No
6.	Were the eligibility criteria (i.e., inclusion and exclusion criteria) for entry into the study clearly stated?	Yes [6,15,22–27,30–32] Partial [14,28,29] No
7.	Did patients enter the study at a similar point in the disease?	Yes [6,14,15,22,24,25,27–32] Unclear No [23,26]
Intervention and co-intervention		
8.	Was the intervention of interest clearly described?	Yes [6,14,23–26,29,30,32] Partial [15,22,31] No [27,28]
9.	Were additional interventions (co-interventions) clearly described?	Yes [6,14,15,23–26,28–30,32] Partial No [27,31]
Outcome measure		
10.	Were relevant outcome measures established a priori?	Yes [6,14,15,23–30,32] Partial [31] No
11.	Were outcome assessors blinded to the intervention that patients received?	Yes [14,15] Unclear No [6,23–32]
12.	Were the relevant outcomes measured using appropriate objective/subjective methods?	Yes [14,23,25,26,29,32] Unclear [6,15,24,27,28] No [22,30,31]
13.	Were the relevant outcome measures made before and after the intervention?	Yes [6,14,23–26,29–32] Unclear [15,22,27,28] No
Statistical analysis		
14.	Were the statistical tests used to assess the relevant outcomes appropriate?	Yes [6,14,15,22–27,29–32] Unclear [28] No

Table A3. Cont.

	Study Objective	
	Results and conclusions	
15.	Was follow-up long enough for important events and outcomes to occur?	Yes [6,15,24–26,28] Unclear [14,27,29,30] No [23,31,32]
16.	Were losses to follow-up reported?	Yes [6,14,15,23–26,28–32] Unclear [27] No [22]
17.	Did the study provided estimates of random variability in the data analysis of relevant outcomes?	Yes [6,14,15,24,26,30] Partial No [22,23,25,27–29,31,32]
18.	Were the adverse events reported?	Yes [6,14,15,22,24,26–32] Partial [23,25] No
19.	Were the conclusions of the study supported by results?	Yes [14,15,22,24–26,30–32] Unclear [23,27–29] No [6]
	Competing interests and sources of support	
20.	Were both competing interests and sources of support for the study reported?	Yes [6,14,15,22,24–29,31,32] Partial No [23,30]

Table A4. Outcomes pooled estimates for the minor size ranges of small and large aneurysms.

	Rupture [a]	Repair Threshold [a]	Aortic Mortality [a]	All-Cause mortality [a]
40–49 mm	n = 294 e = 4 1.0 (0.1–2.6) [24,29]	n = 294 e = 71 24.0 (19.2–29.0) [24,29]	n = 187 e = 4 2.1 (0.6–5.4) [24]	n = 187 e = 20 10.7 (6.7–16.0) [24]
45–50 mm	n = 35 e = 0 0.0 (0.0–10.0) [29]	n = 35 e = 24 68.6 (50.7–83.1) [29]	-	-
45–54 mm	n = 2222 e = 11 0.5 (0.3–0.9) [14]	-	n = 2222 e = 10 0.5 (0.2–0.8) [14]	n = 2222 e = 68 3.1 (2.4–3.9) [14]
50–54 mm	n = 769 e = 3 0.4 (0.1–1.1) [14]	-	-	n = 769 e = 15 2.0 (1.1–3.2) [14]
55–60 mm	-	-	n = 74 e = 31 41.9 (30.5–53.9) [31]	-
61–70 mm	-	-	n = 57 e = 25 43.9 (30.7–57.6) [31]	-
>70 mm	n = 14 e = 8 57.1 (28.9–82.3) [27]	-	n = 23 e = 10 43.5 (23.2–65.5) [31]	n = 14 e = 6 42.9 (17.7–71.1) [27]

n, population available for the specific outcome; e, number of events; ES%, estimate proportion; 95% CI, 95% confidence interval. [a] Data are presented as ES% (95% CI).

References

1. Reimerink, J.J.; van der Laan, M.J.; Koelemay, M.J.; Balm, R.; Legemate, D.A. Systematic review and meta-analysis of population-based mortality from ruptured abdominal aortic aneurysm. *Br. J. Surg.* **2013**, *100*, 1405–1413. [CrossRef] [PubMed]
2. Danish Vascular Registry Report. Database on the Internet. 2020. Available online: https://karbase.dk/onewebmedia/karbase_aarsrapport-2020.pdf (accessed on 5 February 2023).

3. Broda, M.; Eiberg, J.; Taudorf, M.; Resch, T. Limb graft occlusion after endovascular aneurysm repair with the COOK Zenith Alpha abdominal graft. *J. Vasc. Surg.* **2023**, *77*, 770–777. [CrossRef] [PubMed]
4. Powell, J.T.; Brown, L.C.; Forbes, J.F.; Fowkes, F.G.; Greenhalgh, R.M.; Ruckley, C.V.; Thompson, S.G. Final 12-year follow-up of surgery versus surveillance in the UK Small Aneurysm Trial. *Br. J. Surg.* **2007**, *94*, 702–708. [PubMed]
5. Lederle, F.A.; Wilson, S.E.; Johnson, G.R.; Reinke, D.B.; Littooy, F.N.; Acher, C.W.; Ballard, D.J.; Messina, L.M.; Gordon, I.L.; Chute, E.P.; et al. Immediate repair compared with surveillance of small abdominal aortic aneurysms. *N. Engl. J. Med.* **2002**, *346*, 1437–1444. [CrossRef] [PubMed]
6. Cao, P.; De Rango, P.; Verzini, F.; Parlani, G.; Romano, L.; Cieri, E. Comparison of surveillance versus aortic endografting for small aneurysm repair (CAESAR): Results from a randomised trial. *Eur. J. Vasc. Endovasc. Surg.* **2011**, *41*, 13–25. [CrossRef]
7. Wanhainen, A.; Verzini, F.; Van Herzeele, I.; Allaire, E.; Bown, M.; Cohnert, T.; Dick, F.; van Herwaarden, J.; Karkos, C.; Koelemay, M.; et al. Editor's Choice—European Society for Vascular Surgery (ESVS) 2019 Clinical Practice Guidelines on the Management of Abdominal Aorto-iliac Artery Aneurysms. *Eur. J. Vasc. Endovasc. Surg.* **2019**, *57*, 8–93. [CrossRef]
8. Glimåker, H.; Holmberg, L.; Elvin, A.; Nybacka, O.; Almgren, B.; Björck, C.G.; Eriksson, I. Natural history of patients with abdominal aortic aneurysm. *Eur. J. Vasc. Surg.* **1991**, *5*, 125–130. [CrossRef]
9. Darling, R.C.; Messina, C.R.; Brewster, D.C.; Ottinger, L.W. Autopsy study of unoperated abdominal aortic aneurysms. The case for early resection. *Circulation* **1977**, *56* (Suppl. S3), 161–164.
10. Nevitt, M.P.; Ballard, D.J.; Hallett, J.W., Jr. Prognosis of abdominal aortic aneurysm. A population-based study. *N. Engl. J. Med.* **1989**, *321*, 1009–1014. [CrossRef]
11. Powell, J.T.; Greenhalgh, R.M.; Ruckley, C.V.; Fowkes, F.G. The UK Small Aneurysm Trial. *Ann. N. Y. Acad. Sci.* **1996**, *800*, 249–251. [CrossRef]
12. Lederle, F.A.; Johnson, G.R.; Wilson, S.E.; Chute, E.P.; Littooy, F.N.; Bandyk, D.; Krupski, W.C.; Barone, G.W.; Acher, C.W.; Ballard, D.J.; et al. Prevalence and associations of abdominal aortic aneurysm detected through screening. Aneurysm Detection and Management (ADAM) Veterans Affairs Cooperative Study Group. *Ann. Int. Med.* **1997**, *126*, 441–449. [CrossRef] [PubMed]
13. NICE Evidence Reviews Collection. Thresholds for Abdominal Aortic Aneurysm Repair. In *Abdominal Aortic Aneurysm: Diagnosis and Management*; Evidence Review F; National Institute for Health and Care Excellence (NICE): London, UK, 2020.
14. Oliver-Williams, C.; Sweeting, M.J.; Jacomelli, J.; Summers, L.; Stevenson, A.; Lees, T.; Earnshaw, J.J. Safety of Men with Small and Medium Abdominal Aortic Aneurysms Under Surveillance in the NAAASP. *Circulation* **2019**, *139*, 1371–1380. [CrossRef]
15. Lancaster, E.M.; Gologorsky, R.; Hull, M.M.; Okuhn, S.; Solomon, M.D.; Avins, A.L.; Adams, J.L.; Chang, R.W. The natural history of large abdominal aortic aneurysms in patients without timely repair. *J. Vasc. Surg.* **2022**, *75*, 109–117. [CrossRef] [PubMed]
16. Liberati, A.; Altman, D.G.; Tetzlaff, J.; Mulrow, C.; Gøtzsche, P.C.; Ioannidis, J.P.; Clarke, M.; Devereaux, P.J.; Kleijnen, J.; Moher, D. The PRISMA statement for reporting systematic reviews and meta-analyses of studies that evaluate healthcare interventions: Explanation and elaboration. *BMJ Clin. Res.* **2009**, *339*, b2700. [CrossRef] [PubMed]
17. Institute of Health Economics. About Methodology Development. Available online: https://www.ihe.ca/research-programs/rmd/cssqac/cssqac-about (accessed on 5 February 2023).
18. Hozo, S.P.; Djulbegovic, B.; Hozo, I. Estimating the mean and variance from the median, range, and the size of a sample. *BMC Med. Res. Methodol.* **2005**, *5*, 13. [CrossRef] [PubMed]
19. Barendregt, J.J.; Doi, S.A.; Lee, Y.Y.; Norman, R.E.; Vos, T. Meta-analysis of prevalence. *J. Epidemiol. Commun. Health* **2013**, *67*, 974–978. [CrossRef] [PubMed]
20. Der Simonian, R.; Laird, N. Meta-analysis in clinical trials. *Control. Clin. Trials* **1986**, *7*, 177–188. [CrossRef]
21. Higgins, J.P.; Thompson, S.G. Quantifying heterogeneity in a meta-analysis. *Stat. Med.* **2002**, *21*, 1539–1558. [CrossRef]
22. Elmallah, A.; Elnagar, M.; Bambury, N.; Ahmed, Z.; Dowdall, J.; Mehigan, D.; Sheehan, S.; Barry, M. A study of outcomes in conservatively managed patients with large abdominal aortic aneurysms deemed unfit for surgical repair. *Vascular* **2019**, *27*, 161–167. [CrossRef]
23. Buckenham, T.; Roake, J.; Lewis, D.; Gordon, M.; Wright, I. Abdominal aortic aneurysm surveillance: Application of the UK Small Aneurysm Trial to a New Zealand tertiary hospital. *N. Z. Med. J.* **2007**, *120*, U2472.
24. Aortic Wall Inflammation Predicts Abdominal Aortic Aneurysm Expansion, Rupture, and Need for Surgical Repair. *Circulation* **2017**, *136*, 787–797. [CrossRef] [PubMed]
25. Golledge, J.; Morris, D.R.; Pinchbeck, J.; Rowbotham, S.; Jenkins, J.; Bourke, M.; Bourke, B.; Norman, P.E.; Jones, R.; Moxon, J.V. Editor's Choice—Metformin Prescription is Associated with a Reduction in the Combined Incidence of Surgical Repair and Rupture Related Mortality in Patients with Abdominal Aortic Aneurysm. *Eur. J. Vasc. Endovasc. Surg.* **2019**, *57*, 94–101. [CrossRef]
26. Söderberg, P.; Wanhainen, A.; Svensjö, S. Five Year Natural History of Screening Detected Sub-Aneurysms and Abdominal Aortic Aneurysms in 70 Year Old Women and Systematic Review of Repair Rate in Women. *Eur. J. Vasc. Endovasc. Surg.* **2017**, *53*, 802–809. [CrossRef]
27. Al-Thani, H.; El-Menyar, A.; Shabana, A.; Tabeb, A.; Al-Sulaiti, M.; Almalki, A. Incidental abdominal aneurysms: A retrospective study of 13,115 patients who underwent a computed tomography scan. *Angiology* **2014**, *65*, 388–395. [CrossRef] [PubMed]
28. Scott, S.W.; Batchelder, A.J.; Kirkbride, D.; Naylor, A.R.; Thompson, J.P. Late Survival in Nonoperated Patients with Infrarenal Abdominal Aortic Aneurysm. *Eur. J. Vasc. Endovasc. Surg.* **2016**, *52*, 444–449. [CrossRef]
29. Hultgren, R.; Elfström, K.M.; Öhman, D.; Linné, A. Long-Term Follow-Up of Men Invited to Participate in a Population-Based Abdominal Aortic Aneurysm Screening Program. *Angiology* **2020**, *71*, 641–649. [CrossRef] [PubMed]

30. Lim, J.; Wolff, J.; Rodd, C.D.; Cooper, D.G.; Earnshaw, J.J. Outcome in Men with a Screen-detected Abdominal Aortic Aneurysm Who are not Fit for Intervention. *Eur. J. Vasc. Endovasc. Surg.* **2015**, *50*, 732–736. [CrossRef]
31. Noronen, K.; Laukontaus, S.; Kantonen, I.; Lepantalo, M.; Venermo, M. The natural course of abdominal aortic aneurysms that meet the treatment criteria but not the operative requirements. *Eur. J. Vasc. Endovasc. Surg.* **2013**, *45*, 326–331. [CrossRef]
32. Ghulam, Q.M.; Bredahl, K.K.; Lonn, L.; Rouet, L.; Sillesen, H.H.; Eiberg, J.P. Follow-up on Small Abdominal Aortic Aneurysms Using Three Dimensional Ultrasound: Volume Versus Diameter. *Eur. J. Vasc. Endovasc. Surg.* **2017**, *54*, 439–445. [CrossRef]
33. Powell, J.T.; Gotensparre, S.M.; Sweeting, M.J.; Brown, L.C.; Fowkes, F.G.; Thompson, S.G. Rupture rates of small abdominal aortic aneurysms: A systematic review of the literature. *Eur. J. Vasc. Endovasc. Surg.* **2011**, *41*, 2–10. [CrossRef] [PubMed]
34. Parkinson, F.; Ferguson, S.; Lewis, P.; Williams, I.M.; Twine, C.P. Rupture rates of untreated large abdominal aortic aneurysms in patients unfit for elective repair. *J. Vasc. Surg.* **2015**, *61*, 1606–1612. [CrossRef] [PubMed]
35. Patel, P.B.; De Guerre, L.; Marcaccio, C.L.; Dansey, K.D.; Li, C.; Lo, R.; Patel, V.I.; Schermerhorn, M.L. Sex-specific criteria for repair should be utilized in patients undergoing aortic aneurysm repair. *J. Vasc. Surg.* **2022**, *75*, 515–525. [CrossRef] [PubMed]
36. Tomee, S.M.; Lijftogt, N.; Vahl, A.; Hamming, J.F.; Lindeman, J.H.N. A registry-based rationale for discrete intervention thresholds for open and endovascular elective abdominal aortic aneurysm repair in female patients. *J. Vasc. Surg.* **2018**, *67*, 735–739. [CrossRef] [PubMed]
37. Xiong, X.; Wu, Z.; Qin, X.; Huang, Q.; Wang, X.; Qin, J.; Lu, X. Meta-analysis suggests statins reduce mortality after abdominal aortic aneurysm repair. *J. Vasc. Surg.* **2022**, *75*, 356–362.e4. [CrossRef] [PubMed]
38. Wanhainen, A.; Unosson, J.; Mani, K.; Gottsäter, A. The Metformin for Abdominal Aortic Aneurysm Growth Inhibition (MAAAGI) Trial. *Eur. J. Vasc. Endovasc. Surg.* **2021**, *61*, 710–711. [CrossRef]

Disclaimer/Publisher's Note: The statements, opinions and data contained in all publications are solely those of the individual author(s) and contributor(s) and not of MDPI and/or the editor(s). MDPI and/or the editor(s) disclaim responsibility for any injury to people or property resulting from any ideas, methods, instructions or products referred to in the content.

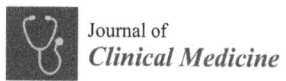

Review

Review of Clinical Applications of Dual-Energy CT in Patients after Endovascular Aortic Repair

Wojciech Kazimierczak [1,2,*], Natalia Kazimierczak [2] and Zbigniew Serafin [1]

1. Collegium Medicum, Nicolaus Copernicus University in Torun, Jagiellońska 13-15, 85-067 Bydgoszcz, Poland
2. Kazimierczak Private Medical Practice, Dworcowa 13/u6a, 85-009 Bydgoszcz, Poland
* Correspondence: w.kazimierczak@cm.umk.pl; Tel.: +48-606670881

Abstract: Abdominal aortic aneurysms (AAAs) are a significant cause of mortality in developed countries. Endovascular aneurysm repair (EVAR) is currently the leading treatment method for AAAs. Due to the high sensitivity and specificity of post-EVAR complication detection, CT angiography (CTA) is the reference method for imaging surveillance in patients after EVAR. Many studies have shown the advantages of dual-energy CT (DECT) over standard polyenergetic CTA in vascular applications. In this article, the authors briefly discuss the technical principles and summarize the current body of literature regarding dual-energy computed tomography angiography (DECTA) in patients after EVAR. The authors point out the most useful applications of DECTA in this group of patients and its advantages over conventional CTA. To conduct this review, a search was performed using the PubMed, Google Scholar, and Web of Science databases.

Keywords: dual-energy computed tomography; endoleaks; abdominal aortic aneurysm; virtual monoenergetic images; metal artifact reduction; diagnostic accuracy; computed tomography angiography

Citation: Kazimierczak, W.; Kazimierczak, N.; Serafin, Z. Review of Clinical Applications of Dual-Energy CT in Patients after Endovascular Aortic Repair. *J. Clin. Med.* **2023**, *12*, 7766. https://doi.org/10.3390/jcm12247766

Academic Editors: Martin Teraa, Constantijn E.V.B. Hazenberg and Alexander Zimmermann

Received: 14 October 2023
Revised: 8 December 2023
Accepted: 16 December 2023
Published: 18 December 2023

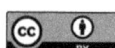

Copyright: © 2023 by the authors. Licensee MDPI, Basel, Switzerland. This article is an open access article distributed under the terms and conditions of the Creative Commons Attribution (CC BY) license (https://creativecommons.org/licenses/by/4.0/).

1. Introduction

Dual-energy CT (DECT) is a rapidly evolving diagnostic method first described by Sir Godfrey Hounsfield in 1973. He observed that dual image acquisition of the same volume at various kilovoltages allows for differentiation between calcium and iodine [1]. DECT enables the simultaneous or nearly simultaneous acquisition of CT images in low- and high-energy spectra, which allows for the differentiation of certain materials. The ability to differentiate elements using DECT stems from their distinct atomic numbers, unique k-edge characteristics, and differing linear attenuation coefficients at high and low photon energies. Some of the primary elements differentiated by DECT include iodine, which enables the creation of virtual noncontrast (VNC) and iodine map reconstructions. Other widely used reconstruction types in DECT are Virtual Monoenergetic Images (VMI), which simulate images acquired with a single-photon energy level.

Abdominal aortic aneurysms (AAAs) affect more than 1 million adults in the United States and result in approximately 15,000 annual deaths, making them the 15th leading cause of death overall [2–4]. Currently, the preferred treatment method for AAAs is endovascular aneurysm repair (EVAR), which carries the risk of a unique complication called an endoleak. This can lead to further aneurysm expansion and potential rupture, with a high mortality rate of 67% [5,6]. As a result, patients require regular imaging examinations to detect and classify endoleaks and identify other life-threatening complications, such as device thrombosis or infection. Various imaging modalities can be utilized during follow-up after EVAR; however, computed tomography angiography (CTA) and duplex ultrasound (DUS) are the basis for EVAR follow-up imaging [3] Despite the heterogeneous results of studies concerning the diagnostic accuracy of DUS [7,8] and its undeniable flaws (significant operator and patient dependencies), CTA is currently the reference standard imaging modality for post-EVAR patients. It allows for the classification of endoleaks and the detection of other potential complications [3,9].

The primary objective of this article was to elucidate the principles of DECTA, outline its advantages in post-EVAR patient follow-up imaging, and offer guidance for incorporating this technique into daily clinical practice.

2. Dual-Energy Acquisition Techniques

2.1. Rapid-Kilovoltage Switching DECT

The rapid-kVp (kilovoltage–peak) switching technique (Revolution GSI, Discovery 750 HD; General Electric Healthcare, Milwaukee, WI, USA) utilizes a single X-ray tube that quickly alternates (approximately every 0.25 ms) between 80 and 140 kVp, along with a single ultrafast registering detector, allowing for nearly simultaneous acquisition of two datasets. A schematic of the rapid kVp switching system is shown in Figure 1.

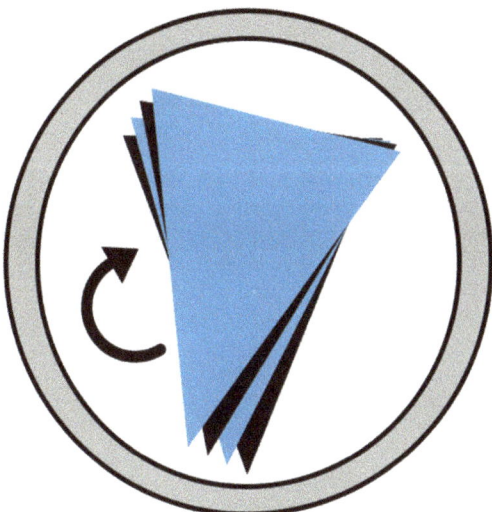

Figure 1. Schematic illustration of the single-source rapid kVp-switching DECT system (GE Healthcare). Dual-energy datasets are acquired by rapidly switching between low- and high-energy spectra. The system employs a unique garnet-based scintillator detector with minimal afterglow and quick sampling abilities.

2.2. Dual-Source DECT

A dual-source, dual-energy CT scanner (Somatom Definition Flash, Somatom Force; Siemens Healthineers, Forchheim, Germany) utilizes two sets of separate detector rings and two X-ray tubes positioned at 90° around the CT gantry. The X-ray tubes operate at low (70–80 kVp) and high (140–150 kVp) energies independently, allowing for the simultaneous acquisition of two datasets. A schematic of the dual-source system is shown in Figure 2.

2.3. Split-Filter DECT

The split-filter system (Somatom Definition Edge and Somatom go.Top; Siemens Healthineers) allows for the simultaneous acquisition of high- and low-energy datasets. In this system, a 120 kVp X-ray beam is prefiltered with gold and tin filters, splitting the beam energy into two spectra before it reaches the patient. The scheme of the split-filter system is shown in Figure 3.

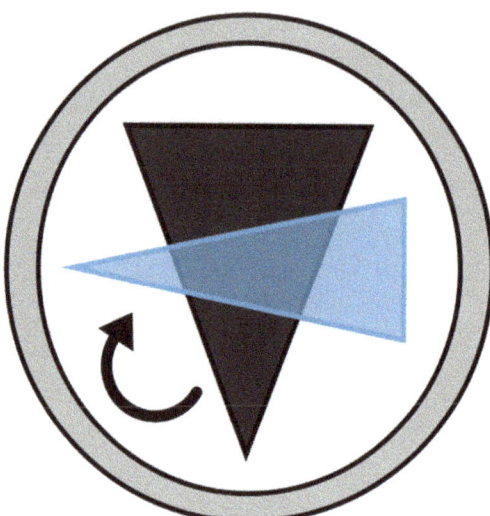

Figure 2. Schematic of the dual-source DECT system (Siemens AG). The system utilizes two dual-source detector–scanner combinations in a nearly orthogonal configuration, allowing for simultaneous volume scanning at the two energies. Typically, the sources operate at 80–100 kVp and 140–150 kVp; other combinations may be used for specific applications. Additional filters that can be used to harden a high-energy beam may be used to achieve better spectral separation. The limited space in the CT gantry, which allows for a smaller second detector, restricts the usable field of view.

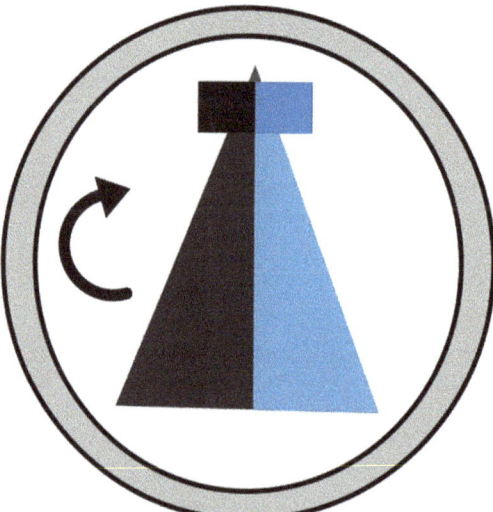

Figure 3. Schematic illustration of the single-source split-filter DECT system (Siemens AG). The filter, which was divided into two parts composed of gold and tin, was positioned at the output of the tube. This causes the beam to separate into low- and high-energy spectra. The respective halves of the detector then facilitate the acquisition of dual-energy datasets.

2.4. Multilayer Detector CT

The dual-layer detector (IQon Spectral CT; Philips Medical Systems, Cleveland, OH, USA) employs a layered or "sandwich" scintillation detector, which allows for the simultaneous collection of two datasets from a single standard X-ray tube operating at 140 kVp. The low-energy data are obtained from the top yttrium-based layer, while the high-energy data are collected from the bottom, a gadolinium-oxysulfide-based layer. A diagram of the multilayer detector is shown in Figure 4.

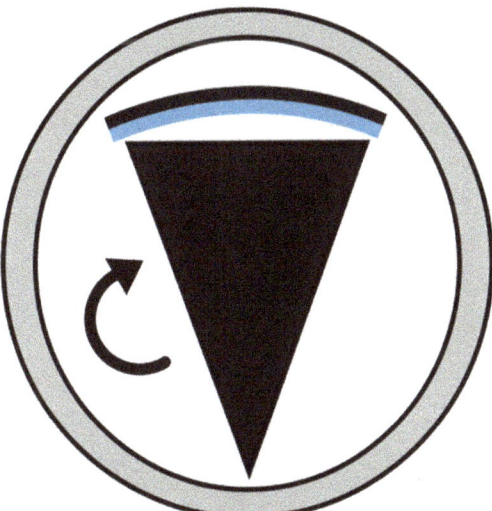

Figure 4. Schematic illustration of the single-source layered detector DECT system (Phillips Healthcare). The dual-energy datasets are achieved via spectral separation at the detector level. This system capitalizes on the polychromatic beam generated at the source and employs specialized dual-layer detectors sensitive to a specific energy spectrum. The superficial layer, which absorbs approximately 50% of the total photons, is designed to primarily absorb low-energy photons. The second layer absorbs the remaining high-energy photons.

3. Dual-Energy CT Postprocessing Techniques

3.1. Material Decomposition

Material-specific information can be obtained by modeling attenuation profiles, material mass density, and atomic number (Z) maps [10,11]. This allows for the reconstruction of images coded with concentrations of certain elements and substances instead of the simple CT attenuation numbers of each voxel in conventional single-energy CT (SECT). Material decomposition facilitates the precise mapping of specific elements, thereby enabling additional reconstructions, such as the virtual subtraction of elements. In vascular studies, the most beneficial images are those from VNC and virtual noncalcium (VNCa) reconstructions.

3.2. Virtual Noncontrast and Iodine Mapping

Dual-energy CT has the potential to generate VNC images via iodine identification and subsequent subtraction. These VNC images mimic the appearance of true noncontrast (TNC) images. Numerous studies in various clinical settings have proven that VNC images can substitute for TNC images and that the TNC phase of multiphasic examinations can be omitted [12–16]. VNC images have been proven to be vulnerable to iodine content, leading to significant differences in CT numbers between TNC and VNC images derived from arterial and delayed examination phases [17,18]. Figure 5 shows the differences between the TNC and the two postcontrast VNC reconstructions.

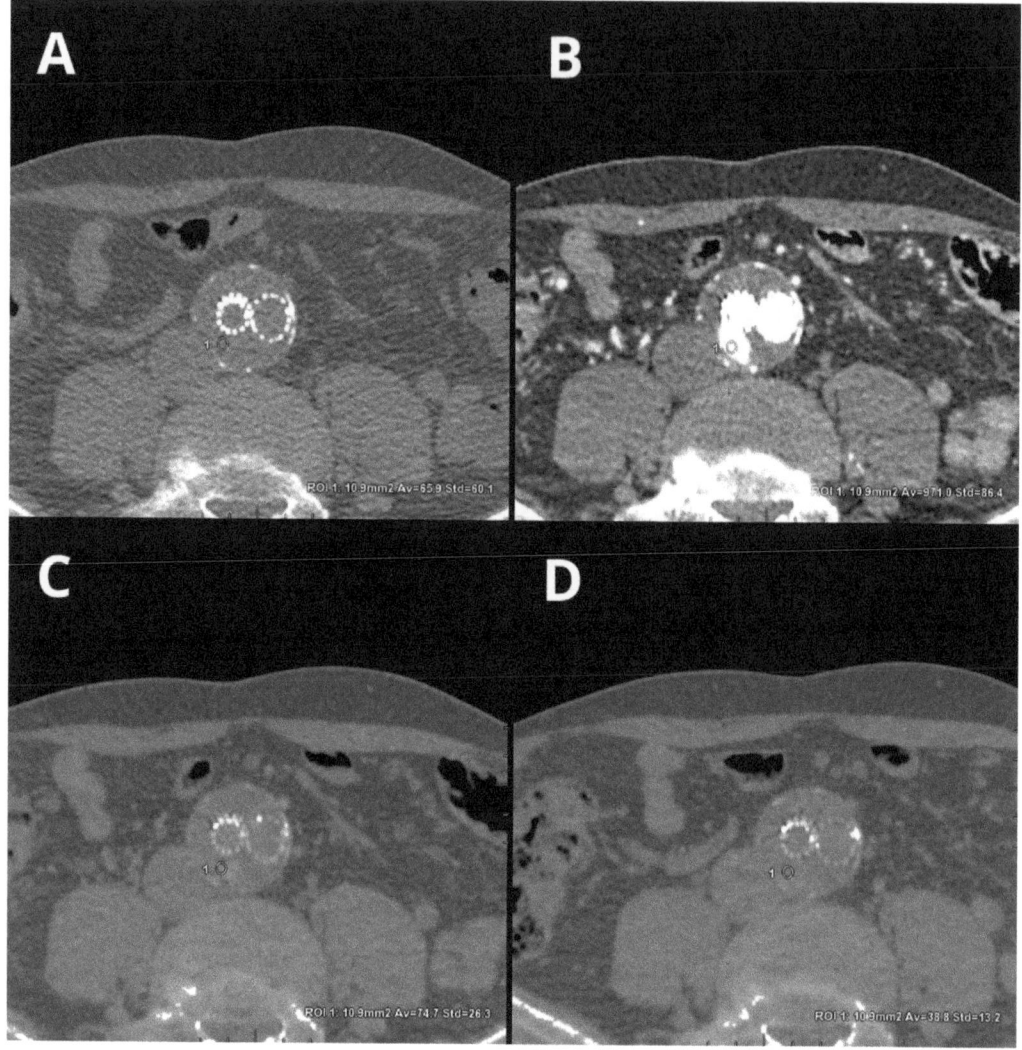

Figure 5. Differences in CT attenuation (average density ± SD) in small endoleak cases with true non-contrast, 40 keV VMI (arterial phase), and two VNC phases. Reconstructions: TNC ((**A**)—65.9 ± 60.1 HU), 40 keV VMI ((**B**)—971 ± 86.4), VNC arterial ((**C**)—74.7 ± 26.3 HU), and VNC delayed ((**D**)—38.8 ± 13.2 HU). An automatic region-of-interest (ROI) propagation tool was used with the same window settings (W 500, L 100).

Another benefit of material decomposition and VNC phase reconstruction is the ability to create iodine maps, which represent the distribution of iodine in tissues [19]. The next step is color coding of iodine, highlighting the iodine content in the grayscale VNC images. Such reconstructions are particularly useful in oncological applications and endoleak detection [20–22].

3.3. Virtual Noncalcium

VNCa algorithms facilitate the removal of calcified plaques without affecting intraluminal iodine-based contrast agent and surrounding soft tissues [23]. VNCa algorithms are particularly useful for imaging narrow vessel stenosis caused by calcified plaques. Furthermore, VNCa algorithms allow for the reduction of streaks and beam-hardening artifacts that obscure the lumen of the vessel and surrounding soft tissues [23,24]. The VNCa algorithm has already proven its value in assessing carotid artery stenosis, reducing blooming artifacts, and mitigating the overestimation of stenosis [23].

3.4. Virtual Monoenergetic Images (VMI), Noise Optimization

Virtual monoenergetic images (VMIs) can be reconstructed from dual-energy CT acquisitions, mimicking the attenuation values of an image obtained using a single energy source. Generally, low-keV images (40–70 keV) are advantageous for increasing iodine contrast but can also lead to higher noise levels [25]. Low-keV datasets can be particularly useful for improving iodine contrast, such as in low contrast volumes at slow injection rates [26], improving the detection and delineation of poorly enhancing lesions [27,28], assessing coronary vasculature, and performing functional evaluation of the myocardium [29,30].

Grant et al. introduced enhancements to the VMI technique to address the challenge of image noise and improve the iodine contrast-to-noise ratio (CNR)-optimized virtual monoenergetic image (VMI+) reconstructions [31]. In addition to noise reduction, the VMI+ technique mitigates artifacts, such as those from beam hardening and photon starvation, that may arise from high-attenuation materials at higher energy levels [32,33].

4. Applications of DECT in Patients after EVAR

4.1. Radiation Dose Reduction

The ionizing radiation dose associated with lifelong diagnostic surveillance is a fundamental problem related to post-EVAR follow-up protocols. The risk of radiation-induced cancer related to repeated CT scans is already well established [34–38]. The basic methods of radiation dose reduction are automatic exposure systems, iterative techniques, and regular service of the tomographic device [39]. One way to reduce the radiation dose is to lower the tube current and voltage; however, this increases the image noise and decreases the diagnostic value of the examination [40].

Among the concerns regarding dual-energy CT examinations, the most significant and recurring are those related to radiation dose. Several studies have demonstrated that the dose delivered during dual-source dual-energy CT acquisition is similar to that of comparable SECT [41–44]. With the advancement of technology, the introduction of iterative techniques, improved detector efficiency, and spectral filtration systems have made it possible to deliver even lower radiation doses with DECT than with SECT [26,45].

Several researchers have highlighted the possibility of using shortened examinations, limited to phases performed after administering a contrast agent, with VNC phase reconstruction without a significant reduction in the sensitivity of CTA for detecting endoleaks [46–51]. The dose reduction obtained in these studies primarily results from skipping the native phase of the examination. The aforementioned studies also pointed out the possibility of dose reduction by additionally skipping the arterial phase of the examination while maintaining the high sensitivity of the single-phase protocol for detecting endoleaks. A summary of these studies is provided in Table 1.

Since cumulative radiation exposure is a fundamental factor influencing post-EVAR diagnostic surveillance protocols, CTA protocols are a compromise between radiation dose and diagnostic accuracy. There is generally a consensus among researchers regarding reducing the number of examination phases by omitting the native phase and reconstructing the VNC. However, the number of examination phases performed after administering a contrast agent is controversial. A few authors have highlighted the importance of the arterial phase in detecting endoleaks, demonstrating a higher sensitivity of multiphasic (VNC + 2 postcontrast DECT acquisitions) examination protocols [48,51]. Potentially life-threatening and requiring treatment, type I and type III endoleaks require the arterial phase of examination for diagnosis [52]. Despite discrepancies in the literature on the necessity of the arterial phase for detecting endoleaks, this phase unquestionably holds value in assessing the potential narrowing of abdominal arteries [53,54]. This issue is particularly significant in the case of post-br/fEVAR procedures due to a higher risk of complications within the target arteries. Furthermore, the arterial phase allows for the evaluation of perfusion disorders of the abdominal organs and potentially the implementation of appropriate treatment. In the general elderly population of EVAR patients, acquiring the arterial phase might be particularly important in assessing additional findings such as tumors. Therefore, the presence of the arterial phase in CTA protocols appears justified. However, the optimal scanning protocol for CT scanning remains controversial [48,49,51,55–57].

Table 1. Reduction in the average radiation dose in DECT studies compared with the triphasic examination protocol.

Research	Protocol		Dose Reduction (%)
	Mono-Phasic (mSv)	Three-Phasic (mSv)	
Chandarana et al., 2008 [47]	11.1	27.8	61
Flors et al., 2013 [48]	9.8	22.4	64.1
Stolzman et al., 2008 [49]	10.9	27.4	61
Buffa et al., 2014 [50]	10.5	27.4	61.7
Kazimierczak et al., 2023 [51]	10.69	27.96	61.37

An interesting study in this context was conducted by Javor et al., who demonstrated the possibility of reducing the radiation dose by 42% via a split-bolus technique with one DE acquisition and VNC reconstruction with 96% sensitivity in endoleak detection [58]. Similar results were achieved by Boos and Iezzi [59,60]. In theory, this technique allows for the optimal contrast of low- and high-flow endoleaks, as well as arterial vessels and parenchymal organs, during a single scan. However, despite promising results, the literature lacks sufficient evidence for the effectiveness of split-bolus protocols in post-EVAR surveillance.

4.2. Contrast Agent Volume Reduction

The use of contrast agents is mandatory in both procedure planning and post-EVAR diagnostic surveillance. The accuracy of delineating three-dimensional vessel structures is crucial for the selection of proper surgical devices and the diagnosis of postprocedural complications. However, high-quality CTA requires the administration of an appropriate volume of iodine contrast agent. The use of contrast agents is associated with adverse effects, such as hypersensitivity allergic reactions, thyroid dysfunction, and nephropathy [61–63]. To minimize the risk of contrast media-induced nephropathy, it is recommended to use as o.w. volume of a contrast agent as possible for diagnostic imaging [64–66]. Therefore, contrast agent volume reduction techniques are used.

The phenomenon of high CT attenuation numbers in low-level virtual monoenergetic images (VMIs) is well established [25,67]. When low-level VMIs are used, CT attenuation of the contrast material can be increased, allowing for the injection of a lower dose of iodine [68]. Low-level VMIs have been shown to boost vascular contrast in several vascular beds, which can reduce the volume of the contrast agent [69–71]. Studies have shown that necessary preprocedural measurements of the aorta can be acquired with low-level VMIs, permitting imaging with an equivalent radiation dose but a lower contrast dose than standard SECT [72,73].

Currently, there is a lack of data in the literature on the diagnostic accuracy of protocols involving reduced contrast agent administration. Despite this, this issue is of significant importance in the context of follow-up CTA of EVAR patients. In clinical practice, there are instances of administering reduced amounts of contrast agents due to staff errors, disconnection of injecting system components, access vessel rupture, or incorrect acquisition timing. Additionally, radiological protection concerns, such as avoiding the repetition of poorly performed examinations, justify the need to implement methods that allow for the assessment of CTA with suboptimal vessel enhancement. Low-energy VMIs may enable a reduction in rejected examinations and provide a reliable assessment of endoleaks in these specific clinical settings. Figure 6 shows the differences between conventional, linearly blended, and low-level VMI reconstructions in type 3 endoleaks.

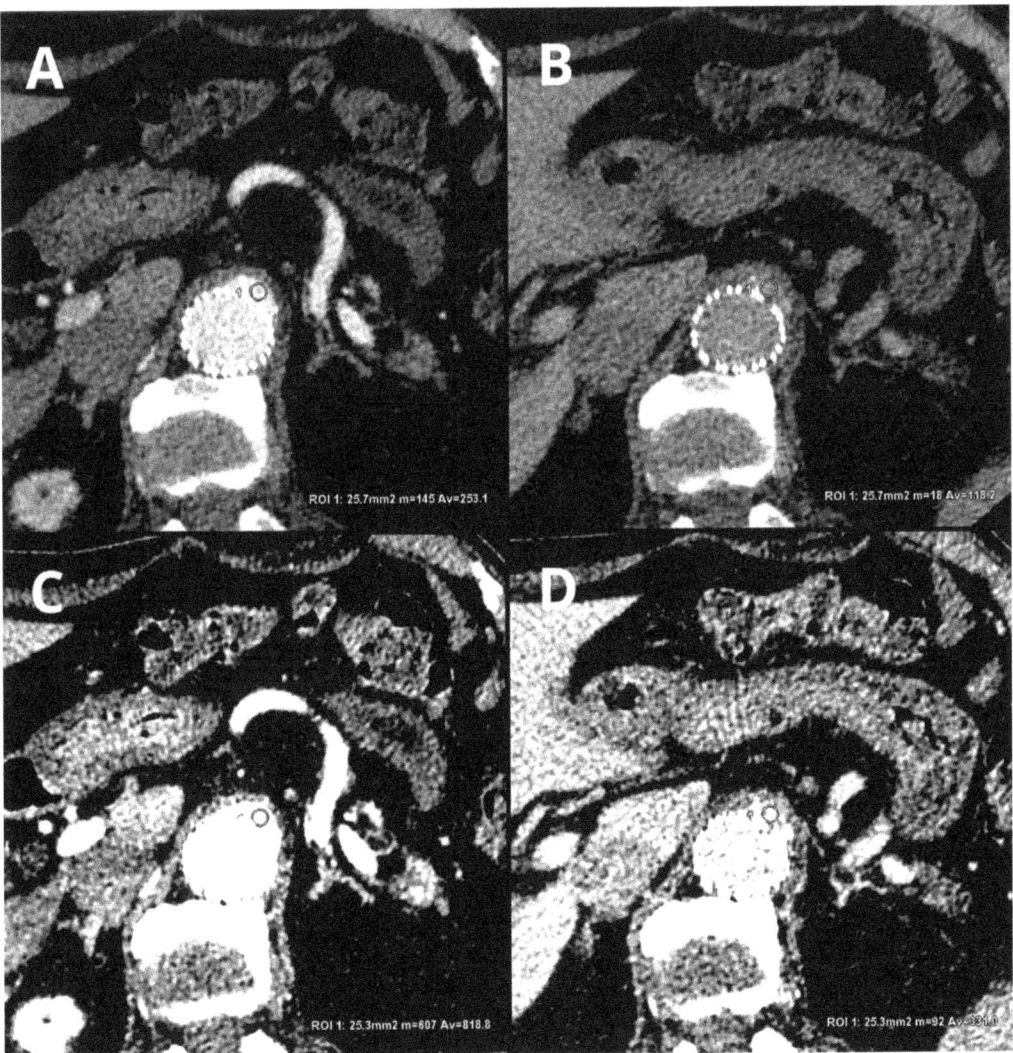

Figure 6. Comparison of LB and 40 keV VMI reconstructions in arterial and delayed phases: LB arterial ((**A**)—253.1 ± 50.2 HU), LB delayed ((**B**)—118.2 ± 25.4), 40 keV VMI arterial ((**C**)—818.8 ± 116.5 HU), and 40 keV VMI delayed ((**D**)—331 ± 53.4 HU). An automatic region-of-interest (ROI) propagation tool was used. The same window settings (W 500, L 100) were used to highlight the differences in the contrast visualization. LB-delayed and 40 keV VMI-delayed images serve as examples of the potential to salvage an examination with a reduced volume of contrast agent.

4.3. Endoleak Detection

Low-level VMIs are a major factor in the superiority of DECT over SECT for detecting endoleaks. To date, few studies have assessed the impact of low-level VMIs on the diagnostic accuracy of endoleak detection [51,74–76]. A study by Maturen et al. [74] showed a higher sensitivity for endoleak detection with a VMI of 55 keV than a VMI of 75 keV. Martin et al. [75] reported a significantly greater rate of endoleak detection in VMI and VMI+ compared to standard linearly blended images (LB). These results were accompanied by a significant improvement in the image quality parameters (contrast-to-noise ratio). Comparable results were achieved by Kazimierczak et al. [51] in a 2023 study, showing a significant increase in the number of endoleaks diagnosed (an increase of almost 30%) and an improvement in image quality parameters with 40 keV VMI compared to LB images. Charalombous et al. reported the use of a 54 keV VMI to enhance the efficiency of endoleak detection efficiency. Moreover, analysis of the normalized effective atomic number and improvised endoleak index was found to have significant power in predicting the aggressiveness of type II endoleaks [77]. However, all of the mentioned studies were conducted on relatively small study groups with fewer than 100 patients and did not influence the current guidelines regarding post-EVAR follow-up. An interesting study by Skawran et al. [76] compared low-level VMIs and single-energy low-kV images (SEIs) in terms of the diagnostic accuracy of six readers in endoleak detection as well as subjective and objective image quality properties. The results of this study indicated that a low-keV VMI+ improved the contrast-to-noise ratio of the aorta. However, the noise level, subjective image quality, and diagnostic accuracy of endoleaks were superior for SEI. Although the results of the present study are related to analyses performed on a phantom, they suggest a promising direction for further research to improve the detectability of endoleaks.

4.4. Metal Artifact Reduction

Materials used in vascular procedures, such as coils, embolization materials, and stent graft materials, can cause artifacts in CT scans, primarily photon starvation and beam hardening artifacts. These artifacts can hamper image quality and significantly decrease the diagnostic value of the examination. Metal artifact reduction (MAR) algorithms theoretically find particular applications in patients after br/fEVAR.

The presence of metallic markers on fenestrations, branches, stents, the metal structure of stent grafts, and previously used coils or embolization materials can result in artifacts that lower the diagnostic value of the examination. Beam-hardening artifacts make it difficult to assess stented vessels, preventing proper evaluation of potential narrowing or occlusion. In the case of significant artifacts, vessel patency assessment must rely on the evaluation of potential collateral circulation, contrast enhancement of the distal branches of the evaluated vessel, and the presence of hypoperfusion/infarction signs in the organ supplied by the studied artery. Early detection of narrowing may allow the implementation of treatment to prevent the development of complete occlusion and, consequently, organ infarction [78]. Additionally, metallic artifacts can mask the presence of small endoleaks in patients after EVAR.

Theoretically, using MAR algorithms can improve the diagnostic value of patients after EVAR [56,59]. However, some studies indicate a significant decrease in the diagnostic value of MAR algorithms compared to that of DECT in a group of patients post-EVAR. In a study by Boos et al., the researchers aimed to assess the effectiveness of MAR algorithms in fast kV-switching DECTA in a group of 24 post-EVAR patients [59]. The primary objective was to determine whether the MAR technique could improve endoleak visualization and reduce the artifacts caused by the metallic components of EVAR stents and coils. The results of artifact evaluation showed an objective decrease in artifacts from EVAR stents in the near field, albeit associated with a subjective increase in artifacts in the near field, far field, and vessels. Furthermore, the MAR algorithm impaired visualization in 60% (n = 6) of patients with endoleaks and improved visualization in 10% (n = 1) of patient with endoleaks. In a recent study, MAR algorithms objectively improved visualization of stents in target vessels in patients after br/fEVAR but surprisingly significantly impaired subjective image quality (rate of 1.57 ± 0.5 on a 5-point Likert scale compared to a mean rate of 4.25 ± 0.44 for adaptive statistical iterative reconstructions) [79]. Additionally, the authors reported hampered endoleak visualization and additional artifacts that could result in false positive diagnoses of endoleaks. However, this topic requires further analysis because the results conflict with a substantial portion of the literature, as well as the very small study groups involved.

The solution to this problem appears to be to use high-keV VMI reconstructions (≥100 keV), which reduce blooming artifacts caused by hyperdense structures, such as calcified plaques and metal stents. This approach has proven particularly useful in cardiac CT scans [80]. Reconstructions in the range of 130–150 keV provide optimal imaging of stent lumens less than 3 mm in diameter, potentially reducing the dose of ionizing radiation [81,82]. Furthermore, these reconstructions enhance the diagnostic value of examinations plagued with artifacts associated with calcified plaques and an influx of contrast material [83,84]. A comparison of the MAR and 140 keV reconstructions is shown in Figure 7.

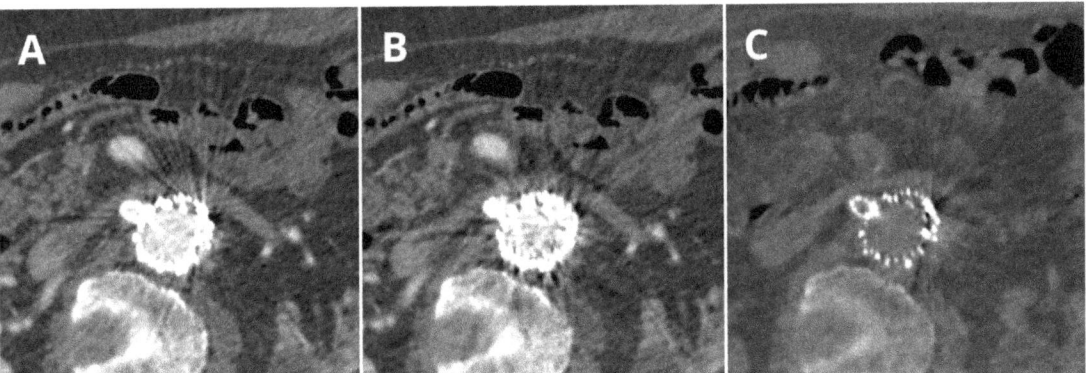

Figure 7. Comparison of the LB (**A**), MAR (**B**), and 140 keV VMI (**C**) reconstructions. Arterial phase: The level of the right renal artery (RRA) in a patient one month after the fEVAR procedure. The same window settings were used (W 500, L 100). It is important to note the additional artifacts in MAR reconstructions that completely prevent the evaluation of the initial segment of the stent to the RRA and the decreased contrast visualization on the 140 keV VMI. Artifact intensity variations between the reconstructions can be observed.

5. Limitations

Despite the numerous advantages of DECT in vascular imaging, concerns have been raised regarding workflow, artifacts, temporal misregistration, radiation exposure, and image quality [85]. A factor that directly affects the utility and frequency of DECT use is its integration into the workflow. Dual-energy CT imaging has been associated with multiple workflow issues, among which the most significant are increased reconstruction time, a large number of images (resulting in increased PACS usage and longer downloading times), and increased interpretation time [86,87]. DECT postprocessing requires exclusive vendor-specific software, which can be costly and vary in capabilities. Postprocessing of spectral data can be very time-consuming for both technologists and radiologists, and additional postprocessing may be impossible without the use of a full spectral dataset [88]. Generally, implementing DECT in a routine workflow requires substantial knowledge of the vendor's scanner and results in a steep learning curve [89]. Moreover, DECT systems are associated with higher costs for specific hardware and software [85].

DECT imaging is susceptible to various artifacts related to scanner design, acquisition protocols, and postprocessing techniques, which may be unique to the platform utilized [85,90]. Image noise can be increased using certain reconstruction approaches (such as low-level VMIs). Patient size, motion, and iodine concentration also contribute to artifacts, potentially leading to nondiagnostic images. Incorrect attenuation thresholds may lead to false positive or false negative results in material decomposition protocols [90]. Additionally, some types of scanners (split-filter scanners) are characterized by a lower temporal resolution [90,91]. Moreover, increased body size can lead to greater image noise and lower quality in DECT abdominal imaging due to reduced photon detection and exacerbated beam-hardening artifacts [85]. Consequently, patient selection criteria based on weight and body dimensions have been suggested [90,92].

Initial concerns regarding the radiation dose combined with DECT have been mitigated by recent advances in technology [88]. Several studies have shown doses comparable to or lower than the delivered SECT radiation doses without compromising image quality [42–44,93,94]. Several techniques leading to significant radiation dose reduction, including VNC imaging, noise reduction algorithms, and limiting the FOV to the area of interest, have been utilized [95–98]. However, radiation doses can vary depending on the scanner model, scan type, body region, and patient factors [88]. Therefore, implementing DECT protocols requires staff to have specialized knowledge that allows for the efficient and safe use of this technology.

6. Conclusions

DECT is an emerging technology that offers additional layers of information inaccessible using conventional CT. DECT enables molecular composition analysis, opening new horizons in imaging that significantly surpasses standard tomographic examinations. With the increasing number of diverse dual-energy systems and their growing availability, we observed a steady increase in the applications of these technologies in various clinical settings. An increasing number of publications demonstrate the significant advantages of DECT over SECT, particularly in angiographic studies.

The application of spectral CT systems in patients after EVAR enhances the diagnostic value of these examinations. The most useful reconstructions were those obtained using material decomposition and VMI reconstruction. Because of the virtual nonenhanced phases, spectral CT angiography can be performed in EVAR patients with a significantly lower effective radiation dose and a potentially reduced contrast agent dosage. VMI reconstruction enhances the visualization of endoleaks and may assist in evaluating images marked by metal artifacts. The benefits of DECT in post-EVAR examinations are summarized in Table 2.

Table 2. Summary of the advantages of DECT over conventional SECT and its clinical applications.

Reconstruction Technique	Advantage	Application
Low-energy VMI	Higher sensitivity for iodine.	Improved endoleak detection. Contrast dose reduction. Salvage of suboptimal contrast examination.
High-energy VMI	Reduction in calcium blooming artifacts. Metal artifact and beam-hardening reduction.	Reduction in artifacts from stentgraft structures and embolization materials. Better visualization of stent lumen. Improved visualization of calcified vessels.
Virtual noncontrast images	Reduction in number of phases of examination.	Reduction in radiation dose. Characteristic of incidental findings in abbreviated examination protocols (without true noncontrast phase).
Material decomposition	Identification of elemental composition of tissues.	Plaque characterization. Improved separation of calcium from iodine.

In summary, the implementation of DECT in patients after EVAR allows for a reduction in ionizing radiation dose and an increase in the diagnostic value of the examination in detecting postprocedural complications. However, implementing DECT acquisitions in clinical practice remains a challenge.

Author Contributions: Conceptualization, W.K.; methodology, W.K.; software, W.K.; validation, W.K., N.K. and Z.S.; formal analysis, W.K.; investigation, W.K.; resources, W.K.; data curation, W.K.; writing—original draft preparation, W.K. and N.K.; writing—review and editing, Z.S.; visualization, W.K.; supervision, Z.S.; project administration, Z.S.; funding acquisition, W.K. All authors have read and agreed to the published version of the manuscript.

Funding: This research received no external funding.

Institutional Review Board Statement: Not applicable.

Informed Consent Statement: Not applicable.

Data Availability Statement: Not applicable.

Conflicts of Interest: The authors declare no conflict of interest.

References

1. Hounsfield, G.N. Computerized transverse axial scanning (tomography): I. Description of system. *Br. J. Radiol.* **1973**, *46*, 1016–1022. [CrossRef]
2. Stather, P.; Sidloff, D.; Rhema, I.; Choke, E.; Bown, M.; Sayers, R. A review of current reporting of abdominal aortic aneurysm mortality and prevalence in the literature. *Eur. J. Vasc. Endovasc. Surg.* **2014**, *47*, 240–242. [CrossRef]
3. Chaikof, E.L.; Dalman, R.L.; Eskandari, M.K.; Jackson, B.M.; Lee, W.A.; Mansour, M.A.; Mastracci, T.M.; Mell, M.; Murad, M.H.; Nguyen, L.L.; et al. The Society for Vascular Surgery practice guidelines on the care of patients with an abdominal aortic aneurysm. *J. Vasc. Surg.* **2018**, *67*, 2–77.e2. [CrossRef]
4. Lederle, F.A.; Johnson, G.R.; Wilson, S.E.; Chute, E.P.; Littooy, F.N.; Bandyk, D.; Krupski, W.C.; Barone, G.W.; Acher, C.W.; Ballard, D.J. Prevalence and associations of abdominal aortic aneurysm detected through screening. *Ann. Intern. Med.* **1997**, *126*, 441–449. [CrossRef]
5. Schlösser, F.; Gusberg, R.; Dardik, A.; Lin, P.; Verhagen, H.; Moll, F.; Muhs, B. Aneurysm Rupture after EVAR: Can the Ultimate Failure be Predicted? *Eur. J. Vasc. Endovasc. Surg.* **2009**, *37*, 15–22. [CrossRef]
6. Schermerhorn, M.L.; Buck, D.B.; O'malley, A.J.; Curran, T.; McCallum, J.C.; Darling, J.; Landon, B.E. Long-Term Outcomes of Abdominal Aortic Aneurysm in the Medicare Population. *N. Engl. J. Med.* **2015**, *373*, 328–338. [CrossRef]
7. Karaolanis, G.I.; Antonopoulos, C.N.; Georgakarakos, E.; Lianos, G.D.; Mitsis, M.; Glantzounis, G.K.; Giannoukas, A.; Kouvelos, G. Colour Duplex and/or Contrast-Enhanced Ultrasound Compared with Computed Tomography Angiography for Endoleak Detection after Endovascular Abdominal Aortic Aneurysm Repair: A Systematic Review and Meta-Analysis. *J. Clin. Med.* **2022**, *11*, 3628. [CrossRef]
8. Mirza, T.; Karthikesalingam, A.; Jackson, D.; Walsh, S.; Holt, P.; Hayes, P.; Boyle, J. Duplex Ultrasound and Contrast-Enhanced Ultrasound Versus Computed Tomography for the Detection of Endoleak after EVAR: Systematic Review and Bivariate Meta-Analysis. *Eur. J. Vasc. Endovasc. Surg.* **2010**, *39*, 418–428. [CrossRef]
9. Wanhainen, A.; Verzini, F.; Van Herzeele, I.; Allaire, E.; Bown, M.; Cohnert, T.; Dick, F.; van Herwaarden, J.; Karkos, C.; Koelemay, M.; et al. Editor's Choice—European Society for Vascular Surgery (ESVS) 2019 Clinical Practice Guidelines on the Management of Abdominal Aorto-iliac Artery Aneurysms. *Eur. J. Vasc. Endovasc. Surg.* **2019**, *57*, 8–93. [CrossRef]
10. Alvarez, R.E.; MacOvski, A. Energy-selective reconstructions in X-ray computerised tomography. *Phys. Med. Biol.* **1976**, *21*, 733–744. [CrossRef]
11. McCollough, C.H.; Leng, S.; Yu, L.; Fletcher, J.G. Dual- and multi-energy CT: Principles, technical approaches, and clinical applications. *Radiology* **2015**, *276*, 637–653. [CrossRef]
12. Connolly, M.J.; McInnes, M.D.F.; El-Khodary, M.; McGrath, T.A.; Schieda, N. Diagnostic accuracy of virtual non-contrast enhanced dual-energy CT for diagnosis of adrenal adenoma: A systematic review and meta-analysis. *Eur. Radiol.* **2017**, *27*, 4324–4335. [CrossRef]
13. Lehti, L.; Söderberg, M.; Höglund, P.; Nyman, U.; Gottsäter, A.; Wassélius, J. Reliability of virtual non-contrast computed tomography angiography: Comparing it with the real deal. *Acta Radiol. Open* **2018**, *7*, 2058460118790115. [CrossRef]
14. Takahashi, N.; Hartman, R.P.; Vrtiska, T.J.; Kawashima, A.; Primak, A.N.; Dzyubak, O.P.; Mandrekar, J.N.; Fletcher, J.G.; McCollough, C.H. Dual-energy CT iodine-subtraction virtual unenhanced technique to detect urinary stones in an iodine-filled collecting system: A phantom study. *Am. J. Roentgenol.* **2008**, *190*, 1169–1173. [CrossRef]
15. Graser, A.; Johnson, T.R.C.; Hecht, E.M.; Becker, C.R.; Leidecker, C.; Staehler, M.; Stief, C.G.; Hildebrandt, H.; Godoy, M.C.B.; Finn, M.E.; et al. Dual-energy CT in patients suspected of having renal masses: Can virtual nonenhanced images replace true nonenhanced images? *Radiology* **2009**, *252*, 433–440. [CrossRef]
16. Phan, C.; Yoo, A.; Hirsch, J.; Nogueira, R.; Gupta, R. Differentiation of hemorrhage from iodinated contrast in different intracranial compartments using dual-energy head CT. *Am. J. Neuroradiol.* **2012**, *33*, 1088–1094. [CrossRef]

17. Lehti, L.; Söderberg, M.; Höglund, P.; Wassélius, J. Comparing Arterial- and Venous-Phase Acquisition for Optimization of Virtual Noncontrast Images from Dual-Energy Computed Tomography Angiography. *J. Comput. Assist. Tomogr.* **2019**, *43*, 770–774. [CrossRef]
18. Kazimierczak, W.; Kazimierczak, N.; Serafin, Z. Quality of virtual-non-contrast phases derived from arterial and delayed phases of fast-kVp switching dual-energy CT in patients after endovascular aortic repair. *Int. J. Cardiovasc. Imaging* **2023**, *39*, 1805–1813. [CrossRef]
19. Heye, T.; Nelson, R.C.; Ho, L.M.; Marin, D.; Boll, D.T. Dual-energy CT applications in the abdomen. *AJR Am. J. Roentgenol.* **2012**, *199*, S64–S70. [CrossRef]
20. Virarkar, M.K.; Vulasala, S.S.R.; Gupta, A.V.; Gopireddy, D.; Kumar, S.; Hernandez, M.; Lall, C.; Bhosale, P. Virtual Non-contrast Imaging in The Abdomen and The Pelvis: An Overview. In *Seminars in Ultrasound, CT and MRI*; Elsevier: Amsterdam, The Netherlands, 2022; Volume 43.
21. Ascenti, G.; Sofia, C.; Mazziotti, S.; Silipigni, S.; D'Angelo, T.; Pergolizzi, S.; Scribano, E. Dual-energy CT with iodine quantification in distinguishing between bland and neoplastic portal vein thrombosis in patients with hepatocellular carcinoma. *Clin. Radiol.* **2016**, *71*, 938.e1–938.e9. [CrossRef]
22. Ascenti, G.; Mazziotti, S.; Lamberto, S.; Bottari, A.; Caloggero, S.; Racchiusa, S.; Mileto, A.; Scribano, E. Dual-energy CT for detection of endoleaks after endovascular abdominal aneurysm repair: Usefulness of colored iodine overlay. *Am. J. Roentgenol.* **2011**, *196*, 1408–1414. [CrossRef] [PubMed]
23. Mannil, M.; Ramachandran, J.; de Martini, I.V.; Wegener, S.; Schmidt, B.; Flohr, T.; Krauss, B.; Valavanis, A.; Alkadhi, H.; Winklhofer, S. Modified Dual-Energy Algorithm for Calcified Plaque Removal: Evaluation in Carotid Computed Tomography Angiography and Comparison with Digital Subtraction Angiography. *Investig. Radiol.* **2017**, *52*, 680–685. [CrossRef] [PubMed]
24. Silvennoinen, H.; Ikonen, S.; Soinne, L.; Railo, M.; Valanne, L. CT angiographic analysis of carotid artery stenosis: Comparison of manual assessment, semiautomatic vessel analysis, and digital subtraction angiography. *Am. J. Neuroradiol.* **2007**, *28*, 97–103. [CrossRef] [PubMed]
25. Hu, D.; Yu, T.; Duan, X.; Peng, Y.; Zhai, R. Determination of the optimal energy level in spectral CT imaging for displaying abdominal vessels in pediatric patients. *Eur. J. Radiol.* **2014**, *83*, 589–594. [CrossRef] [PubMed]
26. Siegel, M.J.; Ramirez-Giraldo, J.C. Dual-energy CT in children: Imaging algorithms and clinical applications. *Radiology* **2019**, *291*, 286–297. [CrossRef]
27. De Cecco, C.N.; Caruso, D.; Schoepf, U.J.; De Santis, D.; Muscogiuri, G.; Albrecht, M.H.; Meinel, F.G.; Wichmann, J.L.; Burchett, P.F.; Varga-Szemes, A.; et al. A noise-optimized virtual monoenergetic reconstruction algorithm improves the diagnostic accuracy of late hepatic arterial phase dual-energy CT for the detection of hypervascular liver lesions. *Eur. Radiol.* **2018**, *28*, 3393–3404. [CrossRef]
28. Zhang, X.; Zhang, G.; Xu, L.; Bai, X.; Lu, X.; Yu, S.; Sun, H.; Jin, Z. Utilisation of virtual non-contrast images and virtual mono-energetic images acquired from dual-layer spectral CT for renal cell carcinoma: Image quality and radiation dose. *Insights Imaging* **2022**, *13*, 12. [CrossRef]
29. Ko, S.M.; Choi, J.W.; Song, M.G.; Shin, J.K.; Chee, H.K.; Chung, H.W.; Kim, D.H. Myocardial perfusion imaging using adenosine-induced stress dual-energy computed tomography of the heart: Comparison with cardiac magnetic resonance imaging and conventional coronary angiography. *Eur. Radiol.* **2010**, *21*, 26–35. [CrossRef]
30. Wichmann, J.L.; Bauer, R.W.; Doss, M.; Stock, W.; Lehnert, T.; Bodelle, B.; Frellesen, C.; Vogl, T.J.; Kerl, J.M. Diagnostic accuracy of late iodine-enhancement dual-energy computed tomography for the detection of chronic myocardial infarction compared with late gadolinium-enhancement 3-T magnetic resonance imaging. *Investig. Radiol.* **2013**, *48*, 851–856. [CrossRef]
31. Grant, K.L.; Flohr, T.G.; Krauss, B.; Sedlmair, M.; Thomas, C.; Schmidt, B. Assessment of an Advanced Image-Based Technique to Calculate Virtual Monoenergetic Computed Tomographic Images from a Dual-Energy Examination to Improve Contrast-To-Noise Ratio in Examinations Using Iodinated Contrast Media. *Investig. Radiol.* **2014**, *49*, 586–592. [CrossRef]
32. Zeng, Y.; Geng, D.; Zhang, J. Noise-optimized virtual monoenergetic imaging technology of the third-generation dual-source computed tomography and its clinical applications. *Quant. Imaging Med. Surg.* **2021**, *11*, 4627–4643. [CrossRef] [PubMed]
33. Wichmann, J.L.; Gillott, M.R.; De Cecco, C.N.; Mangold, S.; Varga-Szemes, A.; Yamada, R.; Otani, K.; Canstein, C.M.; Fuller, S.R.B.; Vogl, T.J.; et al. Dual-Energy Computed Tomography Angiography of the Lower Extremity Runoff. *Investig. Radiol.* **2016**, *51*, 139–146. [CrossRef] [PubMed]
34. Dixon, A.K.; Dendy, P. Spiral CT: How much does radiation dose matter? *Lancet* **1998**, *352*, 1082–1083. [CrossRef] [PubMed]
35. Einstein, A.J.; Henzlova, M.J.; Rajagopalan, S. Estimating risk of cancer associated with radiation exposure from 64-slice computed tomography coronary angiography. *JAMA* **2007**, *298*, 317–323. [CrossRef] [PubMed]
36. de Jong, P.A.; Mayo, J.R.; Golmohammadi, K.; Nakano, Y.; Lequin, M.H.; Tiddens, H.A.W.M.; Aldrich, J.; Coxson, H.O.; Sin, D.D. Estimation of cancer mortality associated with repetitive computed tomography scanning. *Am. J. Respir. Crit Care Med.* **2006**, *173*, 199–203. [CrossRef] [PubMed]
37. Brenner, D.J.; Hall, E.J. Computed Tomography—An Increasing Source of Radiation Exposure. *N. Engl. J. Med.* **2007**, *357*, 2277–2284. [CrossRef] [PubMed]
38. Brenner, D.J.; Elliston, C.D. Estimated radiation on risks potentially associated with full-body CT screening. *Radiology* **2004**, *232*, 735–738. [CrossRef] [PubMed]

39. White, H.A.; MacDonald, S. Estimating risk associated with radiation exposure during follow-up after endovascular aortic repair (EVAR). *J. Cardiovasc. Surg.* **2010**, *51*, 95.
40. Lehti, L.; Nyman, U.; Söderberg, M.; Björses, K.; Gottsäter, A.; Wassélius, J. 80-kVp CT angiography for endovascular aneurysm repair follow-up with halved contrast medium dose and preserved diagnostic quality. *Acta Radiol.* **2016**, *57*, 279–286. [CrossRef]
41. Grajo, J.R.; Sahani, D.V. Dual-Energy CT of the Abdomen and Pelvis: Radiation Dose Considerations. *J. Am. Coll. Radiol.* **2018**, *15*, 1128–1132. [CrossRef]
42. Weinman, J.P.; Mirsky, D.M.; Jensen, A.M.; Stence, N.V. Dual energy head CT to maintain image quality while reducing dose in pediatric patients. *Clin. Imaging* **2019**, *55*, 83–88. [CrossRef] [PubMed]
43. Siegel, M.J.; Curtis, W.A.; Ramirez-Giraldo, J.C. Effects of dual-energy technique on radiation exposure and image quality in pediatric body CT. *Am. J. Roentgenol.* **2016**, *207*, 826–835. [CrossRef] [PubMed]
44. Goo, H.W. Initial experience of dual-energy lung perfusion CT using a dual-source CT system in children. *Pediatr. Radiol.* **2010**, *40*, 1536–1544. [CrossRef] [PubMed]
45. Primak, A.N.; Giraldo, J.C.R.; Eusemann, C.D.; Schmidt, B.; Kantor, B.; Fletcher, J.G.; McCollough, C.H. Dual-source dual-energy CT with additional tin filtration: Dose and image quality evaluation in phantoms and in vivo. *Am. J. Roentgenol.* **2010**, *195*, 1164–1174. [CrossRef] [PubMed]
46. Macari, M.; Chandarana, H.; Schmidt, B.; Lee, J.; Lamparello, P.; Babb, J. Abdominal aortic aneurysm: Can the arterial phase at CT evaluation after endovascular repair be eliminated to reduce radiation dose? *Radiology* **2006**, *241*, 908–914. [CrossRef]
47. Chandarana, H.; Godoy, M.C.B.; Vlahos, I.; Graser, A.; Babb, J.; Leidecker, C.; Macari, M. Abdominal aorta: Evaluation with dual-source dual-energy multidetector CT after endovascular repair of aneurysms-initial observations. *Radiology* **2008**, *249*, 692–700. [CrossRef]
48. Flors, L.; Leiva-Salinas, C.; Norton, P.T.; Patrie, J.T.; Hagspiel, K.D. Endoleak detection after endovascular repair of thoracic aortic aneurysm using dual-source dual-energy CT: Suitable scanning protocols and potential radiation dose reduction. *Am. J. Roentgenol.* **2013**, *200*, 451–460. [CrossRef]
49. Stolzmann, P.; Frauenfelder, T.; Pfammatter, T.; Peter, N.; Scheffel, H.; Lachat, M.; Schmidt, B.; Marincek, B.; Alkadhi, H.; Schertler, T. Endoleaks after endovascular abdominal aortic aneurysm repair: Detection with dual-energy dual-source CT. *Radiology* **2008**, *249*, 682–691. [CrossRef]
50. Buffa, V.; Solazzo, A.; D'auria, V.; Del Prete, A.; Vallone, A.; Luzietti, M.; Madau, M.; Grassi, R.; Miele, V. Dual-source dual-energy CT: Dose reduction after endovascular abdominal aortic aneurysm repair. *Radiol. Medica* **2014**, *119*, 934–941. [CrossRef]
51. Kazimierczak, W.; Kazimierczak, N.; Lemanowicz, A.; Nowak, E.; Migdalski, A.; Jawien, A.; Jankowski, T.; Serafin, Z. Improved Detection of Endoleaks in Virtual Monoenergetic Images in Dual-Energy CT Angiography Following EVAR. *Acad. Radiol.* **2023**, *30*, 2813–2824. [CrossRef]
52. Iezzi, R.; Cotroneo, A.R.; Filippone, A.; Di Fabio, F.; Quinto, F.; Colosimo, C.; Bonomo, L. Multidetector CT in abdominal aortic aneurysm treated with endovascular repair: Are unenhanced and delayed phase enhanced images effective for endoleak detection? *Radiology* **2006**, *241*, 915–921. [CrossRef] [PubMed]
53. Glebova, N.O.; Selvarajah, S.; Orion, K.C.; Black, J.H.; Malas, M.B.; Perler, B.A.; Abularrage, C.J. Fenestrated endovascular repair of abdominal aortic aneurysms is associated with increased morbidity but comparable mortality with infrarenal endovascular aneurysm repair. *J. Vasc. Surg.* **2015**, *61*, 604–610. [CrossRef] [PubMed]
54. Troisi, N.; Donas, K.P.; Austermann, M.; Tessarek, J.; Umscheid, T.; Torsello, G. Secondary procedures after aortic aneurysm repair with fenestrated and branched endografts. *J. Endovasc. Ther.* **2011**, *18*, 146–153. [CrossRef] [PubMed]
55. Sommer, W.H.; Becker, C.R.; Haack, M.; Rubin, G.D.; Weidenhagen, R.; Schwarz, F.; Nikolaou, K.; Reiser, M.F.; Johnson, T.R.; Clevert, D.A. Time-resolved CT angiography for the detection and classification of endoleaks. *Radiology* **2012**, *263*, 917–926. [CrossRef] [PubMed]
56. Stavropoulos, S.W.; Charagundla, S.R. Imaging techniques for detection and management of endoleaks after endovascular aortic aneurysm repair. *Radiology* **2007**, *243*, 641–655. [CrossRef] [PubMed]
57. Iezzi, R.; Cotroneo, A.R.; Filippone, A.; Santoro, M.; Basilico, R.; Storto, M.L. Multidetector-row computed tomography angiography in abdominal aortic aneurysm treated with endovascular repair: Evaluation of optimal timing of delayed phase imaging for the detection of low-flow endoleaks. *J. Comput. Assist. Tomogr.* **2008**, *32*, 609–615. [CrossRef]
58. Javor, D.; Wressnegger, A.; Unterhumer, S.; Kollndorfer, K.; Nolz, R.; Beitzke, D.; Loewe, C. Endoleak detection using single-acquisition split-bolus dual-energy computer tomography (DECT). *Eur. Radiol.* **2017**, *27*, 1622–1630. [CrossRef]
59. Boos, J.; Fang, J.; Heidinger, B.H.; Raptopoulos, V.; Brook, O.R. Dual energy CT angiography: Pros and cons of dual-energy metal artifact reduction algorithm in patients after endovascular aortic repair. *Abdom. Radiol.* **2017**, *42*, 749–758. [CrossRef]
60. Iezzi, R.; Carchesio, F.; Posa, A.; Colosimo, C.; Bonomo, L. *Post-EVAR split-bolus CT angiography using dual-energy CT: All you need in a single scan!* In EuroSafe Imaging; ESR: Vienna, Austria, 2017.
61. Mehran, R.; Nikolsky, E. Contrast-induced nephropathy: Definition, epidemiology, and patients at risk. *Kidney Int.* **2006**, *69*, S11–S15. [CrossRef]
62. van der Molen, A.J.; Thomsen, H.S.; Morcos, S.K. Effect of iodinated contrast media on thyroid function in adults. *Eur. Radiol.* **2004**, *14*, 902–907.
63. Katayama, H.; Yamaguchi, K.; Kozuka, T.; Takashima, T.; Seez, P.; Matsuura, K. Adverse reactions to ionic and nonionic contrast media. A report from the Japanese Committee on the Safety of Contrast Media. *Radiology* **1990**, *175*, 621–628. [CrossRef] [PubMed]

64. Yamamoto, M.; Hayashida, K.; Mouillet, G.; Hovasse, T.; Chevalier, B.; Oguri, A.; Watanabe, Y.; Dubois-Randé, J.-L.; Morice, M.-C.; Lefèvre, T.; et al. Prognostic value of chronic kidney disease after transcatheter aortic valve implantation. *J. Am. Coll. Cardiol.* **2013**, *62*, 869–877. [CrossRef] [PubMed]
65. Kane, G.C.; Doyle, B.J.; Lerman, A.; Barsness, G.W.; Best, P.J.; Rihal, C.S. Ultra-Low Contrast Volumes Reduce Rates of Contrast-Induced Nephropathy in Patients with Chronic Kidney Disease Undergoing Coronary Angiography. *J. Am. Coll. Cardiol.* **2008**, *51*, 89–90. [CrossRef] [PubMed]
66. McDonald, R.J.; McDonald, J.S.; Bida, J.P.; Carter, R.E.; Fleming, C.J.; Misra, S.; Williamson, E.E.; Kallmes, D.F.; Paltiel, H.J.; Gilligan, L.A.; et al. Intravenous contrast material-induced nephropathy: Causal or coincident phenomenon? *Radiology* **2013**, *267*, 106–118. [CrossRef] [PubMed]
67. Huda, W.; Scalzetti, E.M.; Levin, G. Technique factors and image quality as functions of patient weight at abdominal CT. *Radiology* **2000**, *217*, 430–435. [CrossRef] [PubMed]
68. van Hamersvelt, R.W.; Eijsvoogel, N.G.; Mihl, C.; de Jong, P.A.; Schilham, A.M.R.; Buls, N.; Das, M.; Leiner, T.; Willemink, M.J. Contrast agent concentration optimization in CTA using low tube voltage and dual-energy CT in multiple vendors: A phantom study. *Int. J. Cardiovasc. Imaging* **2018**, *34*, 1265–1275. [CrossRef] [PubMed]
69. Carrascosa, P.; Leipsic, J.A.; Capunay, C.; Deviggiano, A.; Vallejos, J.; Goldsmit, A.; Rodriguez-Granillo, G.A. Monochromatic image reconstruction by dual energy imaging allows half iodine load computed tomography coronary angiography. *Eur. J. Radiol.* **2015**, *84*, 1915–1920. [CrossRef]
70. Godoy, M.C.; Heller, S.L.; Naidich, D.P.; Assadourian, B.; Leidecker, C.; Schmidt, B.; Vlahos, I. Dual-energy MDCT: Comparison of pulmonary artery enhancement on dedicated CT pulmonary angiography, routine and low contrast volume studies. *Eur. J. Radiol.* **2011**, *79*, e11–e17. [CrossRef]
71. Nijhof, W.; Baltussen, E.; Kant, I.; Jager, G.; Slump, C.; Rutten, M. Low-dose CT angiography of the abdominal aorta and reduced contrast medium volume: Assessment of image quality and radiation dose. *Clin. Radiol.* **2016**, *71*, 64–73. [CrossRef]
72. Dubourg, B.; Caudron, J.; Lestrat, J.-P.; Bubenheim, M.; Lefebvre, V.; Godin, M.; Tron, C.; Eltchaninoff, H.; Bauer, F.; Dacher, J.-N. Single-source dual-energy CT angiography with reduced iodine load in patients referred for aortoiliofemoral evaluation before transcatheter aortic valve implantation: Impact on image quality and radiation dose. *Eur. Radiol.* **2014**, *24*, 2659–2668. [CrossRef]
73. Martin, S.S.; Albrecht, M.H.; Wichmann, J.L.; Hüsers, K.; Scholtz, J.-E.; Booz, C.; Bodelle, B.; Bauer, R.W.; Metzger, S.C.; Vogl, T.J.; et al. Value of a noise-optimized virtual monoenergetic reconstruction technique in dual-energy CT for planning of transcatheter aortic valve replacement. *Eur. Radiol.* **2017**, *27*, 705–714. [CrossRef] [PubMed]
74. Maturen, K.E.; Kaza, R.K.; Liu, P.S.; Quint, L.E.; Khalatbari, S.H.; Platt, J.F. "Sweet spot" for endoleak detection: Optimizing contrast to noise using low kev reconstructions from fast-switch kVp dual-energy CT. *J. Comput. Assist. Tomogr.* **2012**, *36*, 83–87. [CrossRef] [PubMed]
75. Martin, S.S.; Wichmann, J.L.; Weyer, H.; Scholtz, J.-E.; Leithner, D.; Spandorfer, A.; Bodelle, B.; Jacobi, V.; Vogl, T.J.; Albrecht, M.H. Endoleaks after endovascular aortic aneurysm repair: Improved detection with noise-optimized virtual monoenergetic dual-energy CT. *Eur. J. Radiol.* **2017**, *94*, 125–132. [CrossRef]
76. Skawran, S.; Angst, F.; Blüthgen, C.; Eberhard, M.; Kälin, P.; Kobe, A.; Nagy, D.; Szucs-Farkas, Z.; Alkadhi, H.; Euler, A. Dual-Energy Low-keV or Single-Energy Low-kV CT for Endoleak Detection? *Investig. Radiol.* **2020**, *55*, 45–52. [CrossRef] [PubMed]
77. Charalambous, S.; Perisinakis, K.; Kontopodis, N.; Papadakis, A.E.; Maris, T.G.; Ioannou, C.V.; Karantanas, A.; Tsetis, D. Dual-energy CT angiography in imaging surveillance of endovascular aneurysm repair—Preliminary study results. *Eur. J. Radiol.* **2022**, *148*, 110165. [CrossRef] [PubMed]
78. Ragusi, M.A.A.D.; van der Meer, R.W.; Joemai, R.M.S.; van Schaik, J.; van Rijswijk, C.S.P. Evaluation of CT Angiography Image Quality Acquired with Single-Energy Metal Artifact Reduction (SEMAR) Algorithm in Patients after Complex Endovascular Aortic Repair. *Cardiovasc. Interv. Radiol.* **2018**, *41*, 323–329. [CrossRef] [PubMed]
79. Kazimierczak, W.; Nowak, E.; Kazimierczak, N.; Jankowski, T.; Jankowska, A.; Serafin, Z. The value of metal artifact reduction and iterative algorithms in dual energy CT angiography in patients after complex endovascular aortic aneurysm repair. *Heliyon* **2023**, *9*, e20700. [CrossRef]
80. Albrecht, M.H.; De Cecco, C.N.; Nance, J.W.; Varga-Szemes, A.; De Santis, D.; Eid, M.; Tesche, C.; Apfaltrer, G.; Doeberitz, P.L.v.K.; Jacobs, B.; et al. Cardiac Dual-Energy CT Applications and Clinical Impact. *Curr. Radiol. Rep.* **2017**, *5*, 42. [CrossRef]
81. Mangold, S.; Cannaó, P.M.; Schoepf, U.J.; Wichmann, J.L.; Canstein, C.; Fuller, S.R.; Muscogiuri, G.; Varga-Szemes, A.; Nikolaou, K.; De Cecco, C.N. Impact of an advanced image-based monoenergetic reconstruction algorithm on coronary stent visualization using third generation dual-source dual-energy CT: A phantom study. *Eur. Radiol.* **2016**, *26*, 1871–1878. [CrossRef]
82. Hickethier, T.; Baeßler, B.; Kroeger, J.R.; Doerner, J.; Pahn, G.; Maintz, D.; Michels, G.; Bunck, A.C. Monoenergetic reconstructions for imaging of coronary artery stents using spectral detector CT: In-vitro experience and comparison to conventional images. *J. Cardiovasc. Comput. Tomogr.* **2017**, *11*, 33–39. [CrossRef]
83. De Cecco, C.N.; Darnell, A.; Rengo, M.; Muscogiuri, G.; Bellini, D.; Ayuso, C.; Laghi, A. Dual-energy CT: Oncologic applications. *AJR Am. J. Roentgenol.* **2012**, *199*, S98. [CrossRef] [PubMed]

84. Leithner, D.; Wichmann, J.L.; Vogl, T.J.; Trommer, J.; Martin, S.S.; Scholtz, J.-E.; Bodelle, B.; De Cecco, C.N.; Duguay, T.; Nance, J.W.; et al. Virtual Monoenergetic Imaging and Iodine Perfusion Maps Improve Diagnostic Accuracy of Dual-Energy Computed Tomography Pulmonary Angiography with Suboptimal Contrast Attenuation. *Investig. Radiol.* **2017**, *52*, 659–665. [CrossRef] [PubMed]
85. Borges, A.P.; Antunes, C.; Curvo-Semedo, L. Pros and Cons of Dual-Energy CT Systems: "One Does Not Fit All". *Tomography* **2023**, *9*, 195–216. [CrossRef]
86. Goo, H.W.; Goo, J.M. Dual-energy CT: New horizon in medical imaging. *Korean J. Radiol.* **2017**, *18*, 555–569. [CrossRef] [PubMed]
87. Katsura, M.; Sato, J.; Akahane, M.; Kunimatsu, A.; Abe, O. Current and novel techniques for metal artifact reduction at CT: Practical guide for radiologists. *Radiographics* **2018**, *38*, 450–461. [CrossRef]
88. Forghani, R.; De Man, B.; Gupta, R. Dual-Energy Computed Tomography: Physical Principles, Approaches to Scanning, Usage, and Implementation: Part 2. *Neuroimaging Clin. N. Am.* **2017**, *27*, 385–400. [CrossRef] [PubMed]
89. Toia, G.V.; Mileto, A.; Wang, C.L.; Sahani, D.V. Quantitative dual-energy CT techniques in the abdomen. *Abdom. Radiol.* **2022**, *47*, 3003–3018. [CrossRef]
90. Parakh, A.; An, C.; Lennartz, S.; Rajiah, P.; Yeh, B.M.; Simeone, F.J.; Sahani, D.V.; Kambadakone, A.R. Recognizing and minimizing artifacts at dual-energy CT. *Radiographics* **2021**, *41*, 509–523. [CrossRef]
91. Petritsch, B.; Pannenbecker, P.; Weng, A.M.; Grunz, J.-P.; Veldhoen, S.; Bley, T.A.; Kosmala, A. Split-filter dual-energy CT pulmonary angiography for the diagnosis of acute pulmonary embolism: A study on image quality and radiation dose. *Quant. Imaging Med. Surg.* **2021**, *11*, 1817–1827. [CrossRef]
92. Wortman, J.R.; Sodickson, A.D. Pearls, Pitfalls, and Problems in Dual-Energy Computed Tomography Imaging of the Body. *Radiol. Clin. N. Am.* **2018**, *56*, 625–640. [CrossRef]
93. Wichmann, J.L.; Hardie, A.D.; Schoepf, U.J.; Felmly, L.M.; Perry, J.D.; Varga-Szemes, A.; Mangold, S.; Caruso, D.; Canstein, C.; Vogl, T.J.; et al. Single- and dual-energy CT of the abdomen: Comparison of radiation dose and image quality of 2nd and 3rd generation dual-source CT. *Eur. Radiol.* **2017**, *27*, 642–650. [CrossRef] [PubMed]
94. Schmidt, D.; Söderberg, M.; Nilsson, M.; Lindvall, H.; Christoffersen, C.; Leander, P. Evaluation of image quality and radiation dose of abdominal dual-energy CT. *Acta Radiol.* **2018**, *59*, 845–852. [CrossRef] [PubMed]
95. Harder, A.M.D.; Willemink, M.J.; de Ruiter, Q.M.; Schilham, A.M.; Krestin, G.P.; Leiner, T.; de Jong, P.A.; Budde, R.P. Achievable dose reduction using iterative reconstruction for chest computed tomography: A systematic review. *Eur. J. Radiol.* **2015**, *84*, 2307–2313. [CrossRef] [PubMed]
96. Parakh, A.; Macri, F.; Sahani, D. Dual-Energy Computed Tomography: Dose Reduction, Series Reduction, and Contrast Load Reduction in Dual-Energy Computed Tomography. *Radiol. Clin. N. Am.* **2018**, *56*, 601–624. [CrossRef]
97. Mohammadinejad, P.; Mileto, A.; Yu, L.; Leng, S.; Guimaraes, L.S.; Missert, A.D.; Jensen, C.T.; Gong, H.; McCollough, C.H.; Fletcher, J.G. Ct noise-reduction methods for lower-dose scanning: Strengths and weaknesses of iterative reconstruction algorithms and new techniques. *Radiographics* **2021**, *41*, 1493–1508. [CrossRef]
98. Dunet, V.; Bernasconi, M.; Hajdu, S.D.; Meuli, R.A.; Daniel, R.T.; Zerlauth, J.-B. Impact of metal artifact reduction software on image quality of gemstone spectral imaging dual-energy cerebral CT angiography after intracranial aneurysm clipping. *Neuroradiology* **2017**, *59*, 845–852. [CrossRef]

Disclaimer/Publisher's Note: The statements, opinions and data contained in all publications are solely those of the individual author(s) and contributor(s) and not of MDPI and/or the editor(s). MDPI and/or the editor(s) disclaim responsibility for any injury to people or property resulting from any ideas, methods, instructions or products referred to in the content.

MDPI
St. Alban-Anlage 66
4052 Basel
Switzerland
www.mdpi.com

Journal of Clinical Medicine Editorial Office
E-mail: jcm@mdpi.com
www.mdpi.com/journal/jcm

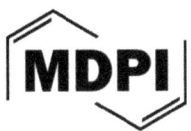

Disclaimer/Publisher's Note: The statements, opinions and data contained in all publications are solely those of the individual author(s) and contributor(s) and not of MDPI and/or the editor(s). MDPI and/or the editor(s) disclaim responsibility for any injury to people or property resulting from any ideas, methods, instructions or products referred to in the content.

www.ingramcontent.com/pod-product-compliance
Lightning Source LLC
LaVergne TN
LVHW070640100526
838202LV00013B/845